Psychosocial Elements of Physical Therapy

The Connection of Body to Mind

Psychosocial Elements of Physical Therapy

The Connection of Body to Mind

Hannah Johnson, PT, DPT, GCS

Routledge
Taylor & Francis Group
NEW YORK AND LONDON

Psychosocial Elements of Physical Therapy: The Connection of Body to Mind includes ancillary materials specifically available for faculty use. Please visit www.routledge.com/9781630915537 to obtain access.

Dr. Hannah Johnson has no financial or proprietary interest in the materials presented herein.

First published 2019 by SLACK Incorporated

Published 2024 by Routledge
605 Third Avenue, New York, NY 10158

and by Routledge
4 Park Square, Milton Park, Abingdon, Oxon, OX14 4RN

Routledge is an imprint of the Taylor & Francis Group, an informa business

Library of Congress Cataloging-in-Publication Data

Names: Johnson, Hannah, 1989- author.
Title: Psychosocial elements of physical therapy : the connection of body to mind / Hannah Johnson.
Description: Thorofare, NJ : SLACK Incorporated, [2018] | Includes bibliographical references and index.
Identifiers: LCCN 2018028906 (print) | ISBN 9781630915537 (alk. paper)
Subjects: | MESH: Physical Therapy Modalities--psychology | Mentally Ill Persons | Mental Disorders--rehabilitation | Case Reports Classification: LCC RM701 (print) | NLM WM 405 | DDC 615.8/2019--dc23
LC record available at https://lccn.loc.gov/2018028906

Cover Artist: Katherine Christie

ISBN: 9781630915537 (pbk)
ISBN: 9781003526063 (ebk)

DOI: 10.4324/9781003526063

CONTENTS

Acknowledgments

Many people have positively influenced the development of this text, some before the idea even emerged.

- Karen Persky (my microbiology teacher): thank you for encouraging me to continue writing stories to bring class material to life and feeding my love of writing and teaching! Maybe I will finish those stories too, someday.
- Bob Barnhart (my doctor of physical therapy [DPT] Program Director and friend): thank you for getting me moving on the idea to start researching and pushing through the book project toward its present form.
- Liz Paly and Lois Harrison (DPT faculty and mentors): thank you for encouraging me to keep going when the going was tough, which certainly helped with the writing of Chapter 1!
- Rachel Pickett and Leah Dvorak (additional faculty members): thank you for answering my questions early on in the process of seeking a publisher, getting my feet wet in trying to get this book out there.
- Neely Sullivan (a physical therapist and author I have yet to meet in person): thank you for letting me reach out to you, guiding me early in the research process, inspiring me to pursue the topic of mental health in physical therapy, and offering yourself as a resource.
- Amy Brinkman, Lori Stevens, Amy Tezak, and Linda Samuel (occupational therapy faculty and clinicians): thank you for offering your perspectives, and a few anecdotes, on the need to bring the mental health needs of patients and clients to the forefront of the reader's mind!
- Cindy Zbytniewski: thank you for your excellent listening skills and for providing a slice of your managerial expertise for Chapter 2.
- Tim Z., Ben D., and my other friends who prayed without me knowing it, you are in the background, but your prayers are in the foreground; I could not have done this without you.
- My parents (who were my first editorial board for content, style, and worldview): your prayers have lifted me up, and your immense English-language skills have made the text a lot better!

About the Author

Hannah Johnson, PT, DPT, GCS is a practicing physical therapist in a skilled nursing facility setting in Wisconsin. Along with patient care focused on geriatric clients and persons with psychological conditions, she enjoys teaching and writing to help the next generation of physical therapy students. She earned her BS in biology and her DPT from Concordia University Wisconsin (Mequon, Wisconsin). Additionally, she has clinical board specialist certification in geriatric physical therapy. Currently, she is working on her PhD in Interdisciplinary Health Sciences, with a focus on carryover of exercise programs for long-term residents of skilled nursing facilities.

Introduction

Why the Physical Therapist Needs This Book

Noble deeds and hot baths are the best cures for depression.

—Dodie Smith[1]

While this book cannot replace a hot bath by any means, I hope it will inspire the noble, or ordinary, work of physical therapists to reach an underserved population in need of better health care. Many textbooks and handbooks already address psychosocial aspects of health care, communicating with patients sensitively, informing the clinician about psychological conditions, and working within an interdisciplinary team/interprofessional team, not to mention adding in the wrinkle of the complex patient over age 65. So, why write a book pulling the concepts together?

As a profession, we are facing what Carole B. Lewis calls the *silver tsunami*, which is the rapidly expanding group of people who are not only aging, but carrying their life's stress, mental health issues, physical illnesses, and limited financial and social resources with them into old age. Without proper training, knowledge, skills, and attitudes, the physical therapist will be ill-prepared to provide cost-effective and evidence-based care to these patients and their younger versions (whether pediatric or adult) who are newly diagnosed. *Psychosocial Elements of Physical Therapy: The Connection of Body to Mind* is my small contribution to shrinking this problem. With a current review of the literature and minimal to no extraneous information, it will make it easier to develop the proper expertise for surfing this tsunami and, for non-geriatric therapists, preparing their younger patients for successful aging.

Goals for the Reader

Originally, my goal for *Psychosocial Elements of Physical Therapy: The Connection of Body to Mind* was to clarify for myself the several intersections of mental health and the practice of physical therapy, focusing on the population over 65 years old, as my area of clinical expertise is in geriatrics. It has morphed into a resource for the DPT student, as well as the newer practitioner who is practicing in any setting with a significant proportion of persons with psychological conditions. My primary goals for the reader are to (1) describe current best practices, as supported by literature and experience, for how the physical therapist can work well with people with mental health issues; and (2) to promote more widespread access to physical therapy, again as supported by literature, for persons with complex medical and psychiatric circumstances. These goals are answered in an intertwined way in the text, but I have attempted to draw out clinical nuggets to better focus reading and studying.

The first of the above goals is supported by the fact that mental function directly impacts movement system function, thus proving relevant to the *Healthy People 2020* vision promulgated by the American Physical Therapy Association. The second goal is driven not only by the need to promote expertise in practice, thus streamlining care even for complex cases, but also by the 2020 vision to reduce health disparities among various populations in the United States and elsewhere. Threaded through both these goals is the importance of an interdisciplinary team/interprofessional team approach, so that the whole person can be treated and treated well.

In most chapters, the reader is invited to reason through several case studies about patients with increasingly complex presentations. Questions for thought and treatment planning are based on the Hypothesis-Oriented Algorithm for Clinicians II.[2] This model begins with initial data gathering, progressing through a formal examination, planning of interventions and resources, and reassessment of existing and anticipated patient problems related to the human movement system. Each step can include consultation with other stakeholders as needed. There is no single right answer to any question; clinical decision-making skills related to case management may benefit from discussion. A useful website for tests and measures, physical and psychiatric, is https://www.sralab.org/rehabilitation-measures.

References

1. Smith D. *I Capture the Castle*. New York, NY: St. Martin's Press; 1948.
2. Rothstein JM, Echternach JL, Riddle DL. The Hypothesis-Oriented Algorithm for Clinicians II (HOAC II): a guide for patient management. *Phys Ther*. 2003;83(5):455-470.

Maintaining the Clinician's Therapeutic Presence

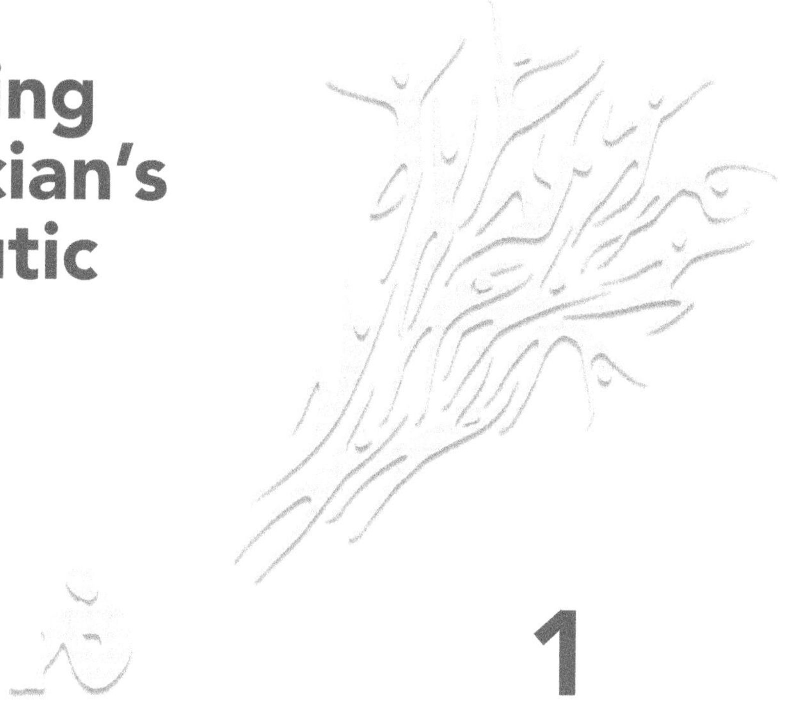

1

Outline

- Physical Therapy Clinical Reasoning and Reflection Tool
- Burnout: Definition, Causes, and Solutions/Prevention
- Physical Therapists' Personal Factors
    - Behaviors of Mental Illness: Putting Ourselves in the Patient's Place
    - Health Behaviors
    - Integrating Professional Development
- Summary
- Key Points
- Review Questions
- Case Studies

Learning Objectives

- State potential uses of the Physical Therapy Clinical Reasoning and Reflection Tool (PT-CRT), or portions thereof, related to current or past clinical cases
- Summarize the appearance and subjective signs/symptoms of burnout
- List ways to decrease or prevent personal burnout

For physical therapists, providing effective patient care goes beyond learning procedural and educational interventions, keeping current on medical conditions and medications, and choosing the best treatment techniques for each patient. Gaining expertise by reflection is not enough either, especially with patient populations where psychiatric and medical complexity is the norm.

Johnson H.
Psychosocial Elements of Physical Therapy: The Connection of Body to Mind (pp 1-13).

These patients and clients can be challenging, whether physically, mentally, or emotionally. Thus, the practitioner needs to be aware of the burnout potential that can detract from one's therapeutic presence.

Therapeutic presence is part of the professional "hat" that therapists wear. Ethical values and personal traits that run against a therapeutic presence include prejudice, indifference, perfectionism, rigidity, de-personalization (treating the patient as an object rather than a person with feelings), patronizing, selfishness, and insecurity.[1] Conversely, an effective clinician shows compassion, valuing of others, scientific problem-solving approaches, acceptance of the other person's individuality, and carefulness of speaking. Compassion is defined as empathy with a concrete response to the other person's condition.[2]

Obviously, a therapist who practices these attributes daily, with every patient or client, is an ideal: one to strive to be but not easy to achieve. Burnout and lack of reflection on practice are 2 reasons for difficulty in maintaining therapeutic presence with a medically and psychiatrically complex patient population. This chapter explores these reasons, as well as the clinician's personal factors that can influence patient care, so the reader can personalize a plan for prevention and management of burnout. It begins by discussing a tool to facilitate development of reflective practice, the PT-CRT,[3] and then explores burnout and therapists' personal factors.

Physical Therapy Clinical Reasoning and Reflection Tool

Developed in 2011, the PT-CRT is structured on the *International Classification of Functioning, Disability and Health* (ICF) model and the *Guide to Physical Therapist Practice*. Its initial application was in a pediatric clinical residency program. The tool was tested and used by several levels of academic and clinical staff, including the resident herself, her mentor, and other staff within the department at the children's hospital. Since then, several sources have referenced the tool, without research on the wider applicability to date.[4-6]

The tool's worksheet (available as an appendix to Atkinson and Nixon-Cave's article) integrates the ICF model, taught in doctor of physical therapy (DPT) programs; the Nagi model of disablement; and the patient management model, appearing in the *Guide to Physical Therapist Practice* (Figure 5-1).[7] Depending on which areas of clinical reasoning the user feels he or she is deficient in, individual sections with their reflection questions may be explored with a mentor, if available; mentorship is critical for professional development and clinical decision-making skills. Use can hone one's clinical reasoning, expertise, and efficiency, regardless of years of practice. Thinking about thinking, or metacognition, is the basis of this improvement.

Per the original article, central purposes of the PT-CRT are to guide the resident and clinician and facilitate the mentoring process. **Clinical decision-making strategies improved by use of the PT-CRT include "prospective or forward reasoning, deductive or backward reasoning, concept mapping, evidence appraisal, and interactive collaboration with the patient and family."**[3] Consistently applied, these strategies can accelerate the development of expertise. As Jensen et al state, experts have "(1) multidirectional and patient-centered knowledge; (2) collaborative and reflective clinical reasoning; (3) observational and manual skill in movement, with a focus on function; and (4) consistent virtues."[8]

Because expert physical therapist practice uses best evidence and available rubrics for applying evidence, the PT-CRT uses the patient management and ICF models. Sections of the PT-CRT include:

- Initial data gathering/interview
- Generation of initial hypothesis (ie, potential treatment diagnosis)
- Examination

- Evaluation (using an ICF-based grid)
- Plan of care (including goals, outcome measures, and dosage of physical therapy services)
- Interventions (emphasizing evidence base for practice)
- Reexamination
- Outcomes (including discharge planning)

Each section of the tool has reflection questions to guide the user and mentor (if available) in reflecting critically on the aspects of patient care that may impair outcomes or efficient use of resources. The author of this text has found individual questions within each section to be helpful when completing entry-level clinical coursework within her DPT curriculum, especially to assist in pulling the entire patient case together for better case management.

Burnout: Definitions, Causes, and Solutions/Prevention

According to renowned geriatric physical therapist, Carole Davis, burnout means "to fail, wear out, or become exhausted by making excessive demands on energy, strength, or resources."[9] Certain practice settings, including acute care and skilled nursing, increase clinicians' risk of burnout due to high demands on staff, low level of control of circumstances, and lack of personal and professional training and support.[10] Especially in one's first several years of practice, the high risk can have serious consequences.

One effect of burnout is loss of therapeutic presence. Three phases of the process are similar to the generalized stress response or "general adaptation syndrome."[11] Selye's model of an organism's response to stress progresses from alarm, to resistance or adaptation, to exhaustion. In physiological terms, alarm means that the central nervous system becomes more active, resistance and adaptation mean a fight or flight response to manage the stressor, and exhaustion means that compensatory mechanisms break down. The first phase of burnout decreases energy, efficiency, memory, humility, and humor. The second phase includes behaviors and attitudes of depersonalization of patients, rigidity, self-isolation, and increased absence from work. By the third phase, the therapist shows cynicism, boredom, poor health behaviors, and potential psychosis related to insomnia. Therapeutic presence can be maintained only in the first phase, but even then, it is with difficulty.

Moreover, symptoms of burnout can be classified into somatic, emotional, and behavioral. Table 1-1 allows the therapist to assess personal burnout potential and approximate phase.[12] If the point total is between 20 and 56, one should consider a health problem as differential diagnosis; between 57 and 103 points indicates a definite issue; and 104 or more points requires professional referral and treatment. Table 1-1 lists symptoms and baseline point values assigned to them; points are added for duration (1 for weeks, 2 for months, 3 for over a year), frequency (sometimes, frequently, or constantly), and intensity (mild, moderate, or severe).

Burnout is closely connected to stress. As clinicians educate patients about how to reduce physical stress via activity and lifestyle modification, they also need to look objectively at their own stressors and the health effects. Stress leads to changes in immune, cardiovascular, central nervous system, endocrine, and metabolic systems with variable coping mechanisms (ie, how the individual interprets stress). Factors influencing coping style, which guides response to stress, include one's locus of control, resilience, and openness to change. Specific stress-induced illnesses include:

- Heart disease: connected to job stress, anxiety, and potentially type A personality
- Hypertension: connected to stress, anger/anxiety, high-status job, gender/ethnicity, and obesity
- Migraine, tension, and cluster headaches: associated with stress and negative emotions
- Asthma: associated with decreased help-seeking and decreased symptom awareness, increased emotional expression, and depression[13]

Table 1-1

Symptoms of Burnout

Physical Symptoms	Personal Symptoms	Behavioral Symptoms
• Fatigue (2 points baseline) • Insomnia (3 points) • Headache (2 points) • Backache (1 point) • Gastrointestinal problems (2 points) • Weight loss or gain (1 point) • Shortness of breath (1 point) • Lingering cold (2 points)	• Boredom (3 points) • Restlessness (2 points) • Stagnation (3 points) • Rationalization (4 points) • Feelings of irreplaceability (5 points) • Obsession (5 points) • Depression (3 points)	• Irritability (4 points) • Cynicism (5 points) • Defensiveness (4 points) • Alcohol dependence (5 points) • Inability to enjoy or compliment colleagues' success (4 points) • Drug dependence (5 points)

Some personality traits can increase burnout risk as well. The Big 5 personality traits seem to have roles in protecting or making volunteer end-of-life counselors vulnerable to burnout. A recent study of physical therapists associated higher levels of neuroticism (the negative side of emotional stability) in therapists with poorer patient outcomes.[14] The positive aspects of these 5 basic personality traits are:

1. Extraversion: marked by high self-confidence, activity, and optimism
2. Agreeableness: marked by "altruism, nurturance, and caring"[15]
3. Conscientiousness: marked by self-discipline, dutifulness, and ability to problem-solve
4. Emotional stability: marked by tendency to experience positive emotions
5. Intellect/autonomy or openness to experience: marked by trying to take lessons from experiences

In someone who lacks adequate extraversion, emotional stability, and intellect/autonomy, burnout risk increases. Davis summarized these negative traits, or risk factors, as "bossiness" with lack of work-life balance.[9] Potentially due to lack of experience, physical therapists who have worked for under 2 years are at moderate burnout risk; mid-career therapists with 5 to 9 years' experience have the greatest risk. While this may relate to work environment, causing many therapists to change jobs vs address the burnout itself, it is critical to internalize and apply knowledge about burnout early on. The author of this text had several cycles of mild to moderate burnout within the first 3 years of clinical practice, associated with high levels of neuroticism and low extraversion, and learned to apply this knowledge to get past the burnout to remain in the position and flourish.

Even when someone avoids burnout, there are still many ways job-related stress can manifest itself. Kerzner,[16] writing to project managers (who have a job description similar to that of many physical therapists), lists 10 additional signs and symptoms of stress:

1. Being tired in the short term
2. Feeling depressed
3. Being physically and emotionally exhausted
4. Being unhappy
5. Feeling trapped
6. Feeling worthless

7. Feeling resentful and disillusioned about people
8. Feeling hopeless
9. Feeling rejected
10. Feeling anxious

Kerzner[16] recommends maintaining work-life balance, changing one's job assignment or position if needed, asking for enough authority to complete required job functions, maintaining dignity, and avoiding perfectionism. While these strategies help, **the clinician should carefully discern the causes of stress and burnout before leaving a position**, as some of the problems may originate within the therapist vs the job itself.

No matter how much therapists may enjoy their jobs, they will still likely experience job-related stress and burnout. To prevent burnout in palliative care workers, for example, self-care is essential; care providers need to self-assess their strengths and weaknesses accurately, pay attention to intuition, allow mental and physical breaks from work (during the day or via vacation time), manage time strictly, seek help as needed, use social support, and maintain a healthy lifestyle.[17] Fischer et al agreed that "mental hygiene," attention to employer support, and training of employees could lessen the incidence and severity of burnout among physical therapists.[18] Mindfulness training can prevent burnout among mental health care providers, being "in the moment" helps to reduce the many individual stresses that otherwise pile up to produce burnout.[19] Finally, reframing demanding or challenging job situations as problems to be solved, via discussion and collaborative decision making that values participants, can help.[20]

Physical Therapists' Personal Factors

This section explores several topics not often covered in the explicit curriculum of many DPT programs.[21] These topics are nonetheless important to a clinician's therapeutic presence. They include experiences of behaviors and feelings similar to those in psychological conditions, the influence of physical activity and health behaviors, level and use of social support, and the therapist's integration of professional and personal development into a busy work and home life.

Behaviors of Mental Illness: Putting Ourselves in the Patient's Place

The true definition of mental illness is when the majority of your time is spent in the past or future, but rarely living in the realism of NOW.

—Shannon L. Alder[22]

By definition, many mental health issues cause certain behaviors or feelings with major effects on the person's life and function. While individual mental illnesses are relatively rare (though cumulatively affecting one-quarter of the population), the underlying behaviors and feelings are common. Examples include test anxiety, situational depression, and difficulty in concentrating when faced with multiple demands. Both students and therapists can cycle through these and other situations, but the effects on therapeutic presence and patient care vary depending on how the clinician deals with them.

When dealing with patients and clients who have diagnosed or suspected psychological illness, it is important to recognize what their symptoms feel like. The website for the National Alliance on Mental Illness (www.nami.org) contains short essays by persons living with various mental illnesses and is worth exploring. Once the clinician realizes the personal impact of a mental health problem, he or she can start to improve the ability to take a "step back," so to speak, while imagining him- or herself in place of a patient.

The following is a list of selected attributes of psychological conditions, as set forth by the American Psychiatric Association. Recall that to be pathological, an attribute or set of attributes needs to be pervasive and drastically affect the individual's function. However, even at a lesser level, the symptoms can adversely affect students or practicing therapists and need to be acknowledged and addressed.

- Anxiety: fatigue, irritability, or restlessness
- Depression: decreased interest in activities, difficulty in concentrating, or feelings of guilt
- Mania (in bipolar disorder): little need for sleep, flurry of ideas, or distractibility
- Personality disorders
    - Antisocial type: irresponsibility, lack of empathy, or impulsivity
    - Avoidant type: high sensitivity to negative feedback, fear of rejection, or low self-image
    - Borderline type: unstable personal relationships, efforts to avoid potential abandonment, or feelings of emptiness
    - Narcissistic type: high self-importance, sense of entitlement, or lack of empathy
    - Obsessive-compulsive type: preoccupation with lists, rules, work/productivity, and ethics
- Substance use disorders: decreased interest in activities and preoccupation with certain behaviors

For the therapist to develop a sense (early on and hopefully during the student years) of how these common feelings and behaviors affect one's own personal life is valuable to the development of the professional and therapeutic self. If clinicians can step into each patient's place, so to speak, they can be more empathetic to establish and maintain rapport. This is critical to improving patients' compliance to therapy treatment programs.[23]

Sometimes, therapists struggle with severe mental illness themselves. Lisa Halpern,[24] the program director for Vinfen Recovery Center (Dorchester, Massachusetts), described her long, arduous cognitive recovery from a diagnosis of schizophrenia, likening it to lengthy physical rehabilitation. In a brief but moving article, she told what it felt like to fight to regain her short-term memory, physical energy, attention span, word-finding abilities, and instrumental skills for daily living. She highlighted the ongoing struggle of chronic illness that drains one's energy but also can be alleviated by an iron will to recover and improve. Her example, and that of others,[25,26] can remind the student and clinician of how to empathize with patients living with multiple medical and mental conditions.

Another example is the large proportion of patients in rehabilitation who have dementia. While organizations, such as the Aging and Disability Resource Center and American Geriatrics Society, actively educate the public about what dementia actually is and how to interact with persons with dementia, stigma still exists for this and other mental disorders.[27,28] Because of the pervasive nature of symptoms, it can be difficult for the care provider to differentiate his or her emotions from challenging situations that arise. Thus, it is important to practice stepping back for a more clinical analysis of such situations to develop professionally and avoid burnout.

Education can affect attitudes of physical therapists and physical therapist assistants toward persons with dementia. A survey of skilled nursing facilities (SNFs) in Indiana unfortunately indicated that increased cognitive symptom severity of dementia, regardless of providers' education and training, was correlated with negative attitudes of the providers about the ability of persons with dementia to benefit from therapy.[29] Despite generally positive results from studies of other types of specially trained health care providers noted in the article, Staples and Killian noted that such "therapeutic nihilism among health care workers would provide a threat to the provision of appropriate care."[29] Thus, gaining a diagnosis-specific knowledge base can be very helpful in minimizing burnout and poor care provision to persons with dementia or other severe conditions. Staples and Killian[30] also published the survey instrument they developed for the study to facilitate therapist self-assessment of potential issues regarding dementia-related attitudes and beliefs.

Yokoi and Okamura[31] took an interesting perspective in their study of persons with dementia about understanding these patients for therapeutic empathy. Combining several models related to metacognitive abilities (thinking about thinking), they analyzed such patients during observed activities of daily living. From this analysis, they determined that the loss of a "theory of mind" or the ability to self-evaluate led to self-care deficits of failing to seek others' assistance, or improperly evaluating an unsafe or illegal situation, such as operating a hot stove or driving without a license. The theory of mind is the ability to hypothesize what state of mind another person might be in; this ability typically develops around 4 years old.

In a similar vein and with the same developed model of self-awareness, Yokoi et al[32] explored the relationship between lack of self-awareness and the dementia-related behavior of wandering. They discovered that "purposeless activity [such as wandering], purposeful actions [such as wanting to use the toilet], irritation, and symptoms of depression" are potentially influencing conditions upon the tendency to wander within or outside of a facility. Commonly, a person with dementia may not be aware that he or she is wandering and may not have a purpose for it either. Thus, by realizing this viewpoint, clinicians can analyze wandering clinically and think of other ways to redirect or prevent development of potentially dangerous wandering behaviors (eg, elopement from a facility, falling due to an obstacle, or going into unauthorized areas).[32]

Mentoring helps the clinician develop the ability to take a step back. Barr and Tichenor[33] explored what mentoring is in the context of residency and fellowship education for physical therapists. A mentor, to help hone the student's or therapist's analysis skills, may give targeted constructive feedback (in person or by email/phone), guide a thought process shift from rigid use of basic knowledge toward flexible use of experience and reflection to make clinical decisions, and answer questions to stimulate further thought and keep communication lines open. Such mentoring most easily takes place within a structured residency, but even informal mentoring in the workplace can help the student or novice clinician.[33]

Health Behaviors

Physical therapists, starting as students, are encouraged by faculty, administration, and values of the profession of physical therapy to model good health behaviors for patients and clients. These behaviors include structured and unstructured physical activity, posture and ergonomics, balanced nutritional intake, and sleep hygiene (Table 1-2). Frequently, the demands of professional training and career place a heavy strain on these behaviors. Thus, the clinician must find a way to maintain a healthy lifestyle for his or her own sake as well as the patients' sake; clients learn the most from observing their therapists.

Because physical therapists specialize in the human movement system, they are aware early on in their education of the importance of physical exercise, including benefits and dosage. Exercise is vital for physical as well as mental health.[34,35] Additionally, a systematic review identified the following ways to reduce occupational stress, especially in health care workers: cognitive behavioral therapy, relaxation techniques for mind and body, and changing one's work schedule to reduce continuous excessive demands.[36]

Mindfulness has been promoted in recent years as a way to improve compassion, automate good listening skills, and enable solid decision making without increasing stress. Hambley[37] noted that mindfulness increased the size and function of the hippocampus (which forms long-term memories) and prefrontal cortex (which guides decision making, regulation of emotions, and focus), while decreasing the size and interconnections of the amygdala (which is sensitive to stress and danger stimuli), as well as improving the function of the immune system. **She recommends the following procedure**[37]:

- Set aside 15 to 30 minutes each day in a quiet, uninterrupted area
- Focus on breathing through the nose and gradually relax the body
- Become more aware of muscle tone and redirect any thoughts back to breathing

Table 1-2

Current Recommendations for a Balanced, Physically Healthy Lifestyle

PHYSICAL ACTIVITY[38]	POSTURE AND ERGONOMICS[39,40]	NUTRITION[41]	SLEEP HYGIENE[42]
• Structured aerobic moderate-intensity exercise (150 minutes per week) • Strength training of major muscle groups (2 to 3 days per week) with 48-hour rest breaks between sessions • Dynamic and static muscle stretching (2 to 3 days per week for 60 seconds per muscle) • Functional fitness training including motor skills and proprioceptive training (20 to 30 minutes per day)	• Limit sitting time • Change position every 30 minutes • Maintain as neutral a spine as possible during sitting, standing, and bending • Use proper squat form to save knees • Use larger muscle groups for tasks (use elbow vs hand to carry a bag) • Limit grip strength used during the clinical day to 30% of maximum	• Balance calories in and calories out • Focus on nutrient-rich foods vs taking supplements: o Vegetables o Fruits o Whole grains o Fat-free or low-fat dairy o Seafood o Lean meats o Eggs/poultry o Beans/peas o Nuts/seeds	• Avoid daytime naps • Avoid stimulants near bedtime (eg, caffeine) • Exercise regularly and earlier in the day • Decrease food intake before bedtime • Expose skin/eyes to natural sunlight • Relaxing routine • Use bed only for sleep

Integrating Professional Development

Advancing one's skills, expertise, and career is another aspect of implicit DPT curricula. While integrating outside reading, seminars, and shadowing or observation may be difficult during student years, it becomes more difficult once the student enters the profession full time. The young professional may be starting a family, paying off loans, maintaining good health behaviors, and staying involved in leisure activities during this time. In this section, the author of this text will offer tips from her personal experience, as well as what is found in the scholarly literature, to aid the student or practitioner in the successful integration of valuable professional development into working life for successful lifelong learning.

While in school, the student may work in conjunction with a faculty advisor or clinical instructor to develop goals of professional development:

- Gain a baseline familiarity with one's intended practice setting (eg, attending workshops at state chapter conferences related to orthopedics if one is seeking a position in orthopedics)
- Remediate deficiencies identified during classwork and faculty advising (eg, supplemental reading in documentation skills if that is a weakness identified on a clinical rotation)
- Satisfy curiosity that is sated by classes within the curriculum (eg, observing neurodevelopmental treatment in clinical practice)

After graduation, the student's goals must be integrated into his or her first job: with additional considerations of state licensure requirements, facility-specific training, industry trends, and especially financial impact (ie, how the clinician can use continuing-education funds, if available, through the company). The American Physical Therapy Association website (Career Management and Career Development sections) has aids for the novice and expert practitioner in planning professional development.

An example is a second-year DPT student who determined that she preferred a practice setting in geriatrics upon graduation. Her 5-year goals at this point included clinical instructor credentialing through the American Physical Therapy Association, Geriatric Clinical Specialist certification through the American Board of Physical Therapy Specialties, and independent reading or continuing education about related interests (adult neurologic disorders, manual therapy, and the biopsychosocial model). Each year, the student updated the plan to reflect achievement of benchmarks. During her final semester, she initially did not pass the entry-level SNF rotation, but after a self-designed remedial course, she did progress, meeting her original short-term goals in the next 4 years.

What is the best way to achieve multiple ambitious goals? While each person learns differently, literature shows that gradual changes can best be maintained. Practically, this means breaking up the work into manageable chunks, reflecting extensively on one's experience to date,[43] and engaging in multiple lines of inquiry to maintain interest in material to be learned and internalized. Multiple ways to facilitate professional development include[44]:

- Writing a journal to reflect on clinical practice or teaching
- Learning a new language for improved communication
- Observing or being observed by a peer
- Maintaining a portfolio of work samples
- Finding or being a mentor to another professional
- Participating in research in partnership with an academic institution
- Attending a course or conference
- Reading professional journals and contributing to the literature via writing or review
- Starting and maintaining a journal discussion club
- Earning a postprofessional degree
- Presenting at a conference or guest lecture within a course
- Providing pro bono services or otherwise volunteering in service organizations

Devoting 15 to 45 minutes per day toward professional goals is one part of a successful strategy for ongoing integrated professional development. Fuhrmann et al[45] described an individualized plan as emphasizing the writing, tracking, and achieving of SMART goals as small as daily items on a to-do list. As many DPT students learn, SMART stands for **specific, measurable, attainable, realistic, and timely**. Patients' goals within each therapy plan of care can be organized by this principle; the same applies to their therapists.

As with motor learning, so also professional skill development requires training, structured and random practice, and integration of feedback from multiple sources. Fuhrmann et al[45] also notes the importance of accountability partners to help the clinician achieve set goals with limited short-term results. Between periods of training, practice, and feedback, the clinician needs to rest, do enjoyable activities, and practice gratitude for balance.

Summary

This chapter has addressed facets of stress management relating to the profession of physical therapy. As the high professional and personal standards of many students and therapists can predispose them to stress and burnout, maintaining a balanced outlook is a priority. On the professional development side, the PT-CRT can develop reflection in and on action, thus enhancing efficient, effective clinical decision making. Thus, clinicians' cognitive resources can be used more effectively. Also, a professional development plan and a manageable daily schedule for integrating achievement of those goals into busy daily life facilitate work-life balance.

On the personal side, clinicians working with more challenging populations, including geriatrics and mental health, should be aware of relationships between their personalities, each patient's needs, each therapist's duties, and risks for stress and burnout. Mental health is challenging to deal with on solely a clinical level because effective patient care requires therapists to step into each patient's place. However, too much personal involvement can also cause burnout and lessen effectiveness of care. This text lists resources to prevent, lessen, or remedy these stressors while facilitating work-life balance.

Key Points

- Use the PT-CRT to develop prospective and deductive reasoning, collaboration skills, evidence evaluation, and concept-mapping skills.
- Before leaving a position due to burnout, the clinician should discern and address the causes.
- Mentorship includes constructive feedback, guidance toward more flexible thought processes, stimulating further questions, and maintaining open lines of communication.
- A simple way to practice mindfulness is to set aside 15 to 30 quiet minutes, focus on breathing through the nose while relaxing the body, and stay aware of muscle tone while redirecting thoughts back to breathing.

Review Questions

- What are some uses of the PT-CRT?
  - Describe the frameworks underlying the PT-CRT and why they were integrated into the tool.
  - Recall a recent challenging patient case from your clinical experience. Using the PT-CRT template,[3] work through the challenging components of patient management from this case and discuss with a coworker or fellow student.
- What are several symptoms from each of the 3 domains relating to burnout?
  - Describe the connections between job-related stress and stress-related illnesses.
  - Given your own personality (related to the Big 5 personality traits), discuss your own risk for job-related burnout and formulate a short list of ways to decrease or prevent this burnout.
- How can your own experience of emotions and behaviors common to psychological conditions improve how you deal empathetically with the patient population of persons with mental illness?
- If you have not done so already, consider using this chapter as a springboard for a professional and personal development plan to strengthen your therapeutic presence.

Case Studies

For each case description below, briefly document or discuss the following:

- Think about your response to stress. After identifying the stressors in the case, state how you would deal with each one in real time and the effects on your stress and patient care.
- What extra information would you like to know about the situation? Why? How would knowing such information help you maintain your therapeutic presence?
- Compare and contrast your ideal response in the situation with how you have responded to a similar situation in the past.

Case 1

In a long-term care setting, you are working alone with a patient with bipolar schizoaffective disorder to improve ambulation enough to transition her to a group home. Yesterday and today, she has demonstrated symptoms of distractibility, medication refusal, insomnia, and yelling at staff. Attempts to redirect her are less and less successful as the session goes by. She is aware of her symptoms but states repeatedly that she feels fine.

Case 2

While working with a patient in the therapy gym in an SNF, you hear an overhead page "code S in the basement." You recognize this as an active-shooter code, knowing also the facility protocol that such codes are to be spread via telephone and not by overhead page. The patient you are working with has hearing deficits, advanced dementia, osteoarthritis, and is restricted to a wheelchair. The rest of the team seems unsure of what to do.

Case 3

You are in an inpatient hospital setting early in the morning. As soon as you walk into work, a nurse calls out to you from inside a patient's room as you walk past it to punch in. You have not seen this patient before, and the nurse asks you for help because the patient is agitated and has dementia. Another nurse and an aide are in the room, and each person is speaking loudly to the patient, who is trying to get off the bed and is also shouting. You have been at this position for a few months and have broad experience with geriatrics in the community.

Case 4

You are in an outpatient setting with your first DPT student in her first rotation. Shortly after a teenage patient's mother calls to cancel the day's appointment due to illness, the same patient comes in with an angry demeanor. He starts swearing at the receptionist and appears to be intoxicated. You were documenting on the previous patient in the back, and your student, scheduled to treat this patient, seems unsure of what to do and where to go.

References

1. Davis CM. *Patient Practitioner Interaction: An Experiential Manual for Developing the Art of Health Care.* 4th ed. Thorofare, NJ: SLACK Incorporated; 2006.
2. Thomas Y, Menage D. Reclaiming compassion as a core value in occupational therapy. *Br J Occup Ther.* 2016;79(1):3-4.
3. Atkinson HL, Nixon-Cave K. A tool for clinical reasoning and reflection using the *International Classification of Functioning, Disability and Health* (ICF) framework and patient management model. *Phys Ther.* 2011;91(3):416-430.
4. Furze J, Kenyon LK, Jensen GM. Connecting classroom, clinic, and context: clinical reasoning strategies for clinical instructors and academic faculty. *Pediatr Phys Ther.* 2015;27(4):368-375.
5. Bakker SE, Painter EE, Morgan BC, et al. Systematic clinical reasoning in physical therapy (SCRIPT): a tool for the purposeful practice of clinical reasoning in orthopedic manual physical therapy. *Phys Ther.* 2017;97(1)61-70.
6. Tucker A, Bradshaw M. Clinical reasoning: action-focused thinking. In: Bradshaw M & Lowenstein A, eds. *Innovate Teaching Strategies in Nursing and Related Health Professions.* Sudbury, MA: Jones & Bartlett Learning; 2014:65-79.
7. American Physical Therapy Association. *Guide to physical therapist practice 3.0.* Guide to Physical Therapist Practice. http://guidetoptpractice.apta.org/. Published November 27, 2016. Accessed January 19, 2018.
8. Jensen GM, Gwyer J, Shepard K. Expert practice in physical therapy. *Phys Ther.* 2000;80(1):28-43.
9. Davis CB. Clinical geriatric neurology. [Course notes.] Great Seminars & Books;2014.
10. Balogun JA, Titiloye V, Balogun A, Oyeyemi A, Katz J. Prevalence and determinants of burnout among physical and occupational therapists. *J Allied Health.* 2002;31(3):131-139.
11. Selye H. The general adaptation syndrome and the diseases of adaptation. *J Clin Endocrinol Metab.* 1946;6(2):117-230.
12. Halenar JF. Doctors don't have to burn out. *Medical Economics.* 1981;58:148-161.
13. Sue D, Sue DW, Sue S. *Understanding Abnormal Behaviors.* 6th ed. Boston, MA: Houghton Mifflin; 2000.
14. Buining EM, Kooijman MK, Swinkels ICS, Pisters MF, Veenhof C. Exploring physiotherapists' personality traits that may influence treatment outcome in patients with chronic diseases: a cohort study. *BMC Health Serv Res.* 2015;15:558.
15. Bakker AB, van der Zee KI, Lewig KA, Dollard MF. The relationship between the Big Five personality factors and burnout: a study among volunteer counselors. *J Soc Psychol.* 2008;146(1):31-50.
16. Kerzner H. *Project Management: A Systems Approach to Planning, Scheduling, and Controlling.* 9th ed. Hoboken, NJ: Wiley; 2006.
17. Rokach A. The dying and those who care for them. *J Pat Care.* 2015;1(1):101.
18. Fischer M, Mitsche M, Endler P, Mesenholl-Strehler E, Lothaller H, Roth R. Burnout in physiotherapists: use of clinical supervision and desire for emotional closeness or distance to clients. *Int J Ther Rehabil.* 2013;20(11):550-558.
19. Felton TM, Coates L, Christopher JC. Impact of mindfulness training on counseling students' perceptions of stress. *Mindfulness.* 2015;6(2):159-169. DOI 10.1007/s12671-013-0240-8.
20. Scanlan JN, Still M. Job satisfaction, burnout and turnover intention in occupational therapists working in mental health. *Aust Occup Ther J.* 2013;60(5):310-318.

21. Jensen GM, Paschal KA, Shepard KF. Curriculum design for physical therapy educational programs. In: Jensen GM, Mostrom E, eds. *Handbook of Teaching and Learning for Physical Therapists.* St. Louis, MO: Elsevier; 2013:2-18.
22. Wride EL. *Your Life User Manual: Practical Insights for Living a Meaningful Life.* Self-published, 2018.
23. Thompson L, McCabe R. The effect of clinician-patient alliance and communication on treatment adherence in mental health care: a systematic review. *BMC Psychiatry.* 2012;12:87.
24. Halpern L. Brain training: an athletic model for brain rehabilitation. *Psychiatric Services.* 2006;57(4):459-460.
25. Magill JH. Connections: stories of recovery from mental illness. *South Carolina Department of Mental Health Steering Committee.* https://www.state.sc.us/dmh/client_affairs/connections.pdf. Published September 11, 2009. Accessed January 19, 2018.
26. Centre for Addiction and Mental Health. Stories of recovery. *CAMH: Centre for Addiction and Mental Health.* http://www.camh.ca/en/hospital/about_camh/newsroom/stories_of_recovery/Pages/default.aspx. Published 2012. Accessed January 19, 2018.
27. Aging and Disability Resource Center. Aging and Disability Resource Centers Consumer Page. *Wisconsin Department of Health Services.* https://www.dhs.wisconsin.gov/adrc/index.htm. Published September 7, 2016. Accessed January 19, 2018.
28. Drench ME, Noonan AC, Sharby N, Ventura SH. *Psychosocial Aspects of Health Care.* 3rd ed. Upper Saddle River, NJ:Pearson; 2012.
29. Staples WH, Killian CB. Education affects attitudes of physical therapy providers toward people with dementia. *Educ Gerontol.* 2012;38(5):350-361.
30. Staples WH, Killian CB. Development of an instrument to measure attitudes of physical therapy providers working with people with dementia. *Am J Al Dis Oth Dem.* 2012;27(5):331-338.
31. Yokoi T, Okamura H. Why do dementia patients become unable to lead a daily life with decreasing cognitive function? *Dementia.* 2012;12(5):551-568.
32. Yokoi T, Aoyama K, Ishida K, Okamura H. Conditions associated with wandering in people with dementia from the viewpoint of self-awareness: five case reports. *Am J Alz Dis Oth Dem.* 2012:27(3);162-170.
33. Barr JB, Tichenor CJ. Post-professional clinical residency and fellowship education. In: Jensen GM, Mostrom E, eds. *Handbook of Teaching and Learning for Physical Therapists.* St. Louis, MO: Elsevier; 2013:259-273.
34. Mortazavi S, Mohammad K, Eftekhar Ardebili H, Dorali Beni R, Mahmoodi M, Keshteli AH. Mental disorder prevention and physical activity in Iranian elderly. *Int J Prev Med.* 2012;3(Suppl 1):S64-72.
35. Fox KR, Stathi A, McKenna J, Davis MG. Physical activity and mental well-being in older people participating in the Better Ageing Project. *Eur J Appl Physiol.* 2007;100(5):591-602. DOI 10.1007/s00421-007-0392-0.
36. Ruotsalainen JH, Verbeek JH, Mariné A, Serra C. Preventing occupational stress in health care workers. *Cochrane Database Syst Rev.* 2015;4:C0028292.
37. Hambley C. The benefits to developing a mindfulness practice. *Physicians Practice.* http://www.physicianspractice.com/articles/benefits-developing-mindfulness-practice. Published June 14, 2017. Accessed January 19, 2018.
38. ACSM Media Room. ACSM issues new recommendations on quantity and quality of exercise. *American College of Sports Medicine.* http://www.acsm.org/about-acsm/media-room/news-releases/2011/08/01/acsm- issues-new-recommendations-on-quantity-and-quality-of-exercise. Published June 28, 2011. Accessed January 19, 2018.
39. Besser B. Materials handling: heavy lifting. *US Department of Labor.* https://www.osha.gov/SLTC/etools/electricalcontractors/materials/heavy.html. Accessed January 19, 2018.
40. Spectrum Health Rehabilitation and Sports Medicine Services. Joint protection principles. *Kwazulu-Natal Department of Health.* http://www.kznhealth.gov.za/occtherapy/jointprotectionprinciples.pdf. Published August 2007. Accessed January 19, 2018.
41. US Department of Agriculture. Dietary guidelines for Americans 2010. *US Dietary Guidelines.* https://health.gov/dietaryguidelines/dga2010/dietaryguidelines2010.pdf. Published December 2010. Accessed January 19, 2018.
42. Thorpy M. Sleep hygiene. *National Sleep Foundation.* https://sleepfoundation.org/ask-the-expert/sleep-hygiene. Published 2003. Accessed January 19, 2018.
43. Wainwright SF, Shepard KF, Harman LB, Stephens J. Novice and experienced physical therapist clinicians: a comparison of how reflection is used to inform the clinical decision-making process. *Phys Ther.* 2010;90(1):75-88.
44. Wong MS. Fifty ways to develop professionally: what language educators need to succeed. *Language Education in Asia.* 2011;2(1):142-155
45. Fuhrmann CN, Hobin JA, Clifford PS, Lindstaedt B. Goal-setting strategies for scientific and career success. *Science Magazine.* http://www.sciencemag.org/careers/2013/12/goal-setting-strategies-scientific-and-career-success. Published December 3, 2013. Accessed January 19, 2018.

The Interdisciplinary Team/ Interprofessional Team

2

Outline

- Rationale for the IDT/IPT Versus Practice in Silos
  - Example: Areas of Counseling
  - Example: Indications for Counseling Provided by a Physical Therapist Within an IDT/IPT Context
- Components of an Effective IDT/IPT
  - General Principles
    - Personnel-Related Principles
    - Resource-Related Principles
    - Communication-Related Principles
  - Communication
  - Models of Effective IDTs/IPTs in Health Care
- Mechanisms of Team Dysfunction and Repair
- Summary
- Key Points
- Review Questions
- Case Study: An IDT/IPT of Mixed Effectiveness

Johnson H.
Psychosocial Elements of Physical Therapy: The Connection of Body to Mind (pp 15-32).

Learning Objectives

- State a clear rationale for an interdisciplinary team/interprofessional team (IDT/IPT) vs each discipline working in silo for a complex patient/client
- Describe the structure and function of an effective IDT/IPT
- Develop potential solutions for common IDT/IPT issues

As health care becomes more complex, a clear understanding of the IDT/IPT concept is vital. Especially in medically complex and geriatric populations, IDTs/IPTs provide more comprehensive and effective care than any single profession working alone. This chapter explores the IDT/IPT in the context of psychiatrically and medically complex patient populations, the physical therapist's role on the team, and problem-solving strategies for common dysfunctions that arise.

Rationale for the IDT/IPT Versus Practice in Silos

Many ideas grow better when transplanted into another mind than the one where they sprang up.

—Oliver Wendell Holmes[1]

Alone we can do so little; together we can do so much.

—Helen Keller[2]

Literature documents adverse effects of individual health care professionals practicing within their own silos, including fragmented patient care, increased costs, worse health outcomes, and inefficiency. Even with the best intentions, no single profession can care for the whole patient due to blind spots and scopes of practice. Renowned physical therapist Alan Jette wrote a thoughtful editorial about team-based, family-centered health care, based on personal experience of extended family caring for his mother, who was then 90 years old, to help her maintain health and independence. Successful team-based care that includes family participation can reduce hospital readmission rates and other adverse outcomes of poor care coordination.[3]

Striving to replace the silo model of health care is the concept of the IDT/IPT:

> Team-based health care is the provision of health services to individuals, families, and/or their communities by at least two health providers who work collaboratively with patients and their caregivers—to the extent preferred by each patient—to accomplish shared goals within and across settings to achieve coordinated, high-quality care.[4]

By these criteria, the IDT/IPT does not have to be large, but rather tailored to the patient's needs, whether medical, psychological, spiritual, emotional, financial, and social, per a consensus statement of the Union of European Medical Specialists.[5]

One national resource in the United States for geriatric care is the National Association of Area Agencies on Aging.[6] This association is made up of each community's local Aging and Disability Resource Center (ADRC), which leverages state and local resources to provide information to persons with disabilities or to those over age 65. ADRCs are access points for long-term care, and can direct patients and caregivers toward the proper resources for information, care, and finances. In tandem with ADRCs, Area Agencies on Aging employ strategies including "working directly with the older adult's family to improve planning; providing additional services including transportation, in-home care services and case management; and providing or paying for home modification [for example, ramps or grab bars]." These strategies target care transitions between health care settings and home.

Smoothly coordinated care transitions are vital to reduce the 20% readmission rate of Medicare beneficiaries (persons over 65 years old and persons with certain qualifying conditions) within 30 days of discharge from acute hospitals. **This high readmission rate to acute hospitals can also be**

lowered by more physical therapist participation in team rounds within the hospital setting, as they help coordinate postdischarge services for complex patients. When therapists do not participate in rounds, readmission risk is almost 4 times higher than when therapists do participate; a discharge directly to home increases readmission risk over twofold vs if the patient is first transitioned to a subacute setting.[7]

In a long-term care setting, patient management by an IDT/IPT is also helpful. When physical and occupational therapy were combined with physical education provided to persons with dementia living in institutions, balance improved and cognitive decline slowed.[8] Resident well-being in skilled nursing facilities is further improved with high staff retention and empowerment.[9]

Outside of long-term and acute care settings lies a continuum of community-based options. For persons with disabilities, remaining in the community as long as possible is best practice, especially when they "have input into the types of services and supports they need."[9] Effective IDT/IPT function for such patients includes knowledge of health issues such as "dementia, visual impairments, hearing impairments, thyroid conditions, osteoarthritis, oral health, and obesity."[9] All team members also need to be familiar with potentially inappropriate medications, such as those in the Beers criteria (see Chapter 4). Finally, practitioners in geriatrics should know about evidence-based treatment of depression, a common mental health issue in older adults and their caregivers.

Clinically diagnosable depression occurs in over one-quarter of patients in the community, and in over one-third of patients in long-term care settings; however, only half of diagnosed depressive disorders are treated, despite known benefits of medications, cognitive interventions, and physical activity. Multiple medical conditions including Parkinson's disease, stroke, dementia, cardiovascular disease, and multiple sclerosis can cause depression. Each provider should be aware of the increased comorbidity and suicide risk if depression is untreated, as well as inappropriate medications for older persons with depression. These medications include the following:

- Reserpine, normally prescribed for hypertension
- Beta blockers, normally prescribed for hypertension
- Most anticancer medications
- Tricyclic antidepressants, if glaucoma, benign prostatic hypertrophy, heart block, or orthostatic hypotension are also present[9]

While the patient's pharmacist and primary care provider are often the best professionals to review medications, the physical therapist may be the first clinician to notice the need for such a review. Side effects and medication interactions often include movement abnormalities, changes in alertness, and pain in various body regions. Through a thorough initial medication review, diligent symptom observation, and prompt reporting, the clinician can help the team identify adverse medication effects for prompt action, including potentially changing or eliminating one or more drugs used.

Example: Areas of Counseling

If it's free, it's advice; if you pay for it, it's counseling; if you can use either one, it's a miracle.

—Jack Adams[10]

A significant part of what physical therapists do is education of patients, clients, family members, health care team members, and other stakeholders in a person's health and wellness. This concept permeates doctor of physical therapy curricula, both in class and in clinical rotations; education is 1 of 18 performance indicators assessed on the physical therapist and physical therapist assistant Clinical Performance Instruments. Part of the education clinicians provide is counseling and referral for various medical and psychosocial issues that may or may not be within the therapist's scope of practice.

The therapist's scope is already extensive, including:

> [A]ssessment of smoking and smoking cessation (or at least its initiation), basic nutritional assessment and counseling, recommendations for physical activity and exercise, stress assessment and basic stress reduction recommendations, and sleep assessment and basic sleep hygiene recommendations.[11]

These areas, as well as lifestyle-related conditions, directly affect the human movement system. Because most patients in physical therapy have more face-to-face time with the clinician than with other medical providers, physical therapists are well positioned to be behavior change counselors in these areas, individually or in an IDT/IPT.[12]

Counseling, broadly defined in a medical context, is "professional guidance of the individual by utilizing psychological methods especially in collecting case history data, using various techniques of the personal interview, and testing interests and aptitudes."[13] Most people may think of counseling as being performed by a pastor, psychologist, or other mental health professional, but in reality all health care professionals counsel patients to some degree. For the purposes of this text, counseling areas encompass promotion of positive behaviors (eg, physical activity, appropriate medication usage) and discouragement of negative behaviors (eg, substance dependence), alleviation of caregiver burden, and using portions of specific psychological therapies including cognitive behavioral therapy (CBT) and remotivation therapy.

Physical activity counseling is a focus of several government initiatives, including *Healthy People 2020*.[14] A review of the previous objectives, from *Healthy People 2010*, noted that the original *Healthy People 2000* objectives were not all met, even for physical activity and fitness.[15] However, leading health indicators in the 2020 objectives are progressing. Several indicators relevant to physical therapists include:

- Percentage of adults meeting objectives for aerobic and muscle-strengthening physical activity (met)
- Adolescents and adults using less alcohol, fewer illicit drugs, or cutting down on cigarettes (target met)
- Percentage of persons with medical insurance (improving)
- Adults with controlled hypertension, obesity, and type 2 diabetes (no detectable change)
- Percentage of adults meeting targets for average daily intake of vegetables (no detectable change)
- Adolescents and adults with a major depressive episode (getting worse)

Medication usage counseling, to decrease risk of side effects and drug interactions, usually needs a pharmacist's knowledge and skill. The therapist working with patients over 65 years old can facilitate this process by knowing and using the Beers criteria for potentially inappropriate medications (see Chapter 4). A related issue is substance dependence because many abused substances are prescription drugs (see Chapter 12). Inpatient and outpatient programs in many communities can best treat the substance use disorder. Smoking cessation counseling, however, is well within the physical therapist's scope of practice; the 5 A's approach can be useful (ask, advise, assist, assess, and arrange follow-up).[16]

Caregiver burden is a topic frequently requiring counseling because the number of people aging with chronic disease (dementia, arthritis, developmental disorders, and others) is rapidly growing, and the fraction who depend on caregivers is growing in tandem. Counseling is one resource for persons with dementia and their caregivers living in the community, along with adult day and respite care, meal preparation assistance, and physical therapy[17]; clinicians can direct patients and caregivers to community resources for better quality of life. In fact, the European Federation of the Neurological Societies and other clinical practice guidelines strongly recommend counseling as part of an IDT/IPT treatment for caregivers and persons with dementia.[18]

Finally, specific methods, including motivational interviewing (MI) and CBT, are tools for counseling (see Chapter 4). One study by orthopedic surgeons described a health behavior change counseling framework that incorporated MI in conjunction with informational phone calls to patients who had undergone lumbar spine surgery. The AIDES format of MI helped to structure the calls to improve patient outcomes, discussed in the following sections[19]:

- A: acknowledge and affirm the person you are meeting
- I: introduce yourself
- D: define the duration of the session
- E: explain the flow of and expectations for the session
- S: set the tone with a stated intention to collaborate (convey the message to the patient that you as the therapist wish him or her to be involved in care planning)

One other psychological technique clinicians may encounter is remotivation therapy, which was developed in the 1940s with the steps of "creating a climate of acceptance, bridge to reality, sharing the world we live in, an appreciation of the work of the world, and [maintaining a] climate of acceptance."[20] Although the evidence base for this method is weak, a valid principle behind it is to treat others based on their inherent worth.

Example: Indications for Counseling Provided by a Physical Therapist Within an IDT/IPT Context

Health promotion, which involves counseling and patient participation, is a major function of physical therapists and other health care professionals. Topics in this area include exercise behaviors; diet and weight management; smoking cessation (since smoking affects multiple movement-related body systems including pulmonary); management of chronic disease and its effects on the human movement system; and mental health as it relates to the *International Classification of Functioning, Disability and Health* domains of participation restrictions, activity limitations, and primary and secondary impairments influenced by mental health issues.[21]

Further rationales for health promotion activities include patient opinions, a growing evidence base, and the complexity of an aging population. Regarding patient opinions, a survey of people in several Midwestern states indicated a need and necessity for physical therapists to be role models and coaches in the promotion of physical activity, smoking cessation, stress management, weight management, and eating of fruits and vegetables.[22] Regarding the growing evidence base, a meta-analysis of 39 clinical trials on various physical activity-related interventions, including exercise counseling, found large effects on depressive and schizophrenia symptoms, and moderate effects on aerobic capacity and quality of life, regardless of the activity intensity.[23]

Finally, the complexity of the aging United States population can be seen in the prevalence of lifestyle-related diseases that cause most deaths and disabilities. Beyond exercise prescription, physical therapist counseling entails "patient consultation aimed at health behavior change" with ongoing research related to the long-term effectiveness of various approaches.[24] Therefore, it is helpful for clinicians to know the basics of CBT interventions and MI. As a group, therapists can increase the effectiveness of health promotion by addressing barriers; effective strategies are a major area for needed research. These barriers include:

- Lack of time
- "Lack of interest or awareness of the patient or client, the public, and other health care providers that physical therapists provide these services"[24]
- Inadequate knowledge and education on the part of the provider
- Lack of resources, including insurance reimbursement

Thus, if a patient has health or wellness needs, the physical therapist should educate himself or herself to meet this need. Health, defined by the World Health Organization, is "a state of complete physical, mental and social well-being and not merely the absence of disease," whereas wellness is "consistent, balanced growth in the physical, spiritual, emotional, intellectual, social, and psychological dimensions of human existence."[24] By integrating these dimensions of health and wellness, clinicians can probe each patient's self-awareness, interest in his or her conditions, perceptions, outlook on life, and social and spiritual support per the clinician's training, comfort level, and experience.

As members of IDTs/IPTs, physical therapists can display self-efficacy related to some areas of health promotion, including physical activity prescription, mental health, and sometimes issues related to nutrition and smoking.[25] Clinicians can and should counsel patients in these areas to the extent allowed by their individual state's scope of practice (found in the practice acts and official websites of state physical therapy associations), personal education, training, and skill set. While there is much room for improvement in these areas to meet *Healthy People 2020* objectives for health and wellness in the United States, most clinicians desire lifelong learning in many areas of knowledge and skill to better help their patients.

Components of an Effective IDT/IPT

Because IDTs/IPTs are diverse in number of members and representation of professions, their structure can be flexible depending on the needs of the patient, facility, and health care system. Jensen and Mostrom[26] emphasize the role of interprofessional education in encouraging current and future health professionals to work with a team mindset in order to strengthen the currently fragmented health care system. In the sections to follow principles for effective IDTs/IPTs are discussed.

General Principles

The secret is to gang up on the problem, rather than each other.

—Thomas Stallkamp[27]

Core values for IDTs/IPTs have been summarized as "shared goals ... clear roles ... mutual trust ... effective communication ... [and] measurable processes and outcomes,"[4] undergirded by honesty, self-discipline, creativity, humility, and curiosity. Core principles of well-functioning IDTs/IPTs relate to personnel, tangible and intangible resources, and communication to improve outcomes and quality of patient care.

Personnel-Related Principles

- Leadership: a clearly identified leader must lead in a democratic way while supporting, supervising, and actively listening to members. Typically, the team leader is the professional with the broadest expertise.
- Skill mix: team members should each bring their training and experience to the table.
- Individual characteristics: team members should have "approachability, appropriate delegation, being able to compromise, confidentiality, decisiveness, empathy, good organisational [sic] skills, initiative; knowing one's strengths and weaknesses; open[ness] to learning; acquiring, demonstrating, and sharing new skills and knowledge, patience, personal responsibility, protective, reflexive [sic] practice, tolerance."[28]

Resource-Related Principles

- Personal rewards for team members: money, career opportunities, autonomy in practice, and ongoing learning challenges that fit individual capabilities
- Training and development: interprofessional education, continuing education, and knowledge-sharing opportunities

- Physical setting: adequate space, privacy for phone calls, and clear policies and procedures
- Clear vision: to steer the team and its interactions with stakeholders. Communication of this vision also reduces detrimental team conflict.

Communication-Related Principles

- Strategies and structures: a climate that supports both listening and speaking out, and limits team size to allow multidirectional communication.
- Supportive climate: camaraderie, mutual support, opportunities for fun, and friendship between members
- Respect and understanding of roles: each professional should understand the other's limitations in scope of practice and define roles accordingly.
- Quality focus: assessment of patient outcomes, facilitation of reflection, and constructive feedback for continuous skill improvement

Communication

Kerzner, exploring communication and team structure and function from a project management perspective, offers valuable insights for the physical therapist.[29] The IDT/IPT may have one of several possible cultural formats; some formats are clearly more advantageous than others:

- Cooperative: this format involves trust and communication, but is also difficult to achieve if members are initially very different in communication styles and underlying values.
- Non-cooperative: this format involves mistrust and individualism; these teams do not succeed.
- Competitive: members are forced to compete with each other for resources; this model is not helpful if members are on multiple teams, but it can work in the short term.
- Isolated: multiple teams are in a large system and interact as a units vs with central management.
- Fragmented: teams are scattered but can telecommunicate.

Regardless of structure and situation faced (related to patient care or not), an effective team will have efficiency, creativity, commitment, interdependence of members, trust, focus on results, flexibility for change, and focus on effective communication especially during conflict management. Conflict can drive results or be detrimental; team members who do not perceive a need to depend on each other tend to have more dysfunctional conflict.

Though conflict can drive results, teams need to know how to resolve conflict, which requires proper atmosphere and information. Methods of conflict resolution include:

- Confrontation/collaboration: gain the best solution via face-to-face meetings, baseline trust, and mutual team member confidence
- Compromise: ensure mutual victory and avoid outright fighting
- Smoothing/accommodating: maintain harmony regardless of how good the solution is
- Forcing/competing: decide rapidly in a dire situation, regardless of relationships injured
- Avoiding/withdrawing: possibly win the argument by delay, or not win at all

Communication barriers include[29]:

- Perception: team members have multiple viewpoints of the same message due to their unique personal characteristics that affect how they receive the message.
- Personality and interests: members pay less attention to topics that do not interest them.
- Attitudes, emotions, and prejudices: members have strong biases that prevent genuine understanding of another member or outside party.

One widely recommended method in medical professions, especially nursing, is the SBAR technique. This stands for situation, background, assessment, and recommendations, and it is most often used for nurse-to-doctor communication of patient status changes. Studies exploring SBAR's application in long-term care, acute care, and undergraduate curricula found that the technique is useful when applied in oral communication, but is typically and incorrectly perceived as written and time-consuming, thus lessening its long-term implementation by nursing staff.[30-32] When SBAR is used as designed, especially with other tools to monitor sudden changes in a patient's medical status, it can improve response time and potential intervention to prevent worsening of the patient's condition.[33]

Models of Effective IDTs/IPTs in Health Care

Several authors have examined IDT/IPT models related to increasing quality of geriatric care. For care transitions, such as between acute care and subacute rehabilitation, one such model is a floating team. This small team consists of a geriatrician and a geriatric nurse practitioner to manage assessment, medical complexity, staff education, facilitation of patient independence, and interprofessional communication. This model can improve patient satisfaction and reduce the risk of delirium, bladder incontinence, and pressure injuries as geriatric patients move from one setting to another.[34]

Another model, for long-term care, reinforces residual cognitive abilities of persons with dementia, based on the Allen cognitive disabilities theory.[35] Team members include rehabilitation staff (physical, occupational, and speech therapists) and all skilled nursing facility employees who interact with patients. These employees, including management, dietary, housekeeping, and nursing, are encouraged to acquire dementia interaction skills by ongoing training.[36] This model does not have published outcomes, but still reinforces the importance of knowledge and skill specific to cognitive and functional losses caused by dementia. The Allen cognitive levels, providing a common set of descriptors for varied health professionals, are summarized in Table 2-1.[35] The Allen Cognitive Level test was developed by Claudia Allen, an occupational therapist in the 1960s. The test assesses a person's functional cognitive abilities via a screen where the person imitates stitches of increasing complexity, along with other craft-based challenges to determine cognitive abilities.

A third model in an assisted-living setting sought to reduce the occurrence of falls and fall-related injury. Nursing staff followed numerous charting guidelines to improve screening and care coordination with physical and occupational therapists, dietitians, pharmacists or primary physicians for medication review, optometrists or audiologists, activities personnel for engaging in pleasurable physical activity, and personal care workers to monitor certain residents more frequently. For success, DeVol[37] emphasized staff training for safe ways to help residents move from place to place, and regular team communication to customize resident care.

A fourth model used technology to involve family caregivers in hospice care supervised by an IDT/IPT.[38] A video-technology–facilitated family caregiver contributes to and benefits from hospice IDT/IPT meetings, to rectify the skill deficits that often occur when a family member is thrust into an end-of-life caregiving role. While the video-phone system increased participation, it did not necessarily increase collaboration between health care professionals and family members. However, this pilot study can spur further investigation to maximize the model's effectiveness.

Benefits of adopting and validating a model of IDT/IPT-based health care go beyond patient safety and outcomes.[5] IDT/IPT-based care increased adherence to management of several chronic conditions, such as type 2 diabetes, and decreased inappropriate utilization of the emergency department vs a less acute care setting. This study did not, however, specify which health care professionals were included in the IDT/IPT.[39]

Table 2-1

Allen Cognitive Levels

ALLEN COGNITIVE LEVEL	SUB-LEVEL	CHARACTERISTICS
1: Automatic Actions	1.0 Withdrawing from stimulus	Very slow response time with small-amplitude movements; individual is non-verbal
	1.2 Responding to stimuli	20-second response delay; use high-contrast cues 14 inches from face; look at face for response
	1.4 Locating stimuli	Head/neck control present; use hand-over-hand assist and very consistent task sequencing
	1.6 Moving in bed	Spontaneous bed mobility; no sense of gravity in sitting; can help with self-cares
	1.8 Raising body parts	Can participate 50% in sit-to-stand; narrow visual field; reduce fatigue by up/down schedule; eats well
2: Postural Actions	2.0 Overcoming gravity	Can sit 20 to 30 minutes in armchair; use universal hand signs (wave, point, clap); fear of falling retained
	2.2 Standing to use righting reactions	Uses unstable objects for support; delayed balance control; can speak in native language; can form new short-term memories
	2.4 Walking	Navigates obstacles on level surfaces; uses swear words; cannot recall weightbearing restrictions; fear of being confined; can bend for bathing/toileting
	2.6 Walking to identified location	Walks to toilet/bed; avoids color changes as obstacles; can sing and dance; can push/throw/catch
	2.8 Using external stable support	Strong grip on railings; may punch unless given object to hold on for painful procedures; use songs with motions; prompt for memory of repetitive actions

(continued)

Table 2-1 (continued)

Allen Cognitive Levels

ALLEN COGNITIVE LEVEL	SUB-LEVEL	CHARACTERISTICS
3: Manual Actions	3.0 Grasping objects	Tunnel vision; responds to name; grasps/releases objects 14 inches away
	3.2 Distinguishing between objects	More adaptive grasp patterns; can distinguish objects by size/color or shape; 1-minute attention span; speak in short phrases
	3.4 Sustaining actions on objects	2 to 3 minute repetitive action; can dress self; can line up objects; can propel wheelchair but not safely
	3.6 Noting effects of actions on objects	Requires 24-hour supervision with verbal cues for next step; can sort objects; use single cue and concept of time (cause/effect)
	3.8 Using all objects for sense of activity completion	Takes 2 to 3 times longer but will complete task; remembers activities and routine in 2 to 3 weeks
4: Goal-Directed Actions (Ability Without Quality)	4.0 Sequencing through steps of an activity	Recognizes but cannot fix errors; keeps track of belongings; does important activities better
	4.2 Differentiating between parts of an activity	Asks for needed objects; places importance on possessions; may retain manners if trained earlier
	4.4 Completing a goal, using drawers (insides of objects)	Imitates others; corrects self if looking in a mirror; can sequence activities through cue cards; tells but cannot recognize a story
	4.6 Scanning the environment	Looks around room but cannot find hidden objects; can recognize impulsivity of actions; tries to fix errors by more physical pressure (eg, handheld eraser)
	4.8 Memorizing new steps	Rigidly adheres to learned steps; slow task performance; benefits from use of checklists
5: Exploratory Actions		Uses trial/error; adjusts with small movements; considers social standards; difficulty in planning ahead for error prevention
6: Planned Actions		Can understand probabilities, pros and cons; plans ahead; can dual task with appropriate attention

Mechanisms of Team Dysfunction and Repair

Coming together is a beginning, staying together is progress, and working together is success.
—Henry Ford[40]

Patient safety and service quality are 2 goals of team-based health care, with instructional methods including classroom sessions and patient simulation good for improving communication, cooperation, and coordination between professionals.[41] However, literature and the reader's experience are filled with examples of team malfunction. Sometimes this dysfunction has life-threatening results. A case from the author's experience involved lack of sufficient documented oral and written communication between speech therapists, dietary staff, and nursing staff that resulted in a resident choking on food too hard to chew. To correct the problem, administration developed all-staff in-services and improved clarity of documentation forms for resident safety.

An IDT/IPT can include family physicians, medical residents, nursing staff, secretaries, social workers, pharmacists, health promoters, as well as rehabilitation therapists, thus creating multiple potential sources of constructive or destructive conflict. These include "role boundary issues; scope of practice; and accountability."[42] Associated barriers to resolution include "lack of time and [excessive] workload; people in less powerful positions; lack of recognition or motivation to address conflict; and avoiding confrontation for fear of causing emotional discomfort." Recommended interventions include team-level protocol implementation and direct action by the team leader, as well as individual-level "open and direct communication; a willingness to find solutions; showing respect; and humility."[42]

These causes, barriers, and solutions are explored further from a business and management perspective in several case studies provided by customer service director Cindy Zbytniewski. One such case study involved a system of long-term care and assisted-living facilities in Ireland, whose parent company found multiple problems in one facility, including budget overrun, poor working environment, impaired resident care, open disrespect for management, inappropriate work relationships and groups, and broken lines of communication. Underlying these problems was strong individualism; each team member, including management, blamed other team members for the problem but was not aware of personal contributions to the situation. Given a year to implement ground rules for self-awareness and constructive communication, the team increased its focus on resident care while maintaining a non-threatening environment.[43] Another survey article lists factors to address during conflicts, with the perspective that individual differences are normal and helpful as long as each member has a team mindset.[44]

Another study examined a large company's team dysfunction.[45] This company had a dictatorial leadership style, which, with poor conflict-management strategies and team member inexperience in self-reflection, produced inefficiency, quarrels, stagnancy, and excessive workplace politics. Since the team members were each experts in their fields and initially had apparently good rapport, they benefited from guided practice in self-awareness, commitment to a common goal of customer service, and effective communication and conflict management.

Case studies and other sources uniformly recommend rules of engagement and a core set of team leader characteristics to bring a team toward optimal functioning.[46] **Rules of engagement** are written or unwritten norms for team member communication. These include:

- Awareness of one's own involvement in a problem yet interdependence on other team members
- Weighting of feedback toward positive vs negative, in a 4:1 ratio
- Dedication toward efficiency by brainstorming solutions for discussion and knowing a meeting's purpose ahead of time
- Establishment of emotional neutrality, if possible, before speaking

Characteristics of an effective team leader include (C. Zbytniewski, email communication, November 1, 2016):

- Ability to self-regulate one's emotions
- Commitment to shift the reference point toward customer service as often as needed
- Wisdom to "focus on the right things in the right way"[46] and reason backward with team members from desired results, to behaviors, to member mindset
- Transparency to model appropriate interpersonal behaviors and remain approachable
- Skill in constructive feedback to manage conflict (includes recommending personality type assessments such as the Myers-Briggs Type Indicator)

In addition to developing core skills and characteristics, the team leader needs to apply them to challenging situations. Some teams may have a so-called toxic member, who produces "a pattern of de-energizing, frustrating, or putting down teammates."[47] Because these behaviors do not directly conflict with established laws, this member can be hard to remove from the team. The leader should analyze the basis of the toxic behavior, offer to help the member, give direct and specific feedback to increase the member's awareness of the behavior's impact on others and self, and document the process including others' complaints and specific behaviors and responses. The toxic member may need to be isolated until the behavior is addressed to reduce collateral damage over time; teams need to do so without compromising patient care.

Another challenge occurs when the team leader inherits a team from another leader.[48] Here, key functions are maintaining stability and establishing a new vision. To do so, the leader needs strong assessment skills for members, current team status, and team dynamics. After assessing, the leader can promote vision revision and be alert for opportunities to "accelerate team development and improve performance."[49] Assessment must be schedule-flexible, efficient, systematic, and prioritized by team members' importance. During reshaping of the vision, the leader may need to replace some members tactfully, or else suggest different roles more suited to individual strengths. Throughout the process, the leader should model and maintain a safe environment for communication between members and leadership.

Table 2-2 summarizes essential team traits, mechanisms of dysfunction, negative impacts of dysfunction, and strategies for repair (C. Zbytniewski, email communication, November 1, 2016).[49] The lists are not exhaustive, and items across columns do not correspond directly to any one item on either side.

While many of these case studies focused on the team leader, other recommended resources for non-leading IDT/IPT members include the following (C. Zbytniewski, email communication, Novemebr 1, 2016):

- *All In: How the Best Managers Create a Culture of Belief and Drive Big Results* by Adrian Gostick and Chester Elton (2012)
- *Walk Awhile in my Shoes: Gut-level, Real-world Messages from Managers to Employees* by Erick Harvey and Steve Ventura (1996)
- *Managing Transitions, Making the Most of Change, 3rd edition* by William Bridges (2009)
- *Good to Great: Why Some Companies Make the Leap ... and Others Don't* by Jim Collins (2001)

Table 2-2

Team Traits, Dysfunctions, Impacts, and Strategies

ESSENTIAL TEAM TRAITS	MECHANISMS OF DYSFUNCTION	NEGATIVE IMPACTS OF DYSFUNCTION	STRATEGIES FOR REPAIR
• Mutual trust • Unfiltered productive conflict • Commitment to action plans and decisions • Mutual accountability • Focus on results for the consumer and company	• Absence of trust • Fear of conflict • Lack of commitment • Avoidance of accountability • Inattention to results	• Stressed budgets and operation • Poor working environment and communication deficits • Low morale and performance • Lack of collaboration and cooperation for results • Loss of customers and poor customer service	• Leader self-disclosure, including personality type and how other members contribute to the team • Illumination of conflict to remind of its necessity • Prioritization of consensus over unanimous agreement, via clear deadlines, firm decisions, and guided practice of conflict management • Publish goals and standards, review progress on a schedule, and reward the team for results • Lead selflessly and publish results and rewards

Summary

Because the IDT/IPT is becoming the norm within health care settings, it is important for the physical therapist to understand its essentials. Physical therapy research about the best ways in which clinicians can contribute to the team is still developing. This chapter has explored common traits of successful and unsuccessful team models, as well as solutions and resources for the team leader and members.

Key Points

- Increase physical therapist participation in discharge planning to reduce readmission rates.
- IDTs should adhere to personnel-, resource-, and communication-related principles for optimal function: leadership, skill mix of individual characteristics, tangible and intangible rewards, clear vision, a good physical setting, and support for team members and the team at all levels.
- Work cultures can be cooperative (preferred), non-cooperative, competitive, isolated, or fragmented.
- Conflict management styles include confrontation/collaboration (preferred), compromise, smoothing/accommodating, forcing/competing, and avoiding/withdrawing.
- Rules of engagement for communication include self-awareness, interdependence, focus on giving positive feedback, dedication to efficiency, and establishment of emotional neutrality.
- An effective team leader should self-regulate emotions, guide a customer-service focus, guide backward reasoning, model good behaviors with transparency and approachability, and give/receive feedback well.

Review Questions

- Based on your experience and the literature reviewed in this chapter, what are some current strengths and opportunities for further research and development of the IDT/IPT concept?
- In your clinical rotations or practice, how are interprofessional models for communication (eg, SBAR) used? How do you measure their effectiveness?
- In your clinical rotations or practice, who comprises the IDT/IPT?
  - Is there a designated leader? If so, which discipline? How does this person display (or not) traits of an effective team leader as noted in the text?
  - Is there team dysfunction? If so, how does this affect communication and patient care?
- How can an IDT/IPT help the patient, especially one with multiple complex medical or psychiatric conditions?
- Based on your experience across practice settings, how has a team approach, or lack thereof, impacted patient care?
- Discuss an example of an ineffective IDT/IPT with a classmate or colleague.
  - Why might it have been ineffective?
  - What were the negative impacts on patient care and team member morale?
  - Suggest potential solutions to implement as a leader or another member.

Case Study: An IDT/IPT of Mixed Effectiveness

Often, IDTs/IPTs do not consistently provide quality patient care, especially if members' roles are not defined and there is insufficient buy in. The following case is adapted from a scenario in an urban short-term rehabilitation facility that employed staff who also worked in the facility's memory care and long-term care units. Formatting of the case is based on the Physical Therapy Clinical Reasoning and Reflection Tool (see Chapter 1).

Patient Description

- An elderly male patient was hospitalized for 2 weeks after an unwitnessed fall at home, resulting in a hip fracture that required open reduction-internal fixation surgery. He was transferred to subacute rehabilitation, at which point his family members stated a desire to take him home prior to day 21 to avoid insurance copays.
- Past social history: he lived at home with family present 24 hours per day, who assisted with laundry, cleaning, cooking, transportation, and other higher-level activities of daily living. He previously walked and negotiated stairs independently. Prior to retirement, he had worked third shift for many years.
- Past medical/psychiatric history: he has advanced dementia, anemia, mild hearing loss, osteoporosis, acute delirium, and remote tobacco and alcohol dependence.

Therapy Evaluation Status (From Physical, Occupational, and Speech Therapy Initial Evaluations)

- Mobility: 25% to 50% assistance for bed mobility depending on momentary level of pain. He required the assistance of 2 people to transfer to wheelchair and was unable to stand or walk due to fear of the floor.
- Cognition/safety: he was able to process information given 3 to 4 times increased time; tolerated a general-consistency diet with thin liquids; demonstrated impaired auditory comprehension, problem solving, short-term recall, and verbal expression, which prevented appropriate response to most cues; unable to express needs in the rehabilitation facility (evidence of incontinence noted at evaluation, without indication of patient awareness to use the call light to request assistance for cleaning up).
- Social: he used foul language in replies to the speech therapist. The patient's daughters visited during the physical therapy evaluation and expressed the desire to be highly involved with care and home exercises.

IDT/IPT Goals (Discussed by Individual Therapists and Nursing Staff)

- Facilitate the patient reaching his prior level of function in mobility and safety skills
- Assess and prescribe an appropriate seating system (wheelchair) for decreased burden of care at home
- Maintain current cognitive and swallow function, as the speech therapist determined that the patient was not appropriate for participation in skilled speech therapy services at time of evaluation
- Facilitate the patient adjusting to the facility routine for participation in care and therapy
- Consistently manage postoperative pain
- Encourage the patient to interact appropriately with other residents and staff

Best Practice Recommendations at Evaluation

- Schedule activities and therapy at times when the patient is most alert
- Train family members at least twice weekly in exercises and safe ways to assist the patient
- Repeatedly practice functional tasks in an environment that simulates the patient's home
- Schedule daily therapy sessions with consistent treating therapists and extend the duration of the total stay to accommodate the patient's learning deficits related to dementia
- Promptly provide necessary equipment to maintain patient safety and skin integrity (fitted manual wheelchair and a heel-offloading shoe to avoid worsening an open area)
- Train staff from nursing and dietary departments in how to prevent undesirable patient behaviors during interactions, with sensitivity to cultural differences (White patient and therapy team, predominantly African American staff, urban setting)

Deviations From These Recommendations During the Patient's Stay

- Treatments were scheduled with several different therapists, without adherence to or documentation of approach at times of the patient's best participation level.
- Family training occurred only at evaluation and at the discharge planning meeting.
- The patient's insurance allowed only 5 times per week of therapy sessions, with copays starting at day 21 of stay that incentivized the family to take the patient home before he had reached his premorbid status.
- Footwear, though ordered at the start of care, was not provided by administration during the patient's stay.
- Staff were not trained in dementia care, though administration intended to provide training in the future.

Outcomes of the Case

- Family members took the patient home prior to day 21 of stay, intending to provide 24-hour care but expressing dissatisfaction with nursing care.
- The patient maintained his cognitive level (Allen Cognitive Level 3.0; see Table 2-1).
- Family and staff needed to provide 75% assistance to the patient for all mobility tasks and daily activities.
- Therapy recommended home physical and occupational therapy services, home nursing for wound care, provision of a tub transfer bench for safe bathing, and provision of a lightweight manual wheelchair for safe patient mobility inside and outside the home.

References

1. Zera R. *Business Wit & Wisdom.* Washington, DC: Beard Books; 2005.
2. Mitchell P, Ramirez S. *Collaboration and Peak Performance.* Fremont, CA: Robertson Publishing; 2013.
3. Jette AM. The revolving hospital door. *Phys Ther.* 2016;96(12):1858-1859.
4. Mitchell P, Wynia M, Golden R, et al. *Core principles and values of effective team-based health care.* [Discussion paper.] Institute of Medicine 2012. www.iom.edu/tbc
5. Neumann V, Gutenbrunner C, Fialka-Moser V, et al. Interdisciplinary team working in physical and rehabilitation medicine. *J Rehabil Med.* 2010;42(1):4-8.
6. National Association of Area Agencies on Aging. Aging and disability resource centers. *N4A.* http://www.n4a.org/adrcs. Published 2016. Accessed January 21, 2018.
7. Kadivar Z, English A, Marx BD. Understanding the relationship between physical therapist participation in interprofessional rounds and hospital readmission rates: preliminary study. *Phys Ther.* 2016;96(11):1705-1713.
8. Christofoletti G, Olani MM, Gobbi S, et al. A controlled clinical trial on the effects of motor intervention on balance and cognition in institutionalized elderly patients with dementia. *Clin Rehabil.* 2008;22(7):618-626.

9. Blackburn JA, Dulmus CN. *Handbook of Gerontology: Evidence-Based Approaches to Theory, Practice, and Policy.* Hoboken, NJ: Wiley; 2007.
10. Price SD. *Best Advice Ever Again: Life Lessons for Success in the Real World.* Guilford, CT: The Lyons Press; 2006.
11. Dean E. Physical therapy in the 21st century (Part I): toward practice informed by epidemiology and the crisis of lifestyle conditions. *Physiother Theory Pract.* 2009;25(5-6):330-353.
12. Frerichs W, Kaltenbacher E, van de Leur JP, Dean E. Can physical therapists counsel patients with lifestyle-related health conditions effectively? A systematic review and implications. *Physiother Theory Pract.* 2012;28(8):571-587.
13. Merriam-Webster dictionary. Counseling. *Merriam-Webster.* https://www.merriam-webster.com/dictionary/counseling. Updated April 10, 2018. Accessed April 13, 2018.
14. Francis KT. Status of the year 2000 health goals for physical activity and fitness. *Phys Ther.* 1999;79(4):405-414.
15. Office of Disease Prevention and Health Promotion (ODPHP). Healthy People 2020. *HelathyPeople.gov.* https://www.healthypeople.gov/. Accessed January 21, 2018.
16. Bodner ME, Rhodes RE, Miller WC, Dean E. Smoking cessation and counseling practices of Canadian physical therapists. *Am J Prev Med.* 2012;43(1):67-71.
17. Weber SR, Pirraglia PA, Kunik ME. Use of services by community-dwelling patients with dementia: a systematic review. *Am J Alzheimers Dis Other Demen.* 2011;26(3):195-204.
18. Hort J, O'Brien JT, Gainotti G, et al. EFNS guidelines for the diagnosis and management of Alzheimer's disease. *Eur J Neurol.* 2010;17(10):1236-1248.
19. Skolasky RL, Riley LH, Maggard AM, Bedi S, Wegener ST. Functional recovery in lumbar spine surgery: a controlled trial of health behavior change counseling to improve outcomes. *Contemp Clin Trials.* 2013;36(1):207-217.
20. Dyer JA, Stotts ML, eds. *Handbook of Remotivation Therapy.* Birminghamton, NY: The Haworth Clinical Practice Press; 2005.
21. Healey WE, Broers KB, Nelson J, Huber G. Physical therapists' health promotion activities for older adults. *J Geriatr Phys Ther.* 2012;35(1):35-48.
22. Black B, Ingman MS, Janes J. Physical therapists' role in health promotion as perceived by the patient: descriptive survey. *Phys Ther.* 2016;96(10):1588-1596.
23. Rosenbaum S, Tiedemann A, Sherrington C, Curtis J, Ward PB. Physical activity interventions for people with mental illness: a systematic review and meta-analysis. *J Sci Med Sport.* 2014;75(9):964-974.
24. Bezner JR. Promoting health and wellness: implications for physical therapist practice. *Phys Ther.* 2015;95(10):1433-1444.
25. Rea BL, Hopp Marshak H, Neish C, Davis N. The role of health promotion in physical therapy in California, New York, and Tennessee. *Phys Ther.* 2004;84(6):510-523.
26. Jensen GM, Mostrom E. *Handbook of Teaching and Learning for Physical Therapists.* 3rd ed. St. Louis, MO: Elsevier; 2013.
27. Brown E. *Take Your Soul to Work: 365 Meditation on Every Day Leadership.* New York, NY: Simon & Schuster; 2013.
28. Nancarrow SA, Booth A, Ariss S, et al. Ten principles of good interprofessional team work. *Hum Resour Health.* 2013;11:19.
29. Kerzner H. *Project Management: A Systems Approach to Planning, Scheduling, and Controlling.* 9th ed. Hoboken, NJ: Wiley; 2006.
30. Renz SM, Boltz MP, Wagner LM, Capezuti EA, Lawrence TE. Examining the feasibility and utility of an SBAR protocol in long-term care. *Geriatr Nurs.* 2013;34(4):295-301.
31. Compton J, Copeland K, Flanders S, et al. Implementing SBAR across a large multihospital health system. *Jt Comm J Qual Patient Saf.* 2012;38(6):261-268.
32. Enlow M, Shanks L, Guhde J, Perkins M. Incorporating interprofessional communication skills (ISBARR) into an undergraduate nursing curriculum. *Nurse Educ.* 2010;15(4):176-180.
33. Ludikhuize J, de Jonge E, Goossens A. Measuring adherence among nurses one year after training in applying the Modified Early Warning Score and Situation-Background-Assessment-Recommendation instruments. Resuscitation 2011. In Ludikhuize J. *Rapid Response Systems: Recognition and Management of the Deteriorating Patient.* University of Amsterdam; 2014:99-114.
34. Arbaje AI, Maron DD, Yu Q, et al. The geriatric floating interprofessional team. *J Am Geriatr Soc.* 2010;58(2):364-370.
35. Johnson CC. Cognition: assessment, treatment, and management. [Seminar.] Therapists Training Therapists;2013.
36. Warchol K. An interprofessional dementia program model for long-term care. *Top Geriatr Rehabil.* 2004;20(1):59-71.
37. DeVol SA. A multidisciplinary fall management program design using home health for elderly residents with dementia residing in an assisted living setting. *GeriNotes.* 2012;20(1):9-13.
38. Wittenberg-Lyles E, Oliver DP, Demiris G, Baldwin P. The ACTive intervention in hospice interprofessional team meetings: exploring family caregiver and hospice team communication. *J Comput Mediat Commun.* 2010;15(3):465-481.

39. Reiss-Brennan B, Brunisholz KD, Dredge C, et al. Association of integrated team-based care with health care quality, utilization, and cost. *JAMA*. 2016;316(8):826-834.
40. Bacon J. *The Art of Community: Building the New Age of Participation*. 2nd ed. Sebastopol, CA: O'Reilly Media; 2012.
41. Weaver SJ, Dy SM, Rosen MA. Team-training in health care: a narrative synthesis of the literature. *BMJ Qual Saf*. 2014;23(5):359-372.
42. Brown J, Lewis L, Ellis E, et al. Conflict on interprofessional primary health care teams - can it be resolved? *J Interprof Care*. 2011;25(1):4-10.
43. McGeough Training Limited. Restoring a dysfunctional team to good health. *McGeough*. http://www.mcgeough.ie/case-studies/restoring-dysfunctional-teams.asp. Published 2014. Accessed January 21, 2018.
44. Liam Healy & Associates. Dysfunctional team intervention. *Liam Healy & Associates*. http://www.psychometrics.co.uk/team.html. Published 2010. Accessed January 21, 2018.
45. Droste Group. Case study: one team's journey from dysfunction to high performance. http://drostegroup.com/wp-content/uploads/2015/09/CASE-STUDY-Team-Development.pdf. Accessed January 21, 2018.
46. Schwarz R. Get a dysfunctional team back on track. *Harvard Business Review*. https://hbr.org/2013/11/get-a-dysfunctional-team-back-on-track. Published November 14, 2013. Accessed January 21, 2018.
47. Gallo A. How to manage a toxic employee. *Harvard Business Review*. https://hbr.org/2016/10/how-to-manage-a-toxic-employee. Published October 3, 2016. Accessed January 21, 2018.
48. Watkins MD. Leading the team you inherit. *Harvard Business Review*. https://hbr.org/2016/06/leading-the-team-you-inherit. Published June 2016. Accessed January 21, 2018.
49. Lencioni P. *The complete summary: the five dysfunctions of a team*. Soundview Executive Book Summaries. 2009.

Cultural Competence

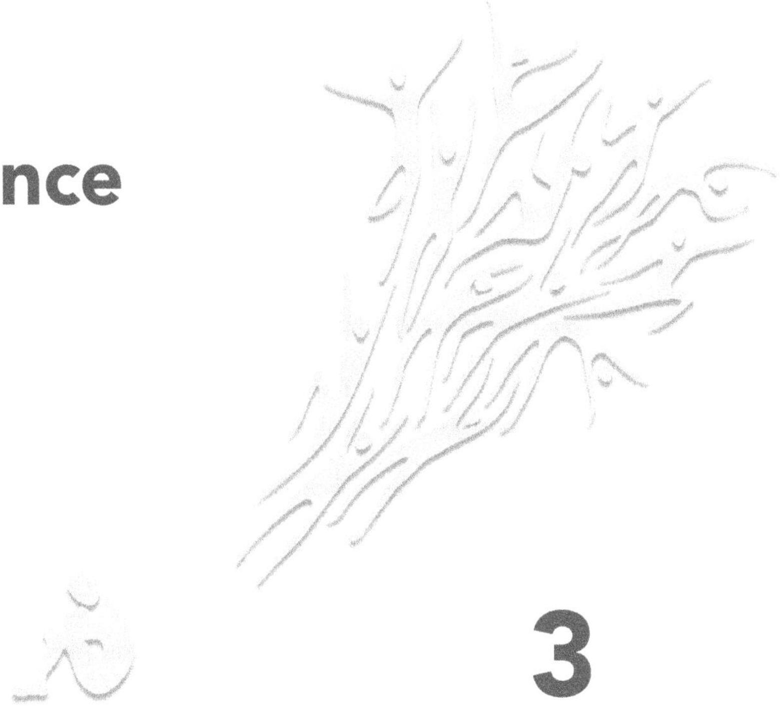

3

Outline

- What Is Culture for the Physical Therapist?
  - The Patient's Culture
  - The Therapist's Workplace Culture
  - Dimensions of Culture
  - Disparities of Culture
- Rationales for Cultural Competence Across Treatment Settings
- How to Increase Cultural Competence
  - Challenges to Cultural Competence
  - Staff Training Models
  - Interpreter Services and Responsibilities
- Emerging Topics
- Special Focus Issues
  - Psychosocial Perspectives on Disability: Applying and Optimizing the ICF model
  - Loss and Grieving: Cultural Considerations at End of Life
  - Sexuality: Encompassing Minority and Mainstream Cultural Groups
  - Motivation and Adherence: Capitalizing on Therapy Culture
- Summary
- Key Points
- Review Questions
- Case Studies: First Impressions

Johnson H.
Psychosocial Elements of Physical Therapy: The Connection of Body to Mind (pp 33-54).

Learning Objectives

- Craft a multidimensional definition of culture applicable across physical therapists' treatment settings
- Demonstrate awareness of several major disparities across cultures in the United States
- Articulate various methods to increase one's own cultural competence, in life and in the clinic

Cultural competence, or cultural sensitivity, is a hotly discussed topic in today's health care industry. Due to global and local diversity, the student and physical therapist will likely work with classmates, colleagues, and patients who have cultural backgrounds, beliefs, and values different from his or her own. Active participatory learning is needed to make interprofessional education and practice effective to serve these diverse patients.[1]

In the context of psychological conditions and substance use disorders (SUDs), cultural awareness is useful in any practice setting. Research yields statistics on how likely one is to encounter a person from a specific population group with psychiatric conditions. Globally, mental disorders affect just under 20% of people by annual diagnosis, and 29% over one's lifetime. Women in any country have a higher risk for mood disorders, while men have a higher risk for SUDs. English speakers have a high risk of any psychiatric condition, while residents of north and southeast Asia and sub-Saharan Africa have an overall lower risk.[2] From an economic perspective, refugees from low- and middle-income countries have a higher risk of epilepsy than of psychotic disorders. In these refugees, overall risk for SUDs and emotional disorders is low.[3]

The author of this book is a native resident of the United States with a German-American background. While reading, students and clinicians are encouraged to think about how their individual cultural background (aspects of culture are discussed later in this chapter) affects how they view and treat patients. The chapter will yield insights about cultural dimensions, disparities, and competence-increasing techniques.

What Is Culture for the Physical Therapist?

A nation's culture resides in the hearts and in the soul of its people.

—Mahatma Gandhi[4]

Since the concept of culture goes beyond a person's age group or ethnicity, this section examines the clinically relevant definition. As stated, culture includes backgrounds, beliefs, values, and ethnicity. There are 2 aspects that will be discussed: a patient's culture and the workplace culture. Being aware of multiple dimensions of one's culture is important for patient dignity, standardized test score interpretation, and interprofessional team function. The following is an example of dignity-related awareness in geriatrics: since many older adults are active and involved in community roles, and since their age cohort is heterogeneous, it is wiser to refer to them as an "older adult/person" and not as "elderly."[5]

The Patient's Culture

Cultural differences affect the development of the therapy plan of care. One such example is US-based therapists working with children and teachers native to Puerto Rico. Teachers in these countries have different normative expectations for children's abilities, influenced by:

> Puerto Rican values of interdependence, pampering or nurturing behaviors, and overprotectiveness that therapists should account for when interpreting Pediatric Evaluation of Disability Inventory scores and establishing plans of care.[6]

Another example is the intended discharge settings for collectivist vs individualistic cultures. Collectivist cultures (where the community comes together to solve problems) may promote home caregiving by extended family, while individualistic cultures (where people prize personal independence) may promote institutionalizing physically or cognitively dependent family members.[7]

A helpful text for courses and research on culture-specific disability and ethnicity in doctorate of physical therapy (DPT) programs is Ingstad and Whyte's *Disability in Local and Global Worlds*.[8] In their book, Ingstad and Whyte survey disability concepts across developed, underdeveloped, and undeveloped countries. Some concepts are country-specific (eg, female genital mutilation in women from certain African countries who then emigrate) or culture-specific (eg, a Brazilian village's belief that a transplanted organ also transplants the donor's personality).

For the student or faculty member, scholarly literature supports several standardized tests of cultural competence and awareness:

- Inventory for Assessing the Process of Cultural Competence Among Health Care Professionals-Student Version: minimal detectable change is 8.57 points.[9]
- Cultural Competence Continuum: an ordinal scale (ie, a scale that ranks items by relative superiority but cannot say how much better one item is than another) that is useful for analyzing reflective writing for its indicators of the writer's cultural competence.[10]
- Cultural Disability Awareness Questionnaire: a measurement tool with good psychometric properties, that is sensitive enough to detect change in faculty members' cultural diversity awareness after a 1-day workshop.[11]

The Therapist's Workplace Culture

How people work together is important for clinicians and faculty to know. Types of workplace culture include cooperative (with trust and communication), non-cooperative (with mistrust and individualism), competitive (where employees are forced to compete for resources), isolated (within a large company), and fragmented (with scattered teams).[12] Non-cooperative cultures are never successful, while competitive cultures work only in the short term. The clinician should be aware of these potential workplace cultures.

Team-based care focuses on improving quality, utilization, and cost of care. It is defined as meeting the 5 components of the Intermountain Mental Health Integration and 3 levels of the National Committee for Quality Assurance. Intermountain Mental Health Integration components are "leadership and culture, clinical workflow, information system, financing and operations, and community resources."[13] While this article did not explore the National Committee for Quality Assurance levels, it found that team-based care—led by a primary medical doctor and monitored by an operations manager—resulted in more depression screening, better adherence to bundled diabetes care, self-care plan documentation, lower emergency department usage, and lower hospital and ambulatory care admissions. Cost savings were unspecified. The system is a work in progress, as shown by mixed results for percentage of patients with controlled hypertension, frequency of documentation of advanced care directives, and urgent care or specialist visits.

Dimensions of Culture

An individual's culture encompasses attitudes, beliefs, values, and customs related to many areas besides ethnicity. This can include history of military deployments,[14] which can affect readjustment to civilian life depending on rank and method of release. Another area is weight and obesity; while some cultures view excess weight as a mark of privilege and wealth, most Western cultural groups view it negatively. Physical therapists address weight due to its effects on the movement system, which include joint loading and chronic pain. Some patients interviewed for a study "perceived negative weight judgments" in the clinic's physical environment and setup, lack of staff knowledge of complex determinants of weight, and lack of collaborative communication techniques.[15]

Age-related social support and spirituality or religion are 2 other dimensions of culture. The *silver tsunami*, as geriatric physical therapist Carole Lewis puts it, means that one-fifth of the US population will be over age 65 by the year 2030. The prevalence of disability will also grow, depending on how prepared the medical community is to address it. However, due to declining birth and marriage rates, family caregivers will be insufficient to cope with this population segment. Family caregivers—the most common for aging persons—can be supported by public policy, professional training, support for stress and mood symptoms, and identification with screening and assessment by therapists. Thus, cultural competence is an essential skill for providers.[16]

Spirituality and religion vary depending on the person's individual and societal background, and affect the success of the person's rehabilitation. Although most therapists recognize the strong impact of a patient's faith beliefs on chronic illness and pain coping strategies, they may hesitate to address faith issues due to insufficient time, training, and comfort level. DPT students, however, tend to believe that faith can positively influence hope and coping skills. In one study, therapists enhanced rapport with patients by both parties knowing the other's faith background. One's own faith background did not necessarily correlate with comfort level in discussing it with patients, but the older the student was, the more comfortable he or she tended to be.[17]

The clinician will encounter many more dimensions in practice, especially in managing chronic disease that is increasingly common in the general population. Since chronic disease management is better done via a team approach than by individual providers, new physical therapists need to learn how to practice collaboratively as well as autonomously. An Australian DPT program curriculum helps students build on foundational skills for management of complex conditions as a teammate, clinician, leader, and clinician-researcher. Many studies mentioned throughout this chapter stress cultural competence as a component.[18]

Disparities of Culture

In the United States, varying education levels, age, sex, social circumstances, and other factors related to different ethnic backgrounds unfortunately correlate with or cause disparities in health status, functional independence, and ability to pursue health and wellness. The *Healthy People 2020* initiative aims to reduce health disparities, which is a goal that also aligns with that of the physical therapy profession. This section surveys studies of health-related disparities relating to culture.

Ethnicity and increasing age can predict functional level. For example, in Hispanic persons (a rapidly aging, prominent minority) functional impairment often comes before age 65 due to earlier onset of diabetes, as well as socioeconomic, educational, and language barriers. Immigrants from these families are more likely to live with their children than are native-born Hispanic adults; while impairments are more severe, better family support decreases institutionalization. Though physician visits are more common, they do not protect health as well, and when Hispanic persons see a physical therapist, it is usually later in the disease and less likely than if the person has a different ethnicity. Strategies for therapists include recruitment of minorities into DPT programs (since patients like to be seen by a clinician of their own culture), increase public awareness of disparities, and steer health care reform toward reducing health disparities.[19]

Other studies have examined older African American women, who have a high risk for osteoarthritis, type 2 diabetes, obesity, heart disease, pain, and other chronic conditions. Authors from 2 studies helped postmenopausal African American women set walking goals with pedometers, to combat health risks associated with high-fat diets and sedentary lifestyles. Individualization helped approximately half of participants meet both personal and the American College of Sports Medicine's recommended step-count goals. Facilitators included small successes and the intent to continue regardless of mood or day of the week; barriers "were related to exercise being tiring, fatiguing, and hard work" and participants lacking "time due to work and family responsibilities."[20,21]

When setting walking goals with African American women over age 45, it is important to emphasize walking speed. This population is more likely to have a speed below 1 m/second, which indicates a threefold higher risk for osteoarthritis than in White women of similar age.[22]

Pain management literature reveals multiple disparities related to culture. Almost half of veterans report pain issues and associated concerns, which require more outpatient health care. Female veterans may need more resources than males for pain management, especially with psychiatric comorbidities such as posttraumatic stress disorder.[23] Management also differs across races, according to increasing evidence, especially regarding opioid medications. White patients are more likely than non-White patients to have opioids prescribed[24]; however, this leads to more issues for patients who become addicted to opioids (see Chapters 12 and 13).

Because HIV spreads through body fluids, certain habits of infected individuals affect their own health and the health of persons with whom they interact. Thus, persons with the infection and syndrome can be considered a cultural group as well. Since HIV-AIDS is considered a chronic disease affecting multiple areas of health, researchers have set the following priorities for study:

> [E]pisodic health and disability; aging with HIV across the life course; concurrent health conditions; access to rehabilitation and models of rehabilitation service provision; effectiveness of rehabilitation interventions; and enhancing outcome measurement in HIV and rehabilitation research.[25]

In the clinic, therapists should screen for comorbid SUDs and psychiatric conditions in persons with HIV infection, who commonly report pain lasting over 3 months. Cognitive behavioral therapy and physical therapy are especially helpful for functional improvement, and doctors should minimize opioid prescription. Statistically, "an estimated 39% to 85% of individuals with HIV infection also suffer from chronic pain compared with only 20% to 30% of the general population."[26] This pain is most often related to musculoskeletal problems, but peripheral neuropathic pain affects 20% to 30% of patients. Chronic pain increases the risk for disability when risk factors such as anxiety, depression, catastrophizing, fear avoidance, poor health, high initial pain severity, and increased age are present.

As noted previously, a person's age alone can be a cultural factor that impacts health care and outcomes. Adults from a different generation than that of the health care provider may have different educational levels, standards and expectations for interpersonal interactions, if and how to use therapy services, and perceived benefits and drawbacks of care. In 2015, about 20% of persons over age 65 in the United States used rehabilitation services. Adults who had more education, chronic medical conditions, frequent falls, pain, and physical performance restrictions received more therapy. However, older adults as a group needed longer episodes of care to achieve their functional goals, related to the therapist-patient differences stated previously as well as the simple facts of physiological aging.[27]

Rationales for Cultural Competence Across Treatment Settings

This section explicitly justifies the need for clinicians to gain cultural knowledge and skill. Ruth Purtilo, the 31st Mary McMillan lecturer, addressed cultural competence as a central topic of her lecture. Because therapists need to focus on care and respect with accountability, she argued that cultural competence should be a graduation requirement from all DPT programs.[28] The American Physical Therapy Association (APTA) responded by making cultural competence a required performance criterion on the 1997 and 2006 versions of the Physical Therapist Clinical Performance Instrument. The culturally competent therapist "adapts delivery of physical therapy services with consideration for patients' differences, values, preferences, and needs."[29]

Literature also encourages cultural competence development beyond graduation. In a consensus-developed *International Classification of Functioning, Disability and Health* (ICF) core set, an "instrument for assessing the physical health and engagement of older adults,"[30] assessment criteria include informal peer relationships, health service use, and a patient's general culture, besides movement-related body structures and functions. Also, the potential health benefits for persons in economically and socially challenged cultural groups (eg, the population of persons over age 65) are enormous if physical therapists are culturally competent. In one study's sample, 85% of persons over age 60 with low socioeconomic status had preclinical risk factors for disability, while half had a moderate risk for disability. A 16-week walking exercise program, prescribed and supervised by physical therapists, significantly improved aerobic and physical function.[31]

One obstacle to cultural competence may be students' attitudes, beliefs, and values. One study of Canadian DPT students found that they placed the highest priority on postoperative and chronic pain rehabilitation, but the lowest priority on addressing geriatrics and cognitive impairment.[32] Since these latter patient populations have a great need for therapy, a values shift needs to occur in students and curricula. To increase the value of rehabilitation, therapists as a group should focus on structure (including provider availability and skill mix), process (technical and interpersonal skills emphasizing cultural competence), and outcome (ICF domain improvements for all patients).[33] In DPT programs that include cultural competence training, students display active learning and consistent individualized patient recommendations.[34]

How to Increase Cultural Competence

As with any other area of professional development, students and physical therapists have multiple ways to improve on deficits in cultural competence and sensitivity. For APTA members, an online self-study course can enhance one's clinical reasoning in diverse populations.[35] Another resource is the ECHOWS tool a checklist for patient interviewing skills, which includes the following areas related to cultural competence and substance use as well as psychosocial considerations[36]:

- E: establishing rapport with the patient
- C: determining the chief complaint (why the patient is coming to physical therapy)
- H: obtaining health history, which includes licit substance use and any abuse history
- O: obtaining the patient's psychosocial perspective of the health issue(s) (ie, how the patient perceives his or her main reason for seeking physical therapy)
- W: wrapping up with pointers to the direction of the episode of care
- S: summary of performance, which includes non-verbal behaviors and attentive listening

A book that the reader may consider is Black Lattanzi and Purnell's[37] *Developing Cultural Competence in Physical Therapy Practice*. Jackson provides a review[38]:

- This book presents a model for increasing one's cultural competence as any health care provider, based on APTA's vision statement toward "culturally sensitive care" by the physical therapist.
- The book is geared toward students, new graduates, and seasoned physical therapists or other allied health professionals, as a reference; 11 physical therapists and 1 registered nurse contributed.
- Each chapter incorporates independent exploration of cultural aspects and introduces the Purnell Model of Cultural Competence (a theory including discipline–non-specific model and framework). Aspects of culture include economy, politics, "communication, family organization, workforce, biological variation, nutrition, death ritual, and health care practice" that can affect a person's culture.[38]

Table 3-1

Acronyms for Goal Writing

SMART	ABCDE
S: specific	A: actor (who does the required action in the goal?)
M: measurable	B: behavior (what is the goal itself?)
A: attainable	C: conditions (including environmental constraints)
R: realistic	D: degree (eg, percent accuracy on a functional task)
T: timely	E: expected time frame (what is the time frame for goal completion?)

- Cultures can be based on country/ethnicity of origin, age group, housing situation, and military service. Individual attention to the person's culture is important, as the Physical Therapist Clinical Performance Instrument emphasizes.
- Final chapters include strategies and resources for culturally competent physical therapy (addressing ethics, diversity, outcomes, accreditation, regulations, patient demographics, DPT curricula, and international service learning [ISL]).

Other areas of cultural competence to consider are health literacy, patient-centered goal writing, and pain assessment in populations including persons with advanced dementia. Health literacy is "the ability to comprehend health information and use that information to make informed decisions about one's health and medical care."[39] Older adults are at high risk for low health literacy, preventing healthy choices and true informed consent. The provider can recognize poor literacy by multiple blank or incorrectly completed areas on forms, lack of ability to name or explain medications taken, and lack of follow-through for a home exercise program or outside referral. In response, the clinician can use simple and clear printed materials, listen actively, speak slowly and concisely, draw out a patient's questions by the teach-back method, use multisensory instruction, and use the Ask Me 3 technique. **These 3 questions are "What is my main problem? What do I need to do? Why is it important for me to do this?"**

Haber[7] offers suggestions for more questions for the patient:

- Where do you go for health care/information?
- What does the family help with?
- What complementary and alternative medicine or traditional methods do you use?
- How are your health beliefs different from those of your doctor?
- When do you seek medical care here?
- Can or do you use traditional foods?
- How would you advise me about your health condition?

Patient-centered goal writing reflects and influences cultural sensitivity. **Therapists can use the SMART and ABCDE acronyms,** along with discussions on what is most meaningful for each patient to accomplish (Table 3-1). Areas for goal writing should encompass the typical day, work routine, dimensions of independence, and burden of care for the patient (especially for patients with more disability).[40]

Pain assessment in some populations is difficult. Especially in persons with advanced dementia, self-report scales such as the 0-10 Numeric Pain Rating Scale and Wong-Baker Faces scale may not be as valid as observational measures. The therapist and institutional staff or caregivers can systematically assess pain in this population using factors from the history and physical as well as observational measures such as the Pain Assessment in Advanced Dementia (see Appendix C).[41]

Finally, perhaps most importantly, a place to start increasing cultural competence is in the student's education and training. One opportunity is in a student-run pro bono clinic. Such clinics develop leadership skills, administrative abilities, clinical skill automaticity, and commitment to the diverse surrounding community by student ownership in the clinic's operations.[42] Literature also supports ISL, where the student will have at least one clinical rotation in a foreign country; such ISL experiences can lessen unconscious ethnocentrism and cultural blindness.[43] Also, social responsibility, a core value of the physical therapy profession, is related to cultural competence which is improved by ISL.[44]

Additional internet resources related to aging minorities include[7]:

- American Society on Aging: http://asaging.org
- Asian & Pacific Islander American Health Forum: www.apiahf.org
- National Association for Hispanic Elderly (Asociación Nacional Pro Personas Mayores): http://anppm.org
- Association of Asian Pacific Community Health Organizations: www.aapcho.org
- The National Caucus and Center on Black Aging: www.ncba-aged.org
- National Hispanic Council on Aging: www.nhcoa.org
- National Indian Council on Aging: http://nicoa.org
- US Department of Health & Human Services Office of Minority Health: www.minorityhealth.hhs.gov

Challenges to Cultural Competence

As with mental health conditions, cultural competence is a complex and difficult topic to master. Challenges to one's cultural awareness and sensitivity include a lack of professional emphasis on related core values; current attitudes, beliefs, values, and skills of clinicians; and the breadth of mental health diagnoses and cultural variants. Personal values shape professional values, with influences on physical therapists including classwork, clinical rotations, and work environment; professional values transcend one's practice setting and career path. Values of "integrity, compassion/caring, and accountability" are integrated well by current clinicians, while social responsibility (related to cultural competence) is not as well integrated.[45]

Perhaps the origin of this limited integration lies in the increasingly diverse academic environments that house DPT programs. For students of a minority culture within a DPT program, one Australian university developed a framework to ensure that all students learned physical therapy skills at a certain level.[46] Stages of this framework included:

- Making potential students aware of course requirements prior to registration (eg, a kinesiology course would require partial disrobing for palpation lab sessions, against which students from some cultures would have a preexisting cultural norm)
- Discussing requirements with students in the first week, educating on administrative criteria, and enabling both reflection and faculty availability for perceived issues
- Maintaining a safe environment for discussion, student-proposed solutions, consultation with appropriate sources of information, and students' written agreement to solutions
- Assessing and reevaluating solutions after implementation

Gaining, maintaining, and respecting the patient's input is another challenging area for both students and practicing clinicians. Most therapists (about two-thirds in one study) want to make decisions on their own, rather than share that power with the patient; however, this paternalistic attitude can result in less patient involvement in therapy.[47] Even in the initial patient interview, another study found that French-speaking physical therapists tended to focus on function-related, closed-ended (yes/no) questions before asking open-ended questions to gain the patient's perspective. The authors of this study noted that, even when adding appropriate nonverbal behaviors such as eye contact and nodding, this sequencing of the initial interview could make it difficult to gain the patient's perspective in the first interaction.[48]

Finally, the breadth of mental health conditions can be daunting for the clinician seeking competence with persons with psychological conditions from various cultures. While statistics and symptoms of major conditions are discussed in Chapters 6 through 12 of this book, the following is a brief summary.

- There are well over 400 defined psychiatric conditions, with 22% of persons in the United States being diagnosed with one or more annually. Diagnosis is heavily affected by cultural norms; for example, "for Native Americans, it is considered normal to hear and speak to dead ancestors," which would otherwise be diagnosed as a schizophrenia spectrum disorder.[49]
- Major families of conditions discussed in this text are anxiety disorders, depressive disorders, bipolar disorders, schizophrenia spectrum disorders, personality disorders, dementias and other neurocognitive disorders, and substance use disorders. A single condition may affect as few as 0.2% of the general population, but many disorders have a significant impact on the physical therapy plan of care and interpersonal approach.[50]
- Various cultures interpret the causes of psychiatric conditions differently. In the predominantly Western culture of the United States, and perhaps in other cultures, professionals may hypothesize that personality disorders, for example, are undesirable variants on the universal Big 5 personality traits (neuroticism, extraversion, openness to experience, agreeableness, and conscientiousness).[51]

Staff Training Models

Clinical internships focused on ISL expose students to different cultures and guide reflection. One school that partnered with an organization that facilitated experiences in global learning increased its students' professionalism and cultural competence.[52] A Delphi consensus study developed guidelines for programs based in the United States, covering norms of professionalism in both participating countries, standards of physical therapist practice, cultural competence, required language skills for successful internship, and conflict management strategies.[53] Per these guidelines, themes for good ISL are "structure, reciprocity, relationship, and sustainability."[54] One school developed its own model in a 2-course sequence that included an ISL experience with academic instruction in the Spanish language, followed by service learning at a Christian orphanage in Ecuador with reflection and reporting on the experience. This model "enabled students to be immersed within a culture, realize the core values in action, develop cultural competence, and solidify their interest in working with ... underserved populations."[55]

Academic programs also use non-ISL training models. The University of Utah (Salt Lake City, Utah) developed the Cultural Competency and Mutual Respect program for all of its interprofessional health science, medicine, pharmacy, nursing, physical therapy, and other student programs. In a 3-year study, students' attitudes, knowledge, and skills related to cultural competence improved significantly, but not to the level that faculty expected.[56] Another school's 3-phase model incorporated "understanding cultural differences through classroom presentations, simulated classroom application through group projects, and clinical application through provision of physical therapy services to patients of various cultures."[57] This model required revision to improve cross-cultural sensitivity and adaptability.

Clinical settings also have training models, with little research support at the time of this book's writing. One diversity training program focused on facilitating therapists changing "their knowledge levels, attitudes, and self-efficacy" regarding the LGBTQ+ population for more confidence in working with the subset of these patients who have a spinal cord injury.[58] The patient-related goal of this program was a decreased risk of "direct physical and mental health consequences" to the patient; the source did not define these consequences. As with all evidence-based practice, the underlying core values, research base, and clinical results of each cultural competence training program need critical evaluation.

One resource for training DPT students is the CIRRIE guide.[59] CIRRIE stands for Center for International Rehabilitation Research Information and Exchange; the website from the University of Buffalo (Buffalo, New York) has files describing ways "to integrate cultural competency education throughout [the program's] curriculum," whether the program is for speech language pathology, occupational therapy, physical therapy, or rehabilitation counseling. The file for physical therapy curricula includes a section on transdisciplinary instruction, which can improve each student's ability to positively influence workplace culture and develop personal competency related to each patient's culture.

Interpreter Services and Responsibilities

Patient-provider language differences can block provision of physical therapy. While some therapists and patients are multilingual, this is not always the case, so the patient needs an interpreter to gain the full benefit from the therapist's instruction and assessment. Also, DPT students often do not think they know enough about translators and sources of information for cultural awareness, despite the knowledge offered by diverse clinical rotations.[60] One option is a medically-focused foreign language course, in an academic or clinical setting. Learning the Spanish language via an elective course transformed DPT students':

> [F]rames of reference (that is, cultural diversity, cultural awareness), beliefs, self-awareness, making and implementing plans related to physical therapy intervention based on this awareness, relationships and rapport with patients, ability to communicate in Spanish, body language awareness, and alternative approaches to living.[61]

Since many patients in the United States speak Spanish, the APTA developed a self-study continuing-education course for basic clinical Spanish vocabulary and communication skills.[62] The course introduction delineates risk management considerations for interpreter services that are encouraged unless the therapist is multilingual. Clinics should choose a medically literate third-party interpreter, consider the use of competent adults and relatives, never use a child to interpret, establish policies and procedures for protecting patients' personal health information, identify needs, and allocate staff to meet and document those needs. Resources for these tasks include:

- Agency for Healthcare Research and Quality: www.ahrq.gov/professionals/systems/hospital/lepguide/lepguidefig5.html
- American Academy of Family Physicians (in Spanish): https://es.familydoctor.org
- Joint Commission on Accreditation of Health care Organizations: www.jointcommission.org
- Center for Medicare & Medicaid Services: www.cms.gov
- US Department of Health & Human Services: www.hhs.gov/ocr

Emerging Topics

Due to cultural diversity in the United States and other countries, without as much diversity in many academic environments, more DPT programs are starting to focus on recruiting and retaining students from minority groups.[63] Having a therapist of the same race or culture can increase a patient's participation and eventually improve outcomes for the population. Current strategies that DPT programs can use, per this study, include preprofessional enrichment courses, ample financial aid information for prospective students, and education in relevant technology skills.

Another emerging topic is the plethora of issues in Hispanic health. Three developing issues are "threats to the health status of elderly Hispanics, mental health, and 'missed opportunities' that occur in clinical and community settings in which conditions or subtle indicators serve as an early warning of an impending widespread threat to community health."[64] One example of such a health indicator is an increase "in such diseases as hepatitis."[64]

A third area is chronic illness (see Chapter 13). A brief from Georgetown University emphasizes the centrality of cultural competence in today's health care arena to improve outcomes.[65] Disparities noted include disproportionate burden of chronic illness borne by racial and ethnic minorities, increasing diversity of those at risk for chronic conditions, varied access to health care due to race and ethnicity, dissatisfaction with services if a professional interpreter or bilingual provider is unavailable, and burden of low health literacy.

The brief also describes aspects of cultural competence, which include:

- Provision of interpreters to communicate complex topics and increase family input into decisions
- Extension of "linguistic competency" to front desk, billing office staff, and printed materials
- Recruitment and retention of minority staff and, by extension, health care students
- Coordination of care with a culture's traditional healers, if applicable
- Incorporation of local health workers/clinics and culture-specific values for health promotion
- Expansion of clinic hours of operation

Training approaches for cultural competence should be process-based and thus ongoing, per government and health care association standards (eg, the American Medical Association). Many professional training programs are also moving toward developing accreditation standards for students. Finally, the government has financial and other incentives for providers to provide culturally competent services to reduce health disparities.

Special Focus Issues

Because this book is meant to be a clinical reference beyond the classroom, it does not include lengthy coverage of introductory topics. In order to save space and weight but also to enable ready reference for the student, this section contains an annotated bibliography of open-access online resources on selected topics.

Psychosocial Perspectives on Disability: Applying and Optimizing the ICF Model

Drew N, Funk M, Tang S, et al. Human rights violations of people with mental and psychosocial disabilities: an unresolved global crisis. *Lancet.* 2011;378(9803):1664-1675.

- In low- and middle-income countries especially, human rights violations affect "basic civil, cultural, economic, political, and social rights" of persons with non-physical disabilities.
- Specifically, affected persons face limited access to mental health services, mistreatment by providers, employment discrimination, and premature denial of legal capacity.

Imrie R. Demystifying disability: a review of the International Classification of Functioning, Disability and Health. *Sociol Health & Illness.* 2004;26(3):287-305.

- The ICF model, developed in 2001 to incorporate a biopsychosocial perspective, emphasized that there are other causes of disability beyond merely biological malfunction. However, as of this 2004 review, the ICF model did not explicate what impairment and disability mean and consist of, thus limiting its educational potential. In this review, impairment is defined from a materialistic worldview.

- Suggestions to improve the ICF include definition of impairment, specifying elements of biopsychosocial theory, and clarifying what the principle of universalization means for how ICF-using countries develop policies on disability.

Jensen MP, Moore MR, Bockow TB, Ehde DM, Engel JM. Psychosocial factors and adjustment to chronic pain in persons with physical disabilities: a systematic review. *Arch Phys Med Rehabil.* 2011;92(1):146-160.

- In chronic conditions that cause disability, including spinal cord injury, amputation, and muscular dystrophy, psychosocial factors were linked with dysfunction and pain. Factors included inaccurate pain-related beliefs such as catastrophization, coping responses such as persisting on a task and guarding, and the level of perceived social support.

Jones MA. Deafness as culture: a psychosocial perspective. *Dis Studies Quarterly.* 2002;22(2):51-60.

- Literature indicates that deafness (or other traits) signifies either a culture or a disability. The concept of "deafness-as-disability" requires hearing as a normal function of individuals in society, thus incentivizing the development of technological and educational advances. However, the concept of "Deafness-as-culture" (with a capital D) indicates that Deaf peers form their own culture, distinct from hearing biological family.
- Theories of group dynamics lend insights to the above referenced discussion. Note that each insight can apply to either the hearing culture or the Deaf culture.
    - Stigma equates to the reduction in personhood as viewed by others. Because each person wants to esteem him- or herself, he or she has the perceived need to stigmatize someone else to maintain that self-esteem.
    - Language has powerful cultural uses, including identification and evaluation.
    - Prejudice is a fluctuating characteristic maintaining group cohesiveness against other persons who are stigmatized.

Kearney PM, Griffin T. Between joy and sorrow: being a parent of a child with developmental disability. *Issues Innov Nurs Pract.* 2001;34(5):582-592.

- Western society commonly assumes that parents of children with developmental disabilities view the child's existence as a "tragedy" and go into crisis mode.
- Six parents of children with severe developmental disability articulated emotions held in balance: "'joy and sorrow,' 'hope and no hope,' and 'defiance and despair.'"
- While this article was written from a nursing perspective, physical therapists can gain insight into how they interact with parents and caregivers of persons with disability.

Leplege A, Gzil F, Cammelli M, et al. Person-centredness: conceptual and historical perspectives. *Dis Rehabil.* 2007;29(20-21):1555-1565.

- The concept of person-centeredness, viewed as essential to holistic rehabilitation, has changed over the years. Earlier definitions, however, did not and do not relate to how the term is used in rehabilitation contexts.
- Practical application of person-centeredness requires embracing its central tenet that a person is much more than his or her disabilities.

Purdue University. Disability Resource Center: Student Success Programs. https://www.purdue.edu/drc/index.html. Published 2016. Accessed February 12, 2018.

- Students, faculty, and staff are welcome to browse resources relevant to disability accommodations, services, documentation, worldview, and other areas.
- The Purdue University Disability Resource Center has the goal of universal student access to the university and educational offerings.

Loss and Grieving: Cultural Considerations at End of Life

Bonanno GA. Loss, trauma, and human resilience: have we underestimated the human capacity to thrive after extremely aversive events? *Amer Psychologist*. 2004;58(1):20-28.

- Since most loss and resilience research up to the 2000s looked at persons with major psychological issues, most theorists had looked at resilience as rare and pathological.
- Resilience is not recovery: the former keeps equilibrium; the latter improves over time.
- Resilience is very common, whether to loss or to violent events.
- Multiple ways to achieve resilience include hardiness, self-enhancement, repressive coping (including emotional dissociation), and positive emotion with laughter.

Bonanno GA, Wortman CB, Lehman DR, et al. Resilience to loss and chronic grief: a prospective study from preloss to 18-months postloss. *J Personal Soc Psychol*. 2002;83(5):1150-1164.

- Patterns of grieving and resilience toward a spouse's death vary based on the relationship they had before the death, as well as basic beliefs about death. Spouses very dependent on each other tended to experience chronic grief for over 1 year. Resilience, the most common pattern of bereavement, was more common in persons who accepted inevitable death and justice as a basic operating principle of the world.

Cowchock FS, Lasker JN, Toedter LJ, Skumanich SA, Koenig HG. Religious beliefs affect grieving after pregnancy loss. *J Relig Health*. 2010;49(4):485-497.

- Authors assessed 103 women who had lost an unborn child regarding religious beliefs' relationship to severity and outcomes of grief at a 1-year follow-up. In the sample, grief was not related to religiosity, frequency of attendance at services, or positive religious coping strategies. However, women who were more attached to their infants had faith-related struggles, negative coping styles, and had more grief.
- From a faith-based analytical perspective, this article highlights (1) the need to listen to and empathize with expressions of grief and (2) the often-necessary nature of grief and grief acceptance after a major loss.

Dumont I, Dumont S, Mongeau S. End-of-life care and the grieving process: family caregivers who have experienced the loss of a terminal-phase cancer patient. *Qual Hlth Res*. 2008;18(8):1049-1061.

- A study of caregivers of a recently deceased family member with cancer identified traits of caregivers who may need intervention from palliative care professionals. Yellow flags include a repressed emotional and psychological load, patient's denial of disease, strained family relationships, and the lack of a calm home setting at the time of death.
- The caregiving experience has 6 main facets: caregiver and patient characteristics, illness symptoms, context of the relationship, support socially and professionally, and circumstances of the death.

Gold KJ. Navigating care after a baby dies: a systematic review of parent experiences with health providers. *J Perinatology.* 2007;27(4):230-237.

- In a hospital setting, a newborn's unexpected death can cause posttraumatic stress symptoms in parents for years, cementing memories of provider interactions as well. While parents usually perceived nurses as supportive and good listeners, they had especially negative reactions toward communication errors (eg, an obstetrician asking about the current health of a dead baby). Also, parents resented caregivers who either avoided newly bereaved parents or made emotionally insensitive comments.
- Helpful provider behaviors included support of emotional reactions, provision of physical assistance, and factual education such as counseling resources.

Kreibig S. Autonomic nervous system activity in emotion: a review. *Biological Psychology.* 2010;84(3):394-421.

- Negative emotions with experimentally demonstrated autonomic nervous system (ANS) involvement
  - Anger: typically alpha-adrenergic activation of sympathetic nervous system (SNS) that increases respiratory rate
  - Anxiety: typically alpha- and beta-adrenergic activation with shallow tachypnea
  - Disgust: contamination- or injury-related stimuli decrease cardiac stimuli, do not change vagal activity, and increase electrodermal activity and respiratory rate
  - Embarrassment: vagal decrease and overall SNS increase in activity
  - Fear: SNS activation increasing heart rate, blood pressure, and sweating
  - Sadness: a mixed pattern of sympathetic and parasympathetic activation
- Positive emotions with experimentally demonstrated ANS involvement
  - Affection: decreased heart rate, with few published experiments
  - Amusement: variable heart rate changes, with beta-adrenergic cardiac deactivation and increased control by the vagus nerve
  - Contentment: decreased SNS activation with increased vagal activity
  - Happiness: increased respiratory rate, vasodilation, and cardiac parameters
  - Joy: increase in vagal, beta-adrenergic, and cholinergic input but inconsistent
  - Anticipatory pleasure: strikingly different depending on seen or imagined stimuli
  - Pride: decreased beta-adrenergic and increased cholinergic input for bradycardia
  - Relief: decreased respiratory rate and SNS vascular parameters
- Neutral emotions with experimentally demonstrated ANS involvement
  - Surprise: spike in SNS cardiac response with tachycardia and pause in breathing
  - Suspense: decreased heart rate and many respiratory parameters

Maciejewski PK, Zhang B, Block SD, et al. An empirical examination of the stage theory of grief. *JAMA.* 2007;297(7):716-723.

- The 5-stage theory of grief posits that sequential stages are disbelief, yearning, anger, depression, and acceptance. In a 2-year study, authors found that while all indicators were at their highest around 6 months postloss, stages were not sequential nor distinct.
- Participants most often had acceptance and yearning throughout the 2 years. Peak values of each indicator did occur in the order predicted by the model.

Richardson M, Cobham V, Murray J, McDermott B. Parents' grief in the context of adult child mental illness: a qualitative review. *Clin Child Fam Psychol Rev.* 2011;14(1):28-43.

- When a child with diagnosed mental illness reached adulthood, parents typically reported strong senses of grief and loss. Earlier in the child's life, parents experienced a slow or sudden realization of the crisis-nature of severe mental illness, occasionally combined with relief that a suspicion has been confirmed by diagnosis.
- Causes of grief can include lost potential, the chronic stress-inducing nature of the illness, and the inability to construct a fully satisfactory meaning from the experience.

Wortman CB, Silver RC. The myths of coping with loss. *J Consult Clin Psychol.* 1989;57(3):349-357.

- Common false expectations of persons with major loss include inevitable depression, ubiquitous distress, the necessity of processing, and full recovery. Current research either lacks support for or contradicts these expectations.
- While many people do experience loss in the above ways, population variability is high, and thus others' responses and advice is less helpful when not accounting for variability.

Sexuality: Encompassing Minority and Mainstream Cultural Groups

Fronek P, Kendall M, Booth S, Eugarde E, Geraghty T. A longitudinal study of sexuality training for the interdisciplinary team. *Sexuality Disabil.* 2011;29(2):87-100.

- Interprofessional therapy providers working with persons with spinal cord injury benefited from individualized team training about sexuality. They retained accurate knowledge, a higher comfort level in discussions with patients, and therapeutic attitudes.

Hinchliff S, Gott M, Galena E. "I daresay I might find it embarrassing": general practitioners' perspectives on discussing sexual health issues with lesbian and gay patients. *Hlth Soc Care Community.* 2005;13(4):345-353.

- In a survey of health care providers in the United Kingdom, attitudes toward persons with non-heterosexual orientations were rarely a treatment barrier. Rather, communication and knowledge gaps prevented proactive addressing of some issues with these patients.

Lindau ST, Schumm P, Laumann EO, et al. A study of sexuality and health among older adults in the United States. *N Engl J Med.* 2007;357(8):762-774.

- From national survey data, surveyors found that older adults who report better health are more sexually active, though a significant portion (about 35%) considered sex unimportant and half reported physical sexual problems. A very small number took function-enhancing substances, and about 30% talk with a medical provider about sex. Providers can become aware of this factual data in their older clients for holistic care.

Moreno JA, Lasprilla JCA, Gan C, McKerral M. Sexuality after traumatic brain injury: a critical review. *NeuroRehabilitation.* 2013;32(1):69-85.

- According to the World Health Organization, sexuality is expressed and experienced via thoughts, words, and actions, influenced by a variety of external factors. After a traumatic brain injury (TBI), impaired function in medical or neuropsychological domains can adversely affect relationship aspects of sexuality in 50% to 60% of persons with TBI. For example, if the partner turned into the caregiver, intimacy was hampered.
- Rehabilitation in the sexual domain after TBI includes psychotherapy, behavioral therapy, psychopharmacology, and tailored information in a biopsychosocial approach.

Norwood K. Grieving gender: trans-identities, transition, and ambiguous loss. *Comm Monographs.* 2013;80(1):24-45.

- When a person begins to identify to family as transgender, members often experience high levels of tension, since the person they knew no longer seems to be entirely present. The making of meaning, one way or another, helps family members to address the grief about the transgender person transitioning.

Penwell-Waines L, Wilson CK, Macapagal KR, et al. Student perspectives on sexual health: implications for interprofessional education. *J Interprof Care.* 2014;28(4):317-322.

- Due to time constraints in school and in later interprofessional teams, most health professions students do not receive sexual health care training. Of note, students tend to use a biomedical rather than biopsychosocial approach in this area. Authors recommend interprofessional education activities to best address this gap.

Schneider MS, Brown LS. Implementing the resolution on appropriate therapeutic responses to sexual orientation: a guide for the perplexed. *Prof Psychol: Res Pract.* 2002;33(3):265-276.

- In 1997, the American Psychological Association recommended certain psychologist responses to patients "struggling with issues surrounding their sexual orientation." This resolution took a neutral stance between attacking unproven therapies for sexual minorities and attacking patients who sought help to try to change their non-heterosexual orientations.
- Questioning one's orientation occurs more typically in adolescents and children, and decreases over time. Regardless of one's stance toward moral, social, and biological aspects of sexual orientation, the American Psychological Association recommends therapists express neutrality, and find and provide facts rather than superimpose personal values to alter facts.

Motivation and Adherence: Capitalizing on Therapy Culture

Brewer BW, Cornelius AE, Van Raalte JL, et al. Age-related differences in predictors of adherence to rehabilitation after anterior cruciate ligament reconstruction. *J Athl Train.* 2003;38(2):158-162.

- In participants 14 to 47 years old with acute sports injuries and surgeries rehabilitating at home, Brewer et al found that patients with higher self-motivation—regardless of age—were more likely to complete their home exercises.

Chan DK, Lonsdale C, Ho PY, Yung PS, Chan KM. Patient motivation and adherence to postsurgery rehabilitation exercise recommendations: the influence of physiotherapists' autonomy-supportive behaviors. *Arch Phys Med Rehabil.* 2009;90(12):1977-1982.

- Study of the relationships between motivation, adherence, and physical therapists' behaviors supportive of patient autonomy revealed that such therapist behaviors predicted patient motivation (specifically autonomous), which in turn predicted treatment adherence.
- Autonomy support training for physical therapists induced them to explain treatment rationales and processes, and provide options to patients.

Dorflinger L, Kerns RD, Auerbach SM. Providers' roles in enhancing patients' adherence to pain self management. *Transl Behav Med.* 2013;3(1):39-46.

- Self-management of chronic disease and pain is more effective over time. Providers' biopsychosocial approaches to facilitate self-management include patient-centered care, empathic responses, and discussion of and education on motivation factors.

Ebben W, Brudzynski L. Motivators and barriers to exercise among college students. *J Ex Physiol.* 2008;11(5).

- Specifically in college students, motivators for exercise included health and wellness, stress management, personal enjoyment, and the positive feedback loop of exercise.
- Barriers included perceived workload, limited free time, lack of energy, and lack of intrinsic motivation that would prioritize exercise above other things.

Grindley EJ, Zizzi SJ. Using a multidimensional approach to predict motivation and adherence to rehabilitation in older adults. *Top Geriatr Rehabil.* 2005;21(5):182-193.

- For geriatric physical therapists, an ICF-based analysis of exercise adherence leads to the following recommendations: (1) include psychosocial measures with an initial orthopedic evaluation to account for the influence of psychosocial variables, (2) periodically assess patient motivation and adherence (though few to no valid measures exist), and (3) center rehabilitation on the patient to tailor intervention.

Hamson-Utley JJ. The comeback: rehabilitating the psychological injury. *Athl Ther Today.* 2008;13(5):35-38.

- Psychological injuries often happen due to physical injury. Impaired adherence is treated by relaxation, mental imagery, and short- and long-term goal setting. Mental imagery has different purposes depending on the stage and symptoms of injury and rehabilitation.

Marks R, Allegrante JP. Chronic osteoarthritis and adherence to exercise: a review of the literature. *J Aging Phys Activity.* 2005;13(4):434-460.

- Because symptoms of osteoarthritis persist, patients given home exercise programs frequently encounter pain and stiffness when completing them. Exercise adherence maintains the beneficial effects of exercise. Therapists can target self-efficacy, long-term progress tracking, and patients' exercise-related social support to improve adherence.

Milroy P, O'Neil G. Factors affecting compliance to chiropractic prescribed home exercise: a review of the literature. *J Can Chiropr Assoc.* 2000;44(3):141-148.

- Milroy and O'Neil found that poor compliance with exercise is common because of influences of attitudes, provider-patient communication, economic constraints, past poor experiences, actual or perceived health, lack of social support, physical resources, time constraints, and lack of patient participation in setting goals.

Yuen HK, Wang E, Holthaus K, et al. Self-reported versus objectively assessed exercise adherence. *Am J Occup Ther.* 2013;67(4):484-489.

- Because many exercise adherence measures are subjective and not standardized, Yuen et al compared subjective exercise logs with objective trackers on a Wii console. Although group estimates were similar, individual logs over-reported duration of exercise.

Zeldman A, Ryan RM. Motivation, autonomy support, and entity beliefs: their role in methadone maintenance treatment. *J Soc Clin Psychol.* 2004;23(5):675-696.

- Examining self-determination theory relating to participants in a methadone maintenance program, Zeldman and Ryan found that adherence required higher internal vs external motivation. Patients who saw their addiction as a fixed trait also saw improved outcomes. Providers can note that if internal motivation is low, successful interventions should not add external at the expense of internal motivators.

Summary

At its core, cultural competence means being sensitive to and respectful of the needs of each individual patient, regardless of differences in cultural background between the patient and provider. Cultural competence and sensitivity are increasingly important regardless of practice area, since the population of countries such as the United States is becoming more diverse in age, ethnicity, and economic factors. This chapter surveyed what cultural competence is, how to improve it, and why it is important.

Key Points

- Demonstrate therapy's value by focusing on structure, process, and outcomes.
- For patients with low health literacy, use the Ask Me 3 questions: "What is my main problem? What do I need to do? Why is it important for me to do this?"
- SMART goals are specific, measurable, attainable, realistic, and timely. ABCDE goals have an actor, desired behavior, condition(s), degree, and expected time frame.

Review Questions

- In your own words, what is cultural competence? How is your definition influenced by where you practice or have practiced? How is it influenced by your own cultural background?
- Explore the CIRRIE website.[59] In your current or past DPT curricula, was the content integrated into the curricula? How did this influence your cultural attitudes, beliefs, and values related to patient care?
- In a potential workplace situation where interpreter services were not offered according to the APTA guidelines described earlier in this text, what are some ways in which you could address that to improve access to quality care for all patients?
- Review the cultural disparities discussed in this chapter. Which ones have you seen in your clinical rotations or jobs so far? How might these have affected customer service and patient care? Discuss with classmates or colleagues.
- How does your academic program or workplace try to increase the cultural competence of students or employees? Do these efforts work? Why or why not? How can you tell?

Case Studies: First Impressions

As you review the following case studies, you may want to consider these questions for thought or discussion:

- What standardized tests and measures (including psychiatric, for example, a depression screen) would you select for this patient? Why?
- Based on available data, what short- and long-term goals would you write for your plan of care? Consider using the acronyms SMART (specific, measurable, attainable, realistic, and timely) or ABCDE (actor, behavior, conditions, degree, and expected time frame) to guide your goal writing.
- What elements (procedures, psychosocial aspects, communication aspects, etc) would you make sure to include or omit in your plan of care for this patient? Why?

- What are your anticipated needs, if any, for consultation and referral for this patient?
- How will you transition this patient toward lasting health behavior change following discharge (eg, recommending a YMCA membership trial)?

Case 1

A 54-year-old female of Japanese-American descent, second-generation, was referred to outpatient physical therapy 3 weeks after a partial rotator cuff tear. Her goals are to resume full-time work as a day care director and complete household management tasks without pain.

- Social history: she lives with her husband and youngest child in an apartment above the day care she manages. Her husband works second shift; her child is attending a local graduate program and works part time.
- Medical/psychiatric history: cyclothymic disorder, osteopenia, hypothyroidism, and prehypertension. She is not on any medications except non-steroidal anti-inflammatory drug pain relievers as needed.
- Impairments, activity limitations, and participation restrictions found on initial interview and examination
    - Pain in shoulder rated 6/10 with active motion and lifting objects
    - Moderate scapular winging on affected side
    - Difficulty reported with dressing and cooking tasks
    - Mildly stooped posture

Case 2

A 63-year-old Jamaican-French-Canadian-American male was admitted to subacute rehabilitation after a 1-week hospitalization for anemia and a series of falls at his apartment. His goal is to go to an assisted living facility.

- Social history: he previously lived in a second-story apartment with 4 hours of daily assistance for light household tasks. He previously was independent in ambulation and stair negotiation.
- Medical/psychiatric history: legal blindness, single-episode major depressive disorder, obesity, hypertension, type 2 diabetes, and history of lower extremity cellulitis
- Impairments, activity limitations, and participation restrictions found on initial interview and examination
    - Speaks rapidly and sometimes does not appear to hear the therapist's questions/answers
    - Marked lower extremity weakness especially in pelvic girdle muscles (hip flexors, extensors, and abductors) noted during sit to stand transfers and ambulation
    - Gait with 2-wheeled walker has a wide base of support and excessive bilateral trunk lurch
    - Requires repeated clarification on the roles of physical, occupational, and speech therapy
    - Standing tolerance limited to 5 minutes with the support of a 2-wheeled walker

Case 3

A 92-year-old German-American male was referred to physical therapy by nursing staff, due to increased difficulty in transfers and wheelchair self-propulsion. His goal is to be able to transfer himself safely and visit his wife, who lives in an assisted living apartment adjacent to the skilled nursing wing.

- Social history: he had served overseas in Russia during World War II, prior to coming to the United States and becoming a naturalized citizen. He formerly worked in a Midwest manufacturing setting to support his wife and daughter, who also lives in the area and visits at least twice monthly.

- Medical/psychiatric history: posttraumatic stress disorder following military service, stroke (20 years prior) with left hemiplegia and expressive aphasia, major depressive disorder (diagnosed 10 years ago), type 2 diabetes (diagnosed 30 years ago), overweight, mild left-sided hearing loss, and coronary artery disease
- Impairments, activity limitations, and participation restrictions found on initial interview and examination
    - Limited ability to follow 2- and 3-step commands
    - Requires assistance of 2 people to transfer (previously required only distant supervision)
    - Experiences bouts of tearfulness and reminiscing in the German language
    - Slides forward and laterally in wheelchair (the staff suspect discomfort, though he does not verbalize pain when asked)

References

1. Purden M. Cultural considerations in interprofessional education and practice. *J Interprof Care.* 2005;19(suppl 1):224-234.
2. Steel Z, Marnane C, Iranpour C, et al. The global prevalence of common mental disorders: a systematic review and meta-analysis 1980-2013. *Int J Epidemiol.* 2014;43(2):476-493.
3. Kane JC, Ventevogel P, Spiegel P, et al. Mental, neurological, and substance use problems among refugees in primary health care: analysis of the health information system in 90 refugee camps. *BMC Medicine.* 2014;12:228.
4. Gandhi M. *The Selected Works of Mahatma Gandhi: The Voice of Truth.* Vol 6. Ahmedabad, India: Navajivan Publishing House; 1968.
5. Avers D, Brown M, Chui KK, Wong RA, Lusardi M. Editor's message: use of the term "elderly." *J Geriatr Phys Ther.* 2011;34(4):153-154.
6. Gannotti ME, Handwerker WP, Groce NE, Cruz C. Sociocultural influences on disability status in Puerto Rican children. *Phys Ther.* 2001;81(9):1512-1523.
7. Haber D. *Health Promotion and Aging: Practical Applications for Health Professionals.* 4th ed. New York, NY: Springer; 2007.
8. Ingstad B, Whyte SR, eds. *Disability in Local and Global Worlds.* Berkeley, CA: University of California Press; 2007.
9. Palombaro KM, Lattanzi JB. Calculating the minimal detectable change for a cultural competency tool. *HPA PTJ-PAL.* 2012;12(2):17-23
10. Wong CK, Blissett S. Assessing performance in the area of cultural competence: an analysis of reflective writing. *J Phys Ther Educ.* 2007;21(1):40-48.
11. Lazaro RT, Umphred DA. Improving cultural diversity awareness of physical therapy educators. *J Cult Divers.* 2007;14(3):121-125.
12. Kerzner H. *Project Management: A Systems Approach to Planning, Scheduling, and Controlling.* 9th ed. Hoboken, NJ: Wiley; 2006.
13. Reiss-Brennan B, Brunisholz KD, Dredge C, et al. Association of integrated team-based care with health care quality, utilization, and cost. *JAMA.* 2016;316(8):826-834.
14. MacLean MB, Van Til L, Thompson JM, et al. Postmilitary adjustment to civilian life: potential risks and protective factors. *Phys Ther.* 2014;94(8):1186-1195.
15. Setchell J, Watson B, Jones L, Gard M. Weight stigma in physiotherapy practice: patient perceptions of interactions with physiotherapists. *Man Ther.* 2015;20(6):835-841.
16. Jette AM. From person-centered to family-centered health care. *Phys Ther.* 2017;97(2):157-158.
17. Sargeant DM, Newsham KR. Physical therapist students' perceptions of spirituality and religion in patient care. *J Phys Ther Educ.* 2012;26(2):63-72.
18. Dean CM, Duncan PW. Preparing the next generation of physical therapists for transformative practice and population management: example from Macquarie University. *Phys Ther.* 2016;96(3):272-274.
19. Mellion LR. Factors that impact functional levels of Hispanic elders: implications for physical therapists. *Issues on Aging.* 2014;24:17-20.
20. Williams B, Bezner J, Chesbro S, Leavitt R. The relationship between achievement of walking goals and exercise self-efficacy in post-menopausal African American women. [Poster presentation.] *J Geriatr Phys Ther.* 2005;28(3):123.
21. Williams B, Bezner J, Chesbro S, Leavitt R. The effect of a walking program on perceived benefits and barriers to exercise in post-menopausal African American women. [Poster presentation.] *J Geriatr Phys Ther.* 2006;29(2):43-49.

22. Kirkness CS, Ren J. Race differences: use of walking speed to identify community-dwelling women at risk for poor health outcomes--osteoarthritis initiative study. *Phys Ther.* 2015;95(7):955-965.
23. Kaur S, Stechuchak KM, Coffman CJ, Allen KD, Bastian LA. Gender differences in health care utilization among veterans with chronic pain. *J Gen Intern Med.* 2007;22(2):228-233.
24. Chen I, Kurz J, Pasanen M, et al. Racial differences in opioid use for chronic nonmalignant pain. *J Gen Intern Med.* 2005;20(7):593-598.
25. O'Brien KK, Ibáñez-Carrasco F, Solomon P, et al. Advancing research and practice in HIV and rehabilitation: a framework of research priorities in HIV, disability and rehabilitation. *BMC Infect Dis.* 2014;14:724.
26. Merlin JS. Chronic pain in patients with HIV infection: what clinicians need to know. *Top Antivir Med.* 2015;23(3):120-124.
27. Gell NM, Mroz TM, Patel KV. Rehabilitation services use and patient reported outcomes among older adults in the United States. *Arch Phys Med Rehabil.* 2017;98(11):2221-2227.
28. Purtilo RB. Thirty-First Mary McMillan Lecture: a time to harvest, a time to sow: ethics for a shifting landscape. *Phys Ther.* 2000;80(11):1112-1119.
29. Roach KE, Frost JS, Francis NJ, et al. Validation of the revised Physical Therapist Clinical Performance Instrument (PT CPI): version 2006. *Phys Ther.* 2012;92(3):416-428.
30. Ruaro JA, Ruaro MB, Guerra RO. International Classification of Functioning, Disability and Health core set for physical health of older adults. *J Geriatr Phys Ther.* 2014;37(4):147-153.
31. Moore-Harrison TL, Speer EM, Johnson FT, Cress ME. The effects of aerobic training and nutrition education on functional performance in low socioeconomic older adults. *J Geriatr Phys Ther.* 2008;31(1):18-23.
32. Laliberté M, Feldman DE. Patient prioritization preferences among physiotherapy entry-level students: the importance of chronic pain. *Physiother Can.* 2013;65(4):353-357.
33. Jewell DV, Moore JD, Goldstein MS. Delivering the physical therapy value proposition: a call to action. *Phys Ther.* 2013;93(1):104-114.
34. May S, Portia TA. An evaluation of cultural competency training in perceived patient adherence. *Eur J Physiother.* 2013;15(1):2-10.
35. American Physical Therapy Association. Clinical decision making in diverse populations. *APTA Learning Center.* http://learningcenter.apta.org/student/MyCourse.aspx?id=e75b603a-9134-4fec-95a9-3c393c092046&programid=dcca7f06-4cd9-4530-b9d3-4ef7d2717b5d. Published February 8, 2017. Accessed February 13, 2018.
36. Boissonnault JS, Evans K, Tuttle N, et al. Reliability of the ECHOWS tool for assessment of patient interviewing skills. *Phys Ther.* 2016;96(4):443-455.
37. Black Lattanzi JF, Purnell LD. *Developing Cultural Competence in Physical Therapy Practice.* Philadelphia, PA: FA Davis; 2005.
38. Jackson V, reviewer. The Internet Journal of Allied Health Sciences and Practice. 2009;7(4). Review of: Black Lattanzi J, Purnell LD. *Developing Cultural Competence in Physical Therapy Practice.*
39. Ennis K, Hawthorne K, Frownfelter D. How physical therapists can strategically effect health outcomes for older adults with limited health literacy. *J Geriatr Phys Ther.* 2012;35(3):148-154.
40. Randall KE, McEwen IR. Writing patient-centered functional goals. *Phys Ther.* 2000;80(12):1197-1203.
41. Hadjistavropoulos T, Fitzgerald TD, Marchildon GP. Practice guidelines for assessing pain in older persons with dementia residing in long-term care facilities. *Physiother Can.* 2010;62(2):104-113.
42. Black JD, Palombaro KM, Dole RL. Student experiences in creating and launching a student-led physical therapy pro bono clinic: a qualitative investigation. *Phys Ther.* 2013;93(5):637-648.
43. Dupre A, Goodgold S. Development of physical therapy student cultural competency through international community service. *J Cult Divers.* 2007;14(3):126-135.
44. Lee ACW, Litwin B, Cheng MS, Harada ND. Social responsibility and cultural competence among physical therapists with international experience. *J Phys Ther Educ.* 2012;26(3):66-74.
45. McGinnis PQ, Guenther LA, Wainwright SF. Development and integration of professional core values among practicing clinicians. *Phys Ther.* 2016;96(9):1417-1429.
46. Bialocerkowski A, Wells C, Grimmer-Somers K. Teaching physiotherapy skills in culturally-diverse classes. *BMC Med Educ.* 2011;11:34.
47. Dierckx K, Deveugele M, Roosen P, Devisch I. Implementation of shared decision making in physical therapy: observed level of involvement and patient preference. *Phys Ther.* 2013;93(10):1321-1330.
48. Opsommer E, Schoeb V. 'Tell me about your troubles': description of patient-physiotherapist interaction during initial encounters. *Physiother Res Int.* 2014;19(4):205-221.
49. Drench ME, Noonan AC, Sharby N, Ventura SH. *Psychosocial Aspects of Health Care.* 3rd ed. Upper Saddle River, NJ: Pearson; 2012.
50. American Psychiatric Association. *Diagnostic and Statistical Manual of Mental Disorders.* 5th ed. Washington, DC: American Psychiatric Association; 2013.
51. Sue D, Sue DW, Sue S. *Understanding Abnormal Behaviors.* 6th ed. Boston, MA: Houghton Mifflin; 2000.
52. Mandich M, Erickson M, Nardella B. Development of an international clinical education extracurricular experience through a collaborative partnership. *Phys Ther.* 2017;97(1):44-50.

53. Pechak CM, Black JD. Proposed guidelines for international clinical education in US-based physical therapist education programs: results of a focus group and Delphi study. *Phys Ther.* 2014;94(4):523-533.
54. Pechak CM, Thompson M. A conceptual model of optimal international service-learning and its application to global health initiatives in rehabilitation. *Phys Ther.* 2009;89(11):1192-1204.
55. Hayward LM, Charrette AL. Integrating cultural competence and core values: an international service-learning model. *J Phys Ther Educ.* 2012;26(1):78-89.
56. Musolino GM, Burkhalter ST, Crookston B, et al. Understanding and eliminating disparities in health care: development and assessment of cultural competence for interprofessional health professionals at the University of Utah—a 3-year investigation. *J Phys Ther Educ.* 2010;24(1):25-36.
57. Shore S. A curricular model of cross-cultural sensitivity. *J Phys Ther Educ.* 2007;21(2):53-59.
58. Burch A. Health care providers' knowledge, attitudes, and self-efficacy for working with patients with spinal cord injury who have diverse sexual orientations. *Phys Ther.* 2008;88(2):191-198.
59. Stone JH. Center for international rehabilitation research information & exchange (CIRRIE). *University at Buffalo: Department of Rehabilitation Science.* http://cirrie.buffalo.edu/culture/curriculum/guides/index.php. Accessed February 13, 2018.
60. Kale S, Hong CS. An investigation of therapy students' perceptions of cultural awareness. *Int J Ther Rehabil.* 2007;14(5):210-214.
61. Masin H, Tischenko AK. Professionalism, attitudes, beliefs and transformation of the learning experience: cross-cultural implications for developing a Spanish elective for non-Spanish-speaking physical therapist students. *J Phys Ther Educ.* 2007;21(3):40-46.
62. Griswold Quijano M, Gonzalez-Lamendola J. *Spanish for Physical Therapists: Tools for Effective Patient Communication.* 2nd ed. Alexandria, VA: American Physical Therapy Association; 2011.
63. Haskins AR, Kirk-Sanchez N. Recruitment and retention of students from minority groups. *Phys Ther.* 2006;86(1):19-29.
64. Iannotta JG, ed.; National Research Council (US) Committee on Population. *Emerging issues in Hispanic health: summary of a workshop.* National Academies Press (US); 2002.
65. Ihara E. *Cultural competence in health care: is it important for people with chronic conditions? Health Policy Institute Issue Brief Number 5.* Georgetown University: Health Policy Institute. https://hpi.georgetown.edu/agingsociety/pubhtml/cultural/cultural.html. Published February 2004. Accessed February 13, 2018.

General Treatment Information and Resources

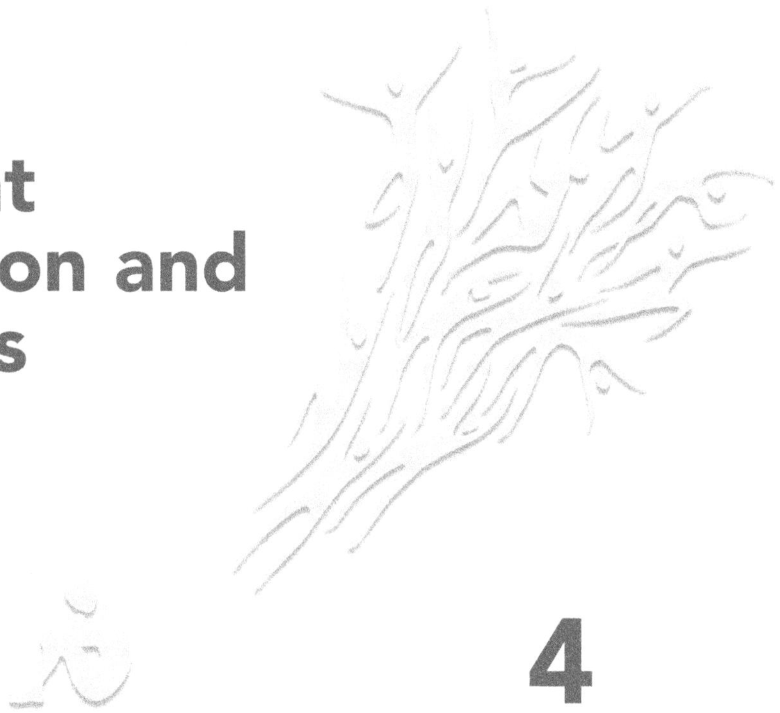

4

Outline

- Ethical Questions in Psychiatric and Geriatric Care
  - Moral Dilemmas and Clinical Decision-Making Models
  - Legal Competency and Other Compliance-Related Factors
  - Addressing Refusals of Treatment
  - Lifespan and Aging Issues
  - End-of-Life Issues
  - Payment Issues
- General Treatment Approaches Validated Across Multiple Psychological Conditions
  - Cognitive Behavioral Therapy With Subtypes
  - Motivational Interviewing
  - Neurolinguistic Psychology
- Legislation and Advocacy
- Geriatric-Focused Resources
  - National Alliance on Mental Illness
  - Academy of Geriatric Physical Therapy
  - International Organization of Physical Therapists in Mental Health
  - Beers Criteria
- Summary
- Key Points
- Review Questions

Johnson H.
Psychosocial Elements of Physical Therapy: The Connection of Body to Mind (pp 55-86).

Learning Objectives

- Gain basic knowledge of ethical and financial issues common in physical therapist practice with populations with mental health diagnoses, especially persons over 65 years old
- Propose applications of cognitive behavioral therapy (CBT), motivational interviewing (MI), and neurolinguistic psychology (NLP) to patient/client management
- List adaptations to the physical therapy plan of care for the **aging** complex patient, especially for impairments secondary to multiple medical and psychiatric conditions and medications
- Summarize available resources for physical therapists practicing in geriatric psychiatric settings

In physical therapy for persons with mental illness, especially in geriatric-focused settings, several approaches and resources apply across nearly all conditions. This chapter explores the basics of several concepts and resources for rapport, patient carry-through and participation in therapy, and promotion of positive behavior change—given complicating factors, such as morally complex situations, refusals of care, end-of-life status, and payment issues. Information on ethical questions, payment issues, general mental health, geriatric physical therapy, and potentially dangerous medications to watch for will be included.

Ethical Questions in Psychiatric and Geriatric Care

In physical therapist education, materials used to shape a common ethical foundation include the *Code of Ethics* for the physical therapist, promulgated through the American Physical Therapy Association (APTA). This document lists ethical principles with examples, based on "seven core values: accountability, altruism, compassion/caring, excellence, integrity, professional duty, and social responsibility."[1] While entry-level coursework or continuing education addresses specific aspects of ethically challenging situations for the clinician, this text focuses on a few aspects pertinent to a geriatric and/or mental health patient population.

Moral Dilemmas and Clinical Decision-Making Models

The clinician will face many situations requiring firm ethical and moral reasoning to make the best decision (these skills are typically taught in introductory courses in doctor of physical therapy [DPT] curricula), but sometimes there will be no one best decision. The APTA *Code of Ethics* for the physical therapist lists guiding principles to facilitate consistent ethical reasoning across the profession. While the physical therapist may not face life-or-death scenarios, complex and sensitive reasoning is still required as the clinician's choices (whether to treat, what treatment approach to use, how and whether to communicate sensitive medical information to various stakeholders) impact the patient's quality of life.

A significant component of such reasoning is the awareness of and respect for the patient's and other stakeholders' cultural values and distinctiveness (see Chapter 3).[2] Another aspect is the choice of whether, and to what extent, to share the clinical decision-making process with the patient. About two-thirds of physical therapists want to make decisions on their own, rather than share that power with the patient. Since patient involvement strengthens adherence to and satisfaction with therapy, clinicians need to avoid paternalism and recognize each patient's desire to decide.[3]

The following is an annotated bibliography to assist the clinician in ethical and moral awareness. These resources outline steps in ethical decision making, core ethical principles, types of situations to avoid in patient care, and ways to minimize an unhealthy role of emotions in reasoning.

Pope KS, Vasquez MT. *Ethics in Psychotherapy and Counseling: A Practical Guide.* 5th ed. Hoboken, NJ: John Wiley & Sons; 2016.

- Ethical education in graduate programs (whether for counseling, medicine, or another profession) is difficult to apply neatly in the working world. Areas of difficulty span appropriate use of information technology and the internet (including patient privacy issues); terminal diseases and the accompanying intense emotions; and keeping novel personal issues out of an objective, patient-centered decision. Influences on the physical therapist include peers, the time urgency of situations, and the perceived need to defend one's own mistakes.
- As with all areas of professional practice, clinicians need the ability to critically evaluate and practice based on evidence.
- The professional, full-time counselor needs to create a directive for the accurate, confidential transmission of patient records to his or her successor. While the physical therapist may not be personally responsible for past patient records, adherence to the Health Insurance Portability and Accountability Act (HIPAA) and other applicable guidelines is still required.
- Licensing and malpractice issues need a calm head, a good attorney, liability insurance, and the readiness to learn from the experience.
- **Steps in ethical decision making include clarifying the issue, determining need for outside resources, reviewing ethical/legal standards and research, actively minimizing bias, accountably implementing the results, and learning from the experience.**

Lo, B. *Resolving Ethical Dilemmas: A Guide for Clinicians.* 4th ed. Philadelphia, PA: Lippincott Williams & Wilkins; 2009.

- Essentials of clinical ethics include informed consent, non-maleficence ("first, do no harm"), confidentiality, avoiding deception, and keeping promises.
- When patients are cognitively unable to participate in shared decision making, an honorable surrogate (whether a family member, friend, or legal guardian) needs to respect the patient's previously expressed preferences. Lo also addresses the issues of persistent disagreements about care and well-informed refusal of treatment.
- Complicating factors to be avoided in the clinician-patient relationship include gift giving, inappropriate use of confidential information, and sexual contact (especially since physical therapy is a high-touch profession). Also, conflicts of interest from superiors, referral sources, colleagues, and financial influences need to be specified and avoided.

Welfel ER. *Ethics in Counseling and Psychotherapy: Standards, Research, and Emerging Issues.* 6th ed. Boston, MA: Cengage Learning; 2016.

- The clinician should be aware of and minimize conflicts of personal and professional values, documenting the stages and outcome of the reasoning process. Also, he or she should patiently seek multiple sources of input and act with a clear conscience.
- Multicultural ethics and counseling require competence with diverse populations, the ability to address prejudiced ideas expressed by patients and colleagues, and the awareness of potential friction between the clinician's religious values and service to various populations.
- Emerging challenges to patient confidentiality include managed care organizations, technological innovations, and institutional violence.
- In urgent situations, be prepared by having a solid ethical base in order to make a rapid, ethically defensible decision with a minimum of stress. For an outline of the ethical decision-making model referenced in the text, see last bullet point under the Pope and Vasquez reference.

Szekely RD, Miu AC. Incidental emotions in moral dilemmas: the influence of emotion regulation. *Cogn Emot.* 2015;29(1):64-75.

- In a realistic example of applied ethical reasoning, Szekely and Miu asked participants to choose between social welfare and harming another person. Common resulting emotions (hypothesized to be central to moral decision making) included fear, sadness, "compassion, guilt, anger, disgust, regret, and contempt." Choices reflect utilitarian (the end justifies the means of action) or deontological (the action is intrinsically right or wrong) thinking; more negative emotions occurred when participants reasoned deontologically.
- Participants were able to reduce their emotional arousal by "acceptance, rumination and catastrophising [sic]." Therapists may consider these strategies to regulate the role of their emotions in complex decision making.

Legal Competency and Other Compliance-Related Factors

In populations with frequent cognitive impairment, whether due to neurocognitive disorders (dementias) or other mental illnesses, clinicians must consider a patient's competence to consent to or refuse treatment. Dimond has written an excellent, freely accessible text on legal aspects of occupational therapy, which can be a reference for all therapy professionals.[4] Indeed, legal competence is only one facet of informed consent and clinical reasoning for the best care for patients and their families.[5] This subject is discussed in greater detail relative to dementia in Chapter 11.

Regardless of the psychological condition present, the clinician should emphasize thorough and sensitive communication with all parties, including patients, family members, significant others, social support systems, and other health care providers. In chronic mental illnesses, such as schizophrenia, inadequate communication on the patient's part can detract from treatment for pain and discomfort if the patient is in palliative care.[6] Within the team of health care providers especially in settings serving geriatric populations, communication deficits may influence moral distress, as well as discomfort regarding decisions the provider must make that risk the patient's health.[7]

Regardless of whether a patient (or power of attorney, if the patient is legally non-decisional) consents to treatment, whether he or she will actively participate depends heavily on personal factors, such as motivation. Since adherence to physical-activity recommendations is fairly low across multiple age groups, **clinicians working in geriatrics or mental health settings need to investigate how patients who are sedentary perceive themselves** (ie, as active or inactive).[8] Geographic location is also important to the goal-setting process for maximal participation; for example, older patients in urban areas tend to select a minimal distance to ambulate as more important for independence than do patients in rural areas.[9]

Finally, factors indirectly related to mental health can influence a patient's participation. In British adults over age 90, a set of surveys found that depressive symptoms, current circumstances, and emotional stability heavily influenced quality of life.[10] Additionally, patients with poor mental health often face stigma, "a negative marking of people just because of a diagnosis of mental illness" that can feed feelings of worthlessness and suicide risk.[11] The clinician needs to be sensitive to these factors and support patients emotionally and with as little bias as possible to make patients feel secure enough to participate fully in sessions and home exercise programs.

Addressing Refusals of Treatment

To complicate these issues, patients with mental health conditions may refuse treatment for reasons that seem illogical to the therapist. Even though cognitive impairments are often present, the therapist can still work around potential refusal by seeking the underlying attitudes, beliefs, and feelings. Factors that affect the likelihood of refusal of treatment—and associated attitudes and outcomes—by persons with chronic fatigue syndrome include communication, appropriate pace and intensity of therapy or home exercises, and the presence or absence of a fallback plan on the therapist's part.[12]

Besides these factors, therapists should, as best practice, promote shared decision making. Not only can this increase active patient involvement in the plan of care, but it can also reduce the likelihood of patient complaints or other actions against the therapist, since responsibility for treatment outcomes does not rest solely on the therapist's judgment, knowledge, and skill. By examining life-affecting decision making in the context of speech therapy (eg, patient refusal of recommended food consistency modifications to reduce risk of aspiration pneumonia), Kaizer et al developed an algorithm to address patient autonomy when it collides with the therapist's need to actively avoid harmful actions. The steps of the algorithm are[13]:

- Evaluation by the interdisciplinary team/interprofessional team (IDT/IPT) to recommend a diet consistency change
- Repeated education of patient and family to ensure understanding of the recommendations and reasons
- Meeting of the IDT/IPT to determine risks to the patient
- Adjustment of the treatment plan by the IDT/IPT, given patient and family input
- Additional meeting with the patient and family to discuss and educate further
- Follow up as needed by the IDT/IPT

This algorithm can be adapted to specific physical therapy issues that affect a patient's safety and quality of life, such as recommended discharge setting, home modifications for accessibility, and appropriate use of an assistive mobility device. As much as possible, patients should be involved in planning and completing their own care, with education by team members on such aspects as advance care planning and the risks of a patient's self-discharge against medical advice.[14,15] When the patient has temporary cognitive impairment, such as delirium, other members of the patient's support system can encourage the patient to avoid "irrational" refusal of treatment in acute and subacute care settings.[16]

Sometimes, however, the best course is for the therapist to document refusal, communicate with the IDT/IPT, and make the best of the situation. Two somewhat humorous examples, from an occupational therapist, relate to refusals that are not attributable to a diagnosed medical or mental health condition, but to the patient's conscious behavior (L. Stevens, oral communication, May 25, 2017). The first example is a patient who would lie in bed and state that he had rigor mortis whenever the therapist approached him for a session. The second patient would disrobe under bed sheets, abruptly removing the sheets and stating "Deal with this!" when the therapist came into the room to complete an activity of daily living training activity. The therapist managed both of these behaviors by adjusting her approach to be direct and firm, telling the patients she would not tolerate the behavior, and maintaining documentation and communication to the IDT/IPT related to the behaviors.

Lifespan and Aging Issues

Some age groups, including pediatrics (those under age 18 or 21) and geriatrics (those over age 65, sometimes subdivided into young-old, middle-old, and old-old), have such starkly different attitudes, beliefs, and values that they are considered their own subcultures. Chapters 2, 4, 5, and 14 explore culture more deeply. However, this section touches on aspects of physical activity counseling for the older adult, since mental health issues are often more complex and ingrained in this age group.

Giangregorio et al[17] published a protocol for 1 year of home exercise for women in Canada and Australia with a vertebral fracture (ie, a geriatric population with osteoporosis). Other studies found that osteoporosis can both facilitate or inhibit physical activity; thus, clinicians should be aware of the patient's medical history. Another sub-population, older women with cancer who are receiving hospice or palliative care, has counseling needs for "social relationships, spirituality, and outlook on mortality" by the physical therapist along with physical activity prescription.[18] Finally, the large proportion of sedentary older adults have unique counseling needs. Despite sedentary and active older adults having similar education and body mass index levels, sedentary older adults "had much lower fitness expectations of a physically active older adult, more perceived barriers to regular PA [physical activity], and required individual tailoring of a PA program" to avoid the feeling of slowing others down in a group fitness setting.[8] Finding out each patient's mindset about physical activity can prompt discussion of motivators and barriers.

Consideration of the older client in designing fitness facilities and clinics maximizes access to equipment and services by the largest possible range of people. Haber[19] suggests the following attributes of aging-friendly facilities:

- Speakers should play softer-volume music similar to what clients listened to growing up.
- Treadmills and other aerobics machines should have display panels easily seen by lower-vision eyes and used by arthritic hands, as well as a low minimum speed to accommodate stiff joints.
- Weight training equipment should have low minimal resistance (in 1- or 2-pound increments).

In addition, clinicians can refer aging clients who use the internet to the following evidence-based websites for reliable health information:

- Healthfinder, general health information: https://healthfinder.gov
- National Institutes of Health: www.nih.gov
- MedlinePlus, information from the National Library of Medicine: https://medlineplus.gov
- US Food & Drug Administration: www.fda.gov
- American Osteopathic Association: www.osteopathic.org/Pages/default.aspx
- Agency for Healthcare Research and Quality: www.ahrq.gov
- National Association of Area Agencies on Aging: www.n4a.org
- American Heart Association: www.heart.org/HEARTORG
- American Diabetes Association: www.diabetes.org
- The Gerontological Society of America: www.geron.org
- National Council on Aging: www.ncoa.org
- Hospice Information: www.hospiceinfo.org
- Caregiver Action Network: http://caregiveraction.org
- Substance Abuse and Mental Health Services Administration: www.samhsa.gov
- National Institute on Drug Abuse: www.drugabuse.gov
- American Association of Retired Persons: www.aarp.org
- WebMD, specific health condition information: www.webmd.com
- Mayo Clinic, high-quality medical care: www.mayoclinic.org

End-of-Life Issues

Physical therapists may not encounter people facing the end of their lives in every care setting. However, clinicians in pediatrics, long-term care, palliative care, and other settings with very young, aging, or medically-complex clients benefit from background knowledge of end-of-life issues. Such issues include advance directives, competency (see previous section on legal competency), and withdrawal of nutrition or ventilation from a person. **At the heart is the clinician's ethical disposition toward what constitutes life and quality of life, as well as the authority of the patient and health care provider to prolong life vs delay dying**. An example could involve a patient in a minimally conscious state vs persistent vegetative state. Since this patient has some level of consciousness, this creates more difficult ethical questions of how to decide whether the patient would wish a particular life-sustaining treatment to be administered or withdrawn, and where the line is for euthanasia.[20] See Hamel and Walter,[21] and Jennett[22] for a more thorough discussion of persistent vegetative state.

Advance directives have several variations and became more common in public discussion after Terri Schiavo's death in 2005, following withdrawal of a feeding tube during her persistent vegetative state. Their basic purpose is to express the person's treatment-related intent, should he or she become unable to communicate these preferences or give informed consent. Persons with mental health issues, cancer, or life-shortening illnesses in palliative care often create such advance directives.[23,14,15] Of note, persons with psychological conditions may, between exacerbations, choose to create advance directives to ensure that they will receive the treatment they need and want, despite their frequent refusal during a mental health crisis. These treatment choices can apply for long periods of time, not just at end of life.

The patient's autonomy, or right to choose regardless of how others perceive the rationality of those choices, is central to advance care planning. While choices reflect values, the person's circumstances and feelings can change over the course of a disease such as cancer.[14] An ethical model to facilitate relevant and sensitive decision making regarding palliative care at late stages of disease involves these components[15]:

- An approach undergirded by a humanistic and holistic (whole-person) worldview
- A method of decision making tailored to the patient's abilities
- Involvement of a multidisciplinary medical team
- Clear documentation throughout the decision-making process
- Awareness of current evidence regarding medical conditions, current laws, and professional standards

For clinicians working with persons with advanced dementia, an additional aspect requires ethical grappling. These patients may not require medical treatment, such as mechanical ventilation, a feeding tube, or hemodialysis, to prolong their lives. However, "they have the same rights [as patients who do require these treatments], but there is simply no life-sustaining medical treatment to refuse" even when the patient may wish to die rather than prolong life.[24] In such cases, some patients who are still decisional, or sometimes non-decisional, can choose to stop eating and drinking. This option is legal and supportable, as it does not legally constitute abuse, neglect, or assisted suicide. Each health care provider and team member supporting a patient towards the end of his or her life will wrestle with these and other questions; this text seeks to stimulate the thought process and give suggested references.

On the opposite end of the lifespan, parents coping with a child's health issues (perhaps terminal) have their own set of considerations for members of the IDT/IPT that include physical therapists. Such aspects of pediatric end-of-life care include treatment setting, specific medical conditions and available treatment modalities, purposes of treatment, and cultural or other psychosocial dimensions. In sharing and using knowledge and skill, physical therapists and other care providers need to balance expertise with psychosocial sensitivity, as a child dying is often more difficult to handle than an older adult dying.

Most pediatric deaths in the United States take place in hospitals, therefore involving nurses and therapists primarily. A survey of pediatric intensive care unit nurses indicated that key barriers to good care "were language barriers and parental discomfort in withholding and/or withdrawing mechanical ventilation."[25] However, since the parents held final responsibility for their children's care, these same nurses indicated that a way of supporting them during the child's end of life was to give them alone time, a precious commodity in many hospital settings.

In a hospital or other setting, with patients of any age, physical therapy addresses the movement system to maximize health, wellness, and quality of life. Therapists who practice in palliative care and hospice focus more on quality of life and managing movement-related symptoms. In hospice, therapists see patients with cancer (any age), HIV-AIDS, multiple sclerosis, altered mental status, amyotrophic lateral sclerosis (Lou Gehrig's disease), or other conditions limiting life expectancy. Although the patient may not be expected to return to a more independent setting, therapists can still use assistive device training for energy conservation, therapeutic exercise and manual therapy for ease of movement, and modalities (biofeedback, electrical, mechanical, and thermal) for pain management. Since cancer and infection are precautions, also sometimes contraindications, to electrical or thermal modality use, the therapist should consider the patient's goals and medical status in choosing treatment.[26]

Psychosocial aspects of palliative and hospice care, especially for pediatric patients, are multiple with significant impacts. Palliative care can go in 2 directions: a cure, or hospice care if the condition is diagnosed as terminal. In most cases, pediatric palliative care centers around cancer. Communication, a key aspect, is often difficult due to language differences (including provider jargon), ethnic worldviews (including non-verbal signs being misinterpreted by provider and parent), and complexity of care (including parents keeping track of team members' roles). Care models used should focus on the family and its needs, and team-family conferences should be carefully planned, managed, and coordinated to maximize good communication for responsible and sensitive care.[27-29]

Payment Issues

In the United States, stakeholders are still developing awareness of the implications of the Affordable Care Act (ACA), signed into law in 2010 and, at the time of this book's writing, under scrutiny for potential modification or repeal. While this law seeks to bring affordable health care insurance to more individuals, it is fraught with complexity, in addition to the regulations of Medicare (Title XVIII) and Medicaid (Title XIX), which cover many older individuals and persons with chronic illness. This book sketches background for reimbursement issues related to these populations. Instructors may further prepare students for integrating insurance policy and regulations into their practice by using realistic patient cases.[30]

One feature of the ACA is a push towards reimbursement to health care professionals based on the true value of services vs a set amount of payment for each procedure performed ("fee-for-service"). Physicians have worked toward this by developing close relationships with hospital systems that bridge the gap between acute care, subacute, home health, and outpatient services. However, the Stark Law, a tool to minimize health care fraud, can conflict with this way of increasing value and decreasing costs. The law "prohibits physician referrals for designated health care services to organizations to which that provider has a qualified financial relationship."[31] These "designated health care services" include physical and occupational therapy, outpatient speech-language therapy, home health care, and others. Although the conflict may be questionable, it can prevent partnership from economic feasibility.

Another approach is integrated care management, including a team and infrastructure for a health care system for patients in a certain geographic area, often rural.[32] The ACA has designated funds for investigating this and other alternative payment and care delivery models. However, "not all payment models reimburse for coordinated care across a care team."[33] Two models of payment are modified fee-for-service, which charges each patient a monthly fee regardless of procedures performed (thus incentivizing the provider to increase quality and decrease quantity of services); and risk-based, which sets upper limits on payments to providers (with a similar incentive). When older adults are eligible for both Medicare and Medicaid, models such as PACE (Program of All-Inclusive Care for the Elderly, started in 1997) improve communication and coordination between the 2 insurance providers due to their very different policies and otherwise minimal incentive for coordinating care.

Under Medicare part A, commonly billed in skilled nursing facilities (SNFs), a daily fee is charged to Medicare based on the weekly amount of therapy and other skilled medical services.[34] Medicare developed resource utilization groups (RUGs) for classifying patients to determine the

Table 4-1

Resource Utilization Groups (RUGs) in Medicare

RUG LEVEL	THERAPY MINUTES PER WEEK	MEDICARE DAILY AVERAGE REIMBURSEMENT (FINANCIAL YEAR 2013)
Ultra high (RU)	720 or more	$476 to $751, depending on level of non-therapy services
Very high (RV)	500 to 719	$421 to $668
High (RH)	325 to 499	$337 to $605
Medium (RM)	150 to 324	$289 to $555
Low (RL)	Under 150	$234 to $488

payment amount. Two large RUG categories encompass therapy services, and within these categories the daily payment varies based on the weekly total minutes of skilled therapy provided. As shown in Table 4-1, therapy providers have significant financial incentive to categorize as many patients in the higher RUG levels as possible; the physical therapist should determine the appropriate level for the patient's medical complexity and activity tolerance, but due to institutional and organizational pressure this does not always happen.

One reason for Medicare reform, both before and after the ACA, is fraud (inappropriate overpayments to health care providers, defined as intentional deception by the provider or billing office for an establishment such as an SNF). In 2009, the Office of the Inspector General found that a quarter of claims submitted by SNFs to Medicare for time-based therapy services were erroneous; this resulted in $1.5 billion of overpayment. Almost 47% of reporting of amounts of therapy provided and functional abilities of patients treated (in the minimum data set) were also in error.[35] A follow-up study found significant pressure exerted on therapists to provide services at the highest-paying level regardless of whether the patient needed or could tolerate that amount of therapy.[36]

DeBoer[37] investigated 5 main effects of the ACA on Medicare and reform efforts, since Medicare spending continues to grow by about 6% per year from 12% of the 2010 federal budget.

1. The ACA does not directly affect Medicare costs, but will influence them in the long term.
2. The ACA preserves the Medicare coverage requirement of medical necessity: "to diagnose or treat illness or injury or to improve the function of a malformed body member."[37]
3. The ACA increased Medicare coverage and benefits regarding preventive services and care management; this is consistent with promoting health, wellness, and IDT/IPT-based functioning.
4. The ACA seeks to facilitate outcomes and effectiveness research, to help stakeholders empower patients to maintain a healthy lifestyle.
5. The ACA includes funding for preventive care as well as other health-related initiatives, which were approved by both sides of the House and Senate.

Other effects remain to be seen, depending on the legislation in the coming years.

Some physical therapy practices have tried to eliminate insurance denial and red tape by becoming cash-based. However, for Medicare beneficiaries (who would use Part B for these services), legal issues may sprout up. These issues include negligence, malpractice, privacy, and payment concerns. Negligence is "a failure to exercise care toward another person that a reasonably prudent person would do in similar circumstances," while malpractice is "negligence in exercising a standard of care or standard of conduct established by a profession."[38]

Because of clinicians' unique education and training on exercise prescription, they may offer fitness services without marketing themselves as providing physical therapy. Regardless of the name of the service, the physical therapist is generally held to a higher practice standard than a non-therapist for the same services, and thus is more liable for malpractice should any ill effects occur, such as falls, injuries, or adverse medical events if participants are not cleared to exercise safely. While the therapist may choose not to, conducting a thorough assessment on each participant before the fitness class is prudent, depending on the specifics of each state's physical therapy practice act.

Privacy is another potential issue for fitness services provided by a physical therapist. Patient health information is protected under HIPAA, and includes the person's name, medical history, and any other information that could personally identify the individual. Whatever information the physical therapist collects needs to be kept confidential; this practice or any deviation from it needs to be spelled out in a written agreement that the participant must comprehend for informed consent.

Payment issues for Medicare beneficiaries are a third major issue, as Medicare determines on a regular basis which services are covered and by which providers. If the fitness services are considered covered by Medicare part B, the physical therapist cannot charge the participant in cash, even if the therapist is not an approved Medicare provider. Simons notes that "physical therapists may only bill for *covered* services that Medicare doesn't pay for if the physical therapist obtains the patient's signature on an Advanced Beneficiary Notice" which "informs the patient in advance that Medicare is not likely to pay for the service."[38] However, if there are solely fitness services involved, the service is not covered by Medicare, thus allowing cash pay and negating the need for an Advanced Beneficiary Notice.

General Treatment Approaches Validated Across Multiple Psychological Conditions

Feelings don't try to kill you, even the painful ones. Anxiety is a feeling grown too large. A feeling grown aggressive and dangerous. You're responsible for its consequences, you're responsible for treating it.

—Patrick Ness[39]

Since communication is an essential function of physical therapist practice,[40] and because the number of persons over age 65 or with mental health concerns are growing, the clinician needs strong background knowledge and skills for communicating with these patients. Communication allows the clinician to listen to the patient's true concerns, motivate for participation and better outcomes, and maintain a professional and empathetic demeanor in more challenging situations. The strategies suggested by CBT, MI, and NLP form a useful foundation. For further reading, *The Validation Breakthrough* by Naomi Feil (most recently revised in 2012) is geared toward dementia and delirium, but may be helpful with multiple populations.

Cognitive Behavioral Therapy With Subtypes

CBT, encompassing several types of psychotherapy, is recommended for various psychosocial issues related to life stressors and mental illnesses. Developed in the 1960s by Dr. Aaron Beck and others,[41] the approach includes several subtypes. Dobson has written an excellent handbook of the therapies, their evidence base, and applicability for mental health.[42] For older adults, principles of CBT subtypes can be used in rehabilitation to "help older adults to see how thoughts guide their exercise behavior."[43] **The clinician's overarching goals for using any type of CBT are to train patients to be more aware of their thoughts, think more positively about exercising, and increase adherence to good exercise habits (Table 4-2).**

Table 4-2

Subtypes of Cognitive Behavioral Therapy and Conditions Treatable by Cognitive Behavioral Therapy

SUBTYPES OF COGNITIVE BEHAVIORAL THERAPY	CONDITIONS TREATABLE BY COGNITIVE BEHAVIORAL THERAPY
• Problem-solving therapy (PST) • Rational emotive behavior therapy (REBT) • Cognitive therapy (CT) • Schema therapy (ST) • Dialectical behavior therapy (DBT) • Mindfulness interventions	• Depression • Bipolar disorder • Phobias • Social anxiety • Obsessive-compulsive disorder • Panic disorder • Chronic posttraumatic stress disorder (PTSD) • Generalized anxiety disorder • Schizophrenia • Borderline personality disorder (BPD)

PST, one subtype of CBT, trains attitudes and skills, especially in the maintenance stage of behavior change. Persons with many stressors and poor coping skills can benefit from PST. The following is a list of general sequential steps of the therapy:

- Development of rapport
- Therapist assessment of the patient's stressors
- Identification of obstacles
- Changing the idea of a problem to that of a challenge
- Channeling of the patient's emotions
- Proposing of alternate solutions
- Instruction in real-time decision making
- Implementation and checking of solutions
- Guided practice for speed and automaticity

The therapist also focuses on the patient's self-efficacy, recognition of problems, definition of problems, and the use of the STOP & THINK technique.[44] Visser et al[45] applied PST clinically in a study protocol for stroke rehabilitation, where patients learned 4 basic problem-solving steps to decrease their stress related to the stroke's impact on their lives:

- Problem and goal definition
- Solution brainstorming
- Analysis of potential consequences to choose the best solution
- Attempt the solution and repeat the cycle if choosing a better solution is needed

REBT, another subtype of CBT, "opposes ... a dogmatic and rigid belief in faith ... [but] shares [with] the philosophy of Christianity the view that we would do better to condemn the sin but forgive (or, more accurately, accept) the sinner."[42] Based on a rationalistic worldview, then, REBT seeks to guide the patient toward correction of irrational thought patterns, termed *cognitive distortions*. Cognitive distortions are as follows:

- Jumping to conclusions
- Focusing on the negative aspects of a situation
- Personalizing the problem to apply to oneself when it actually does not
- Perfectionism, rejecting anything less than perfect
- Thinking in extremes without gray area

Besides sharing portions of a Christian worldview, REBT emphasizes philosophy, humanism, self-acceptance, allowing some healthy negative emotions, and the therapist's level-headed demeanor. In a psychotherapeutic setting, this technique is typically applied diagnostically by evaluating the patient's medical diagnosis, finding the root cause of cognitive problems, developing a problem list, and conceptualizing the problems by their underlying beliefs and consequences.[42] While the physical therapist has different training and so cannot apply the theory in the same way, clinicians can still be aware of cognitive distortions to gently point them out to the patient as applicable, to increase adherence to the therapy plan of care.

CT, a third subtype of CBT, addresses "distorted information processing" with a collaborative, patient-centered emphasis.[42] Techniques of CT include:

- Assignment of written activity and mood logs. This increases the patient's awareness of how he or she processes information, including patterns of cognitive errors.
- Scheduling of challenging activities at specific times. This decreases the burden of decision making on the patient by building habits.
- Changing of task structure to develop a "just-right challenge." This decreases the likelihood that the patient will avoid the situation.
- Use of more open-ended than closed-ended questions. This can improve the flow of sessions.

Therapists may recognize similarities between some of these techniques and other psychosocial interventions, such as graded exposure to create a "just-right challenge" for a patient who avoids movements or activities due to fear. Within a mental health rehabilitation context, the clinician may choose techniques at his or her discretion, since evidence supports each subtype of CBT.

ST, another subtype, is specifically recommended for personality disorders, which have worse outcomes when other types of CBT are applied. The main constructs of ST are:

- "Schemas," which "are core psychological themes (ie, inner influences on behavior)" or thought patterns, that guide how the individual perceives and organizes new information from the environment[42]
- "Coping styles," which "are characteristic behavioral responses to schemas"[42]
- "Modes," which "are the schemas and coping styles operating at a given moment"[42]

Examples of undesirable schemas include abandonment, mistrust, shame, alienation, dependence, failure, entitlement, impaired self-control, approval seeking, pessimism, and increased criticalness.

ST hypothesizes that each of these is an ineffective reaction to a painful aspect of the patient's life. Goals for ST sessions fall under cognitive, experiential, behavioral, and rapport domains, with the psychotherapist functioning as a "healthy adult" to help the patient's underlying "vulnerable child."[42] Steps of ST in a psychiatric context, adaptable to physical rehabilitation, include:

- Identification of modes
- Exploration of each mode
- Linking of each mode to signs and symptoms
- Emphasizing benefits of changing undesirable modes
- Integration and generalization of the patient's understanding of his or her own pathological modes

DBT, the final subtype of CBT, is mainly applied to BPD and suicidality. Based on the idea that behavior change is cyclical, it uses the concepts of thesis, antithesis, and synthesis. Thesis refers to an original idea in a session; combining this with the antithesis, or negation of that idea, will in theory produce a synthesis that guides the discussion in the session toward progressively healthier modes of thinking and relating to others.[46] Presently, there is limited to no evidence available on the application of DBT to physical therapy.

Mindfulness and acceptance interventions span multiple types of CBT. To be mindful is to be in each moment and observe thoughts neutrally. Skills specific to its practice include:

- Observing
- Describing
- Participating "unconsciously" (when one "loses oneself" in an activity)
- Keeping a non-judgmental stance
- Engaging in one task at a time
- Being effective

The therapist reminds the patient practicing mindfulness that thoughts are only thoughts. With this and other CBT subtypes, the therapist must consider cultural aspects such as the patient's health beliefs, characteristics of self-identification (including but not limited to ethnic background), whether the patient is from an individualistic or collectivistic culture, communication styles, therapy goals, immigrant or refugee status, and family structure.[42]

In practice, physical therapists commonly use principles of these therapies in health behavior change counseling for exercise habits. Some therapists develop health contracts with their patients for exercise; these can include the patient's motivator for movement, the specific exercise modality, the patient's baseline (to help the patient see incremental change), the specific health goal, the problem behavior and anticipated solution, both parties' signatures, and a health calendar for tracking. Regardless of whether such a contract is used, 10 tips for encouraging patients to change are: "motivation, modest, measurable, memory, positive thoughts, reinforcement, environmental support, stress management, social support, [and] problem solve [sic]."[19]

While the previous section provides only essential background for the non-psychotherapist seeking to apply principles of CBT with patients, the Beck Institute website offers specific training and more information.[41] All types of CBT have good absolute efficacy, and most types are superior to other psychotherapies. Several are superior to medications; the fewer medications patients take, the fewer side effects and medication interactions will worsen physical therapy outcomes and health-related quality of life.

Motivational Interviewing

Commonly used by counselors and psychologists but also applicable to non-specialists, such as clergy or allied health care providers, MI is a communication technique developed to advance patients through the stages of behavior change.

> Motivational interviewing is an approach designed to help clients build commitment and reach a decision to change. It draws on strategies from client-centered counseling, cognitive therapy, systems theory, and the social psychology of persuasion.[47]

The stages of the transtheoretical model of change in the background of MI sessions are as follows:

- Precontemplation: the 4 R's of "reluctance, rebellion, resignation, and rationalization" about changing an addictive behavior.[19] The patient is unaware that the behavior is a problem.
- Contemplation: ambivalence, analyzing risks and rewards. Here, the patient knows that there is a problem but has not decided to change it for the better. The best response is for the provider to give more information on both sides of the behavior.
- Determination: a commitment to change, and not just an adamant statement of intent to change. True commitment, then, is proportionate to the patient's insight into the difficulty of changing and a "calm dedication to [prioritize change]."[19]
- Action: a sustained demonstration of change, usually taking 3 to 6 months. The provider's role here is to give the patient information on models of change.
- Maintenance, relapse, and recycling: Maintenance can be thought of as a new habit, whereas in relapse the person slips back into the old habit of behavior. Recycling is a repeated cycle of behavior change. Note, however, that the stages are not necessarily linear, but the patient can move back and forth between stages depending on circumstances.

In contrast, MI does not equate to:

- The transtheoretical model of change itself[48]
- "A way of tricking people into doing what you want them to do"[49]
- Decisional balance: where the patient weighs the pros and cons of a potential or current behavior change[48]
- Assessment feedback: a psychological process including reflection on constructive feedback to improve the clinician's assessment skills[50]
- CBT
- Client-centered therapy
- Easy to learn
- Practice as usual
- A cure-all

What is a behavior that should be changed (also termed an *addictive behavior*)? According to Miller and Rollnick:

> [A] defining characteristic of addictive behaviors is that they involve the pursuit of short-term gratification at the expense of long-term harm. Often the person is quite aware of the damaging consequences, and has resolved to control or abandon the addictive behaviors, yet time and again returns to the old familiar pattern.[47]

Examples of such behaviors include smoking, a sedentary lifestyle, an unhealthy diet, and poor sleep hygiene. Therapists should educate patients on these health-related behaviors and also be role models for positive, effective behavior change.

As clinicians model desirable health behaviors and educate patients, they may be tempted to use their knowledge and skills in an authoritarian way. However, in MI, "the counselor does not assume an authoritarian role ... Responsibility for change is left with the individual."[47] This can be difficult to implement initially, but it is a valuable way to gain buy-in. In avoiding authoritarianism, therapists increase the patient's identification of his or her own problems and use of personal choice, which is consistent with an ethical value of patient autonomy. More strategies include therapist reflection on the sources of a patient's resistance and amplification of discrepancy in the patient's mind between the current and desired behavior.

The acronym DEARS summarizes the central principles of MI[47]:

- D: develop discrepancy. Especially in precontemplation, the patient is unaware or unwilling to admit that the behavior is a problem; the therapist should gently question the benefits of continuing the behavior.
- E: express empathy. Here, therapists take an interest in their patient's feelings and use strategies of active listening to let patients know they are there for them.
- A: avoid argumentation. A person's natural response to contradiction or opposition is to solidify one's own position and push back. While arguing with a patient may be an automatic response, it is not beneficial to help the patient change for the better.
- R: roll with resistance. Therapists can choose to ask permission for giving advice, emphasizing the patient's choice, or offer advice from their own experience (for example, asking "Have you ever thought of this?).
- S: support self-efficacy. Therapists can build up the patient's confidence, reframe previous unsuccessful attempts to change as learning experiences, and ask how the patient feels about progress to date and confidence level.

While these strategies are useful during an episode of care, it is important to set the stage early on for positive continued rapport with the patient. During the patient interview or second treatment session, the therapist can ask open-ended questions about details of the problem behavior or behaviors; what the patient's typical day is like; lifestyle and stressors; health and related behaviors; good and less-good aspects of the undesirable health behavior; and, after any advice or information, the question "What do you think?"

During this and other sessions, the clinician should avoid[47]:

- Question-answer patterns, where the therapist asks all the questions and the patient gives all the answers. This can set a tone that is less than collaborative, and may decrease rapport.
- Confrontation-denial patterns, where the therapist repeatedly brings up negative aspects of the patient's undesirable health behavior, since people resist when they perceive an attack.
- Acting as the "expert." While physical therapists have knowledge and skills about many health behaviors and interventions, patient-centered care means that the patient's goals and perspective take precedence, with the therapist acting as more of a coach or cheerleader.
- Labeling the patient or behavior, which can depersonalize the problem, decrease rapport and patient involvement, and decrease therapist empathy necessary for effective practice.
- Focusing prematurely on the behavior to be changed. Autonomous patients need to come to their own conclusions, which may need more time at the beginning to explore the patient's experiences and issues.
- Blaming the patient for the behavior. While in cases it may seem that the patient is directly responsible for the negative health behaviors and their consequences, pointing this out is often counterproductive. Also, many behaviors have multifactorial causes and effects.

In place of the poor strategies listed previously, early-use strategies include:

- Open-ended questions, to increase the percentage of time that the patient spends talking
- Reflective listening, in which the therapist responds to the patient by guessing the meaning
- Affirmations, to encourage the patient forward through the stages of change
- Summaries, delivered periodically and with a collaborative tone
- Eliciting of self-motivational statements, relating to the patient's recognition of the problem, concerns, intent to change, and level of optimism

After the first session, it is critical to follow up with the patient, whether by phone or at the next treatment. Behavior change is ongoing and difficult, and therapists can be a consistent source of support.

Resistance to change can take many forms, including argument, interruption, denial, and ignoring the therapist. To roll with resistance, common especially in mental health settings, use[47]:

- Reflective listening, where the therapist avoids resisting back and instead listens actively
- Amplified reflection, to tactfully exaggerate what the patient seems to be saying, without sarcasm
- Double-sided reflection, where the therapist adds an "on the other hand" perspective to create or increase the patient's ambivalence
- Shifting of focus, around vs against the perceived barriers
- Agreeing with a twist, where the therapist slightly changes the direction of the discussion
- Emphasizing the patient's choice and control
- Reframing of the resistance, to give a new form or meaning to the problem behavior at hand

Finally, Miller and Rollnick[47] provide a brief description of ways to address some challenging situations:

- If a patient comes in with a significant other and "destructive communication patterns" are evident, the therapist may gently ask to speak with each person separately to get both sides of the story and potentially improve the patient's social support.[47]
- If the patient feels pressured into therapy, the clinician can choose to detach him- or herself from the situation as possible, maintaining a frank and matter-of-fact tone. This can decrease the patient's perception of any ethically questionable coercion, and can increase the patient's respect for the therapist as someone who is trying to help.
- If the patient is showing strong emotions, crying, sidetracked, or indicating that his or her life is too chaotic to deal with, it is wisest for the therapist to listen reflectively, redirect politely, and discern whether to explore the source or to be silent for up to a minute to allow the patient to self-calm.

Neurolinguistic Psychology

NLP, developed in the 1970s, is a contested framework to improve communication by the principle that "the meaning of communication is based on the response that you get."[51] The 3 basic principles of NLP can establish and improve rapport or, in certain situations, break rapport consciously by doing the opposite of what the principles recommend. Several older studies concluded that this approach is dramatically effective in emergency medicine, dentistry, and stress management, but other newer sources note conflicting results.[52-54] A systematic review of 5 randomized controlled trials and 5 pre- and poststudies applying NLP to anxiety disorders, substance abuse, and claustrophobia, found that all studies had a high or uncertain risk of bias, and 4 of the 5 randomized controlled trials did not report superior outcomes for NLP or the control intervention. Sturt et al[55] recommended high-quality research into the framework prior to funded clinical applications. A background and research review of NLP explored its terminology and noted a lack of rigorous research to defend its core ideas.

> If NLP encourages people to learn ways of communicating more effectively then that is a noble endeavour [sic] and not particularly problematic ... yet the medical literature is devoid of any published evidence to substantiate these claims [of dramatic success with serious disorders]. This creates a serious ethical problem.[56]

Thus, given studies opposing NLP as a framework but allowing it as a communication system, 2 rapport-related principles can be useful, especially with patients who are agitated or with limited verbal abilities:

1. Matching: the therapist models aspects of the other person's posture, breathing pattern, and voice. This does not mean exact mimicry, but matching allows body language similarity to help the clinician empathize with the other person's feelings.
2. Pacing and leading: the clinician pays attention to the rapport gained, and then gradually changes his or her own "behavior so that the other person can follow. However, one must have rapport *before* one can pace and lead."[51]

The author of this text has found these principles useful in situations involving high emotions, severe behaviors (especially related to dementias), and the need to establish rapid respect between parties. In mental health contexts, practicing these skills for automaticity can be invaluable to one's therapeutic approach. Despite the lack of established evidence to support the framework as a whole, the 2 aspects listed earlier are supported by research in other areas, including communication.[57,58]

Legislation and Advocacy

Two major pieces of legislation to benefit persons with disabilities are the Americans with Disabilities Act (ADA) and Individuals with Disabilities Education Act (IDEA). The ADA was introduced in 1990 to fill gaps in protections for persons with disabilities left by the Social Security Act of 1935 and 1956, the Civil Rights Act of 1964, and the Rehabilitation Act of 1973. Building on a foundation of disability insurance, prohibition of discrimination against basic protected classes, and the requirement for physical accessibility of health care facilities, the ADA has 5 main areas. These were in "employment, public services, public accommodations and services operated by private entities, telecommunications and information technology, and miscellaneous provisions and technical assistance."[59] Residual gaps relating to education, workforce, and community integration were filled by the New Freedom Initiative in 2001. However, insurance gaps still exist for persons with disabilities, leading to lack of proper medical care and medication access.[60]

Particularly affecting pediatric physical therapists, IDEA regulates each state's development and implementation of early intervention services for high-risk children. IDEA recognizes 13 categories of disability and, supported by more accurate assessment tools, can help teenage students with disabilities transition into adult life.[61] The Individual Family Service Plan and Individualized Education Program are 2 components mandated by IDEA and implemented by schools, while the level and intensity of services are determined by individual states. Because many affected children have Medicaid as a primary insurance, rehabilitation services typically need third-party coverage.[62]

To promote the concepts of health and wellness via access to and payment for services, physical therapists advocate at multiple levels for their patients. The American Physical Therapy Association (APTA) has many resources even for association non-members. Such resources address public education; upcoming legislation and legislative action days; emerging issues for physical therapist practice, including multistate licensure compacts; and other areas.

- www.apta.org/Advocacy/Involvement
- www.apta.org/StateAdvocacy
- www.apta.org/FederalAdvocacy
- www.apta.org/PreventionWellness

Geriatric-Focused Resources

For the practitioner in any setting with geriatric patients, several resources are particularly useful. Since poor mental health is more prevalent as people age, the National Alliance on Mental Illness (NAMI) offers research and anecdotes to lend a more personal angle. To span the aging spectrum, the Academy of Geriatric Physical Therapy (AGPT) website offers—especially for APTA members—professional research and opportunities for student involvement to improve the health of persons over age 65 via physical therapy in an interprofessional context. Globally, the International Organization of Physical Therapists in Mental Health (IOPTMH) focuses on developing the research base for therapists to directly impact mental illnesses and their secondary impairments. Finally, the Beers criteria for potentially inappropriate or hazardous medications for geriatric patients provides useful background, especially when the patient is in a home or skilled nursing setting where polypharmacy is common.

National Alliance on Mental Illness

NAMI,[63] founded in 1977, is a nonprofit advocacy group in the United States, supporting state and local organizations and leaders to advocate for better understanding and legislation for persons with psychological conditions. It seeks to reach people via educational materials and programs, social media (eg, the promotion of Mental Illness Awareness Week in the first full week of October), legislative advocacy, and support to health care providers working with persons with mental health issues. A section for personal stories from those experiencing illnesses, such as depression, bipolar disorder, and schizophrenia, shares what the illness actually feels like.

One such story, posted on October 6, 2016, takes the form of a letter written by a woman with combined BPD, PTSD, and major depressive disorder.[64] She traces the development of her conditions and how she deals with them:

> The PTSD is due to my childhood trauma. My father was incredibly abusive in many different ways. I endured that until I was twelve. My mother was in and out of the hospital with her own mental illness. She had multiple personality disorder, now known as dissociative identity disorder, because of her own childhood abuse. Her personality was split into different aspects, called alters. She would dissociate, meaning she'd lose track of her [sic] who she was, her thoughts, feelings, sense of identity, essentially, she'd blackout mentally but still be functioning physically as one of her alters.
>
> All of that was traumatic and it's what caused the PTSD. I experience flashbacks at times, an experience where I am reliving a past event like I'm really there. I have nightmares and lots of anxiety. I get triggered sometimes, like something will happen right now and it will remind me of past events and that triggers anxiety, flashbacks or nightmares. It's gotten a lot better, but that took an awful lot of work. I did exposure therapy, which is where you purposefully relive the event to desensitize you to it. The results have been immense.
>
> The borderline personality disorder emerged from the childhood events. I had a predisposition to it. It's not something you are born with, but rather something you acquire. Aspects of my personality left me susceptible to BPD. It's not something that be cured. There's no pill to treat it. The meds I take, however, help with the symptoms. I take a mood stabilizer because I have intense and sudden mood swings. I take anti-anxiety medication and antidepressants. I also take two antipsychotics because BPD has some dissociative symptoms and I have experienced them. I take a medication that prevents

me from self-harming. Up until fifteen months ago, I burned myself pretty regularly. I've since stopped. The med doesn't stop it completely, like the rest of my meds. It only makes things easier, taking the edge off my experience.

> The other symptoms of BPD that I struggle with are the intense emotions and abandonment issues. Abandonment issues are the worse. I'm afraid that people will get sick of dealing with me and get up and leave. I'm worried that I might do something, even slight, and they're out the door. It's because, in part, my mom wasn't around when I was younger. My dad also had a new girlfriend that was going to be my new mom every six months or so. And I've scared a lot of people away with the borderline. It's mellowed out as I've gotten older, even without therapy. Don't get me wrong: therapy has helped so much. But, I used to be a lot more like the borderlines everyone know [sic] from popular culture, even though I'm on the mild end of the spectrum. I drank, did drugs, self-harmed. I had horrible mood swings. I tried not to get close to people so I wouldn't lose them. And I was angry. I never expressed it externally; rather, I took it out on myself in forms of self-harm.

> I have a hard time with normal, healthy attachments because of the borderline. I am super attached to Karen and my doctor because of this. I'm proud to say that these are the only two borderline relationships in my life. I still experience a lot of ups and downs with them, though. It physically hurts to be apart from them at times. I'm very clingy and have an almost childlike attachment to them. I'd do anything for them and am not sure how I'd live without them. You learn to have [healthy] attachments through your relationships with your parents and because my relationships were so convoluted, I never learned how to have healthy attachments. I'm learning now and even though I better understand them, I can't really change the way I feel about Karen and my doctor. They're both cool with it, thank goodness. I'm very, very lucky.

> I struggle when they are gone. It's not something I bring on myself. It's fact. I used to be afraid they wouldn't come back. Now, I know better. There have been times when I'd rather die than live through the pain of separation. Historically, I've been hospitalized three times while one of them was away. I have issues with object permanence. That's when a child knows his or her parent exists even if they aren't physically there. Sometimes, I think I've made them up. It's why my bedroom is covered with pictures, to remind myself they exist. I know it sounds crazy, but a lot of times it doesn't get better until I'm with them. And since I see them both regularly, I have a hard time when I'm supposed to see them and I don't. It's all part of the borderline.

> The depression is a chemical process in my brain. It's frustrating because my life is pretty good. I found a family that loves and accepts me. I have a decent job, even if it is stressful at times. I don't really have much interaction with my bio family. I have great professional help. I'm going to school so I can do something I love. There isn't a whole lot to complain about. And yet, I'm still very sad. There's only so much I can do about it. Meds help. Talking helps. But, nothing takes it all away. There's no getting over this stuff. It's what I have to put up with for a lifetime. I wish I didn't, but it isn't my choice. What I can do is amass coping skills to help me through it.[64]

Accounts like these, and other resources, enable the therapist to glimpse the inner world and worldview of persons with mental health problems. This can increase empathetic interaction, facilitate individualized adjustments to approach and plans of care, and educate the general public as part of the physical therapist's professional duty of social responsibility. One resource of particular value to the layperson is Mental Health First Aid,[65] which teaches people of all ages to recognize signs of severe mental illness and refer appropriately.

Academy of Geriatric Physical Therapy

The APTA has several sections for specific practice areas, including acute care, neurology, orthopedics, and geriatrics; the section on geriatrics was recently rebranded as the AGPT.[66] As with many section websites, this site focuses on members-only content, but also has resources available to the public. It seeks to promote best physical therapist practice for persons over the age of 65, the age group termed the *silver tsunami* by geriatric specialist Carole Lewis.[67]

Member-focused resources include:

- *Journal of Geriatric Physical Therapy*, a scholarly publication to increase the practice evidence base
- Email-based LISTSERVs for the Special Interest Groups, including Cognitive & Mental Health, Bone Health, Balance & Falls, and Residency & Fellowship
- Information to provide to media outlets to increase accuracy and coverage of related issues

Public-focused resources include:

- Brochures created by students in DPT and physical therapy assistant programs for consumer education
- Project ideas to facilitate additional DPT and physical therapy assistant student involvement
- Details pertinent to the pursuit of the Geriatric Clinical Specialist and Certified Exercise Expert for the Aging Adult certifications
- Details helpful to the completion or development of a geriatric residency or fellowship
- Open-access publication, *Australian Physiotherapy Association's Journal of Physical Therapy*, promulgated by the International Association of Physical Therapists working with Older People

While section membership cost is on top of the APTA membership dues, it is valuable for many practitioners working with geriatric populations, since, as Lewis said in her Mary McMillan lecture, "Therapists working in geriatrics have to practice at the top of their game to get results ... We need to think ahead, plan ahead, and take steps now to practice at the top of our license. We need to be ravenous life-long learners."[67] Use of the AGPT resources can facilitate this process.

International Organization of Physical Therapists in Mental Health

The IOPTMH, recognized since 2011, is primarily composed of therapists outside the United States and is a subgroup of the World Confederation of Physical Therapy. As its website states, "People suffering from mental health problems often have somatic [ie, related to the body and not to the mind] symptoms, representing a major group of patients seeking help from physical therapists over the globe."[68] As such, key components of care include an interprofessional team, biopsychosocial approach, and specific knowledge of mental health conditions, associated secondary impairments, and risk factors for other health conditions.

The IOPTMH has a growing list of scholarly literature on specific treatments for persons with mental illnesses, particularly schizophrenia and eating disorders.[69] While there is currently no specific database for articles written by IOPTMH members, many articles are open-access and reference the organization, facilitating retrieval. Also, the organization sponsors an international conference in even-numbered years to disseminate research (information is available at www.icppmh.org).

Beers Criteria

Originally developed in 1991 by Dr. Mark Beers and subsequently revised, most recently in 2012, the Beers criteria are "a consensus list of medicines considered to be inappropriate for … patients age 65 and older" in multiple care settings, including long-term care, outpatient, and inpatient acute care.[70] Components include contraindicated or cautioned drugs, potential side effects, and alternative drug choices for each indication. In Table 4-3, note that since low acetylcholine levels underlie some dementia symptoms, any anticholinergic drug for persons with dementia is cautioned. Consider also the recent effort by the APTA to encourage physical therapy as an alternative to opioid prescription to curb the increase in opioid-related morbidity and death.[71]

As part of the IDT/IPT, physical therapists have the privilege and responsibility of being aware of the medications that their patients are taking, and how these medications can affect performance and participation in therapy sessions. Particularly with persons with dementia or Parkinson's disease (PD), it is easy to see how important a medication review can be because of potential adverse effects that may be masked by underlying medical conditions.

Table 4-3

Drugs to Be Questioned on Medication Review, per the 2012 Beers Criteria

DRUG	CONCERN(S)	CONSIDERATIONS
Analgesics: meperidine, pentazocine, tramadol (in patients with seizures)	Central nervous system (CNS) effects including: • **Delirium** • Cognitive impairment • **Confusion** • Lower seizure threshold	• Mild-moderate pain: codeine, short-term NSAIDs, acetaminophen • Moderate-severe pain: combined hydrocodone or oxycodone-acetaminophen • Neuropathic pain: duloxetine, venlafaxine, pregabalin, gabapentin, topical lidocaine, capsaicin, desipramine, nortriptyline
Antidepressants: bupropion (if seizures), mirtazapine, paroxetine (if cognitive impairment/dementia), selective serotonin reuptake inhibitor (SSRIs)/serotonin/norepinephrine reuptake inhibitor (SNRIs; if fall history), selected tricyclic antidepressants (if cognitive impairment/dementia, fall history, or delirium risk)	• Lower seizure threshold • Syndrome of inappropriate antidiuretic hormone (SIADH) • Worse constipation and urinary retention • Delirium • **Unsteady gait** • **Syncope and falls** • **Sedation** • **Orthostatic hypotension** • Psychomotor impairment	• Check sodium levels when starting or changing dose • Nortriptyline, trazodone for depression; trazodone, ramelteon, zolpidem for insomnia; see above for neuropathic pain alternatives *(continued)*

Bold: potential side effects most directly impacting the physical therapy plan of care

Table 4-3 (continued)

Drugs to Be Questioned on Medication Review, per the 2012 Beers Criteria

DRUG	CONCERN(S)	CONSIDERATIONS
Antihistamines: anticholinergic (brompheniramine, carbinoxamine, clemastine, dexchlorpheniramine, oral diphenhydramine, doxylamine) or loratidine (if dementia, cognitive impairment, delirium, benign prostatic hyperplasia, or chronic constipation)	• **Confusion** • Cognitive impairment • **Delirium** • Dry mouth • Constipation • Reduced metabolic clearance in elderly • Worsening of medical condition	• Diphenhydramine in severe allergic reaction; cetirizine, fexofenadine, loratadine, desloratadine, levocetirizine as alternative antihistamines
Antihypertensives: alpha blockers, clonidine, guanabenz, guanfacine, methyldopa, nifedipine, reserpine > 0.1 mg, triamterene (if creatinine clearance < 30 mL/min), vasodilators (if history of syncope)	• **Orthostatic hypotension** • Urinary incontinence • **Bradycardia** • CNS compromise • **Myocardial ischemia** • Kidney injury • Increased **syncope**	• Thiazide, angiotensin-converting enzyme (ACE) inhibitor, angiotensin receptor blocker (ARB), beta blocker, calcium channel blocker, or combination antihypertensives
Anticoagulants and antiplatelet agents: aspirin (> 80 years old), dabigatran (> 75 years old), oral short-acting dipyridamole, prasugrel, ticlopidine	• Lack of demonstrable efficacy for primary prevention in the very old, especially if kidney impairment • Bleeding risk • **Orthostatic hypotension**	• Warfarin, clopidogrel, aspirin-dipyridamole, cilostazol, ticagrelor, or prescribe with caution *(continued)*

Bold: potential side effects most directly impacting the physical therapy plan of care

Table 4-3 (continued)

Drugs to Be Questioned on Medication Review, per the 2012 Beers Criteria

DRUG	CONCERN(S)	CONSIDERATIONS
Antipsychotics: any (especially chlorpromazine, clozapine, fluphenazine, loxapine, olanzapine, perphenazine, pimozide, thioridazine, thiothixene, or trifluoperazine) if dementia with behaviors, cognitive impairment, history of falls, PD, or risk of delirium	• **Stroke** • Death • SIADH • **Unsteady gait** • **Syncope and falls** • **Worse PD symptoms** • **Orthostatic hypotension** • **Bradycardia** and abnormal cardiac electrical activity • Lower seizure threshold • Worse urinary retention and constipation	• Check sodium levels • Try behavioral strategies • Try quietapine or clozapine for persons with PD • Aripiprazole, asenapine, haloperidol, iloperidone, lurasidone, paliperidone, ziprasidone (less-anticholinergic alternatives)
Anxiolytics: benzodiazepines (for agitation or delirium, if dementia or fall history) or meprobamate	• Cognitive impairment • **Delirium** • **Unsteady gait** • **Fall and syncope** • Fracture • Physical dependence • **Sedation**	• SSRI, SNRI, buspirone for anxiety, benzodiazepines only for severe anxiety or other severe disorders • Restrict, if possible, to end-of-life care and perioperative anesthesia

(continued)

Bold: potential side effects most directly impacting the physical therapy plan of care

Table 4-3 (continued)

Drugs to Be Questioned on Medication Review, per the 2012 Beers Criteria

DRUG	CONCERN(S)	CONSIDERATIONS
Cardiac drugs: amiodarone, dofetilide, flecainide, ibutilide, procainamide, propafenone, quinidine, sotalol, cilostazol (if congestive heart failure [CHF]), digoxin > 0.125 mg/day (if CHF), diltiazem (if systolic CHF), disopyramide, dronedarone (if atrial fibrillation or CHF), spironolactone > 25 mg/day (if CHF), verapamil (if CHF)	• Additional **arrhythmias** • Thyroid impairment • Pulmonary or renal toxicity • **Worsened CHF** • Dry mouth • Urinary retention • Hyperkalemia (spironolactone); prefer to control rate vs rhythm in geriatric patients	• Control rate in atrial fibrillation • Try pentoxifylline for intermittent claudication, clopidogrel/aspirin for secondary cerebrovascular accident prevention • Alternatives for CHF (diuretic, ACE inhibitor, ARB, titrated beta blocker) or for hypertension (thiazide, ACE inhibitor, ARB, beta blocker, calcium channel blockers) • Monitor kidney function
CNS agents: ACh inhibitors (if syncope), anticonvulsants (if fall history), carbamazepine, dimenhydrinate or meclizine (if dementia or cognitive impairment/delirium)	• **Orthostatic hypotension** • **Unsteady gait** • **Bradycardia** • **Syncope and falls** • Psychomotor impairment • SIADH • Worse **delirium**, urinary retention, cognitive impairment, constipation	• Try memantine (for persons with dementia) • Check sodium, restrict sodium, or use diuretics for persons with Meniere's disease
Chemotherapeutic agents: carboplatin, cisplatin, vincristine	• SIADH	• Check sodium when starting or changing dose
Diabetes: chlorpropamide, glyburide, sliding scale insulin, pioglitazole (if CHF)	• Prolonged hypoglycemia • Poor insulin efficacy if sliding scale • Edema may **worsen CHF**	• Glimepiride, glipizide, gliclazide, basal insulin or premixed 1 to 2 times daily, metformin (if CHF is stable) *(continued)*

Bold: potential side effects most directly impacting the physical therapy plan of care

Table 4-3 (continued)

Drugs to Be Questioned on Medication Review, per the 2012 Beers Criteria

DRUG	CONCERN(S)	CONSIDERATIONS
Gastrointestinal: antispasmodics (belladonna alkaloids, clidinium, dicyclomine, hyoscyamine, scopolamine), H2 blocker or prochlorperazine (if dementia, cognitive impairment, or delirium), metoclopramide, oral mineral oil, promethazine, trimethobenzamide	• Anticholinergic effects (dry mouth, **confusion**, constipation) • **Delirium** • Extrapyramidal symptoms (eg, **tardive dyskinesia**) • **Aspiration** (mineral oil) • **Worse PD** • Poor efficacy for several medications	• Constipation: fiber, fluids, psyllium, polyethylene glycol, lactulose • Diarrhea: loperamide, aluminum hydroxide, cholestyramine • Nausea: prochlorperazine, ondansetron, granisetron, dolasetron • Gastroesophageal reflux disease: antacid, proton pump inhibitor
Hormones: corticosteroids (if risk or delirium), estrogen, growth hormone (except if pituitary gland removed), megestrol, testosterone, dessicated thyroid	• Cause or worsen **delirium** • Incontinence • Breast or uterine cancer (estrogen does not protect heart or brain) • Growth hormone causes **edema, joint pain, carpal tunnel syndrome, and insulin resistance** • Megestrol causes **thrombosis** and death • Testosterone and thyroid increase cardiac events	• Hot flashes: layer clothing, SSRI, gabapentin, venlafaxine • Bone density: calcium with vitamin D, raloxifene, bisphosphonates • Appetite: feeding assistance, freer food choices, snacks, nutritional supplements, mirtazapine for depression • Try levothyroxine for hypothyroidism *(continued)*

Bold: potential side effects most directly impacting the physical therapy plan of care

Table 4-3 (continued)

Drugs to Be Questioned on Medication Review, per the 2012 Beers Criteria

DRUG	CONCERN(S)	CONSIDERATIONS
Hypnotics: benzodiazepines (if insomnia), barbiturates, chloral hydrate, eszopiclone/ zaleplon/ zolpidem/tizanidine (if fall history or dementia), benztropine, muscle relaxants (carisoprodol, cyclobenzaprine, metaxalone, methocarbamol), trihexyphenidyl	• **Delirium** • Worse cognitive impairment • **Extrapyramidal symptoms** • **Sedation** • **Fractures** • **Confusion** • Dry mouth • Many drugs are ineffective in persons with PD	• Muscle spasms: treat etiology • **Physical therapy recommended**, including local heat or cold, optimized seating and positioning, and footwear • Nerve blocks, baclofen or antispasmodics for spasticity • Decrease or stop antipsychotic drug dose
NSAIDs: aspirin (> 325 mg/day chronic), celecoxib (if CHF), indomethacin, ketorolac, non–COX-2 selective (if chronic kidney disease)	• Gastrointestinal bleeding, peptic ulcers • **Edema** (worsens CHF), • Kidney injury if stage IV or V renal disease	• Pain: see previous recommendations • Coronary event: daily 81 mg aspirin • Acute gout: try alternative NSAID • Can add a gastroprotective drug
Respiratory: anticholinergics (if benign prostatic hyperplasia), atropine (if dementia or cognitive impairment), theophylline, phenylephrine or pseudoephedrine (if insomnia)	• Urinary retention • Dry mouth • **Confusion** • Worse **delirium** or cognitive impairment • Last 3 drugs in list stimulate CNS	• Chronic obstructive pulmonary disease: albuterol, long-acting beta-2 agonist, corticosteroid (inhaled) • Saline nasal spray, nasal steroids *(continued)*

Bold: potential side effects most directly impacting the physical therapy plan of care

Table 4-3 (continued)

Drugs to Be Questioned on Medication Review, per the 2012 Beers Criteria

DRUG	CONCERN(S)	CONSIDERATIONS
Stimulants: amphetamines or methylphenidate if insomnia	• CNS stimulation	• Weight: diet and lifestyle • Depression: mirtazapine, trazodone
Urinary tract: nitrofurantoin (chronic if <60 mL/min creatinine clearance), antimuscarinics (if dementia, delirium, or cognitive impairment)	• Pulmonary toxicity • Delirium • Worse cognitive impairment or constipation	• Select alternative drug for urinary tract infection antibiotics or drugs for overactive bladder

Bold: potential side effects most directly impacting the physical therapy plan of care

Summary

Especially in settings serving persons with mental health concerns or medically complex geriatric clients, physical therapists have many resources available to them to improve communication, motivation during the episode of care, medication safety, and evidence-based practice. To improve communication and motivation with patients, clinicians can use principles of CBT, MI, and NLP. With persons with psychological conditions, clinicians can refer to the NAMI and IOPTMH websites as educational tools for themselves and their patients.

To improve evidence-based practice, especially for the patient with multiple medical conditions and associated medications, therapists must know the evidence base for physical therapy interventions and potentially inappropriate medications for the geriatric patient. The AGPT website and the Beers criteria are 2 important resources. As with the other websites mentioned in this chapter, The AGPT offers both public and members-only resources for practitioner and patient education. Using the Beers criteria, the clinician can educate patients on potential cognition- and exercise-related medication effects, communicate with other health care providers to minimize use of inappropriate medications, and monitor for adverse effects and exercise intolerance.

Key Points

- Ethical decision-making steps include clarifying issues, finding and reviewing outside resources and ethical/legal standards, minimizing bias, implementing results, and learning from the experience.
- Clinicians may ask how sedentary or active patients perceive themselves to start discussions of health behavior change.
- Overarching goals for CBT include increasing patients' self-awareness of their thoughts, positive attitude toward exercise, and adherence to good exercise habits.
- Stages of the transtheoretical model of change are precontemplation; contemplation; determination; action; and maintenance, relapse, or recycling.
- MI includes activities in the acronym DEARS: develop discrepancy, express empathy, avoid argumentation, roll with resistance, and support self-efficacy.
- Physical therapy is an effective way to stem the opioid epidemic.

Review Questions

- Reflect on your personal and professional values, both ethical and moral, as well as the code of ethics.
  - What ethical concerns might you have with a patient approaching the end of life?
  - What guidance can you find in the code of ethics for your profession to address these concerns?
- Briefly describe the subtypes of CBT as you understand them from the text: PST, REBT, CT, ST, and DBT.
  - Under what conditions might you as a physical therapist choose to apply principles of CBT, or one of its subtypes, in the management of a patient with mental health conditions?
  - Describe a challenging clinical scenario in which one or more types of CBT might be beneficial.
  - Do you notice any of the principles of CBT in your current practice? Are there areas in which your patient care could benefit from further learning about these principles?

- Review the section on MI.
  - What are important dos and don'ts of MI?
  - When might it be advantageous or less advantageous to use MI in a clinical setting?
  - What good and less-good patterns do you notice in your own clinical communication?
- Despite NLP's limited evidence base, several of its communication principles are valid for patient use.
  - Describe a clinical scenario where you or a colleague may have used matching, pacing, and leading.
  - Did this use help the patient? Why or why not?
- Referring to the Beers criteria summary (see Table 4-3), brainstorm potential secondary impairments that might stem from side effects of each category of medication.
- What patient education resources can you use in the clinic from the NAMI and AGPT websites?

References

1. American Physical Therapy Association. Code of ethics for the physical therapist. *APTA*. https://www.apta.org/uploadedFiles/APTAorg/About_Us/Policies/HOD/Ethics/CodeofEthics.pdf. Published 2013. Accessed February 15, 2018.
2. Purtilo RB. Thirty-First Mary McMillan Lecture: A time to harvest, a time to sow: ethics for a shifting landscape. *Phys Ther.* 2000;80(11):1112-1119.
3. Dierckx K, Deveugele M, Roosen P, Devisch I. Implementation of shared decision making in physical therapy: observed level of involvement and patient preference. *Phys Ther.* 2013;93(10):1321-1330.
4. Dimond BC. *Legal Aspects of Occupational Therapy.* 2nd ed. Oxford, United Kingdom: Blackwell; 2004.
5. Criss M, Heitzman J, Wharton MA. Legal and ethical reasoning to enhance compassionate care in patients experiencing cognitive decline. *GeriNotes.* 2016;23(6):18-22.
6. Terpstra TL, Williamson S, Terpstra T. Palliative care for terminally ill individuals with schizophrenia. *J Psychosoc Nurs Ment Health Serv.* 2014;52(8):32-38.
7. Penny NH, Ewing TL, Hamid RC, Shutt KA, Walter AS. An investigation of moral distress experienced by occupational therapists. *Occup Ther Health Care.* 2014;28(4):392-393.
8. Costello E, Kafchinski M, Vrazel J, Sullivan P. Motivators, barriers, and beliefs regarding physical activity in an older adult population. *J Geriatr Phys Ther.* 2011;34(3):138-147.
9. Brown CJ, Bradberry C, Howze SG, Hickman L, Ray H, Peel C. Defining community ambulation from the perspective of the older adult. *J Geriatr Phys Ther.* 2010;33(2):56-63.
10. Brett CE, Gow AJ, Corley J, Pattie A, Starr JM, Deary IJ. Psychosocial factors and health as determinants of quality of life in community-dwelling older adults. *Qual Life Res.* 2012;21:505-516.
11. Babic D. Stigma and mental illness. *Materia Socio Medica.* 2010;22(1):43-46.
12. Gladwell PW, Pheby D, Rodriguez T, Poland F. Use of an online survey to explore positive and negative outcomes of rehabilitation for people with CFS/ME. *Disabil Rehabil.* 2014;36(5):387-394.
13. Kaizer F, Spiridigliozzi AM, Hunt MR. Promoting shared decision-making in rehabilitation: development of a framework for situations when patients with dysphagia refuse diet modification recommended by the treating team. *Dysphagia.* 2012;27(1):81-87.
14. Michael N, O'Callaghan C, Clayton J, et al. Understanding how cancer patients actualise, relinquish, and reject advance care planning: implications for practice. *Support Care Cancer.* 2013;21(8):2195-2205.
15. Loh AZH, Tan JSY, Puvanendran R, Menon S, Kanesvaran R, Krishna LKR. The ramifications of at-own-risk discharges in the palliative care setting. *J Palliat Care Med.* 2015;5:4.
16. Lorenzi S, Füsgen I, Noachtar S. Acute confusional states in the elderly - diagnosis and treatment. *Dtsch Arztebl Int.* 2012;109(21):391-400.
17. Giangregorio LM, Thabane L, Adachi JD, et al. Build better bones with exercise: protocol for a feasibility study of a multicenter randomized controlled trial of 12 months of home exercise in women with a vertebral fracture. *Phys Ther.* 2014;94(9):1337-1352.
18. Mackey KM, Sparling JW. Experiences of older women with cancer receiving hospice care: significance for physical therapy. *Phys Ther.* 2000;80(5):459-468.
19. Haber D. *Health Promotion and Aging: Practical Applications for Health Professionals.* 4th ed. New York, NY: Springer; 2007.

20. Demertzi A, Ledoux D, Bruno MA. Attitudes towards end-of-life issues in disorders of consciousness: a European survey. *J Neurol.* 2011;258(6):1058-1065.
21. Hamel RP, Walter JJ. *Artificial Nutrition and Hydration and the Permanently Unconscious Patient: The Catholic Debate.* Washington, DC: Georgetown University Press; 2007.
22. Jennett B. *The Vegetative State: Medical Facts, Ethical and Legal Dilemmas.* Cambridge, United Kingdom: Cambridge University Press; 2002.
23. Morrissey F. Advance directives in mental health care: hearing the voice of the mentally ill. *Medico Legal Journal of Ireland.* 2010;21(16).
24. Pope T, Anderson LE. Voluntarily stopping eating and drinking: a legal treatment option at the end of life. *Widener Law Review.* 2011;17:363.
25. Beckstrand RL, Rawle NL, Callister L, Mandleco BL. Pediatric nurses' perceptions of obstacles and supportive behaviors in end-of-life care. *Am J Crit Care.* 2010;19(6):543-552. DOI: 10.4037/ajcc2009497
26. Kumar SP, Jim A. Physical therapy in palliative care: from symptom control to quality of life: a critical review. *Indian J Palliat Care.* 2010;16(3):138-146.
27. Foster TL, Lafond DA, Reggio C, Hinds PS. Pediatric palliative care in childhood cancer nursing: from diagnosis to cure or end of life. *Semin Oncol Nurs.* 2010;26(4):205-221.
28. Michelson KN, Emanuel L, Carter A, Brinkman P, Clayman ML, Frader J. Pediatric intensive care unit family conferences: one mode of communication for discussing end-of-life care decisions. *Pediatr Crit Care Med.* 2011;12(6):e336-e343.
29. Davies B, Contro N, Larson J, Widger K. Culturally-sensitive information-sharing in pediatric palliative care. *Pediatrics.* 2010;125(4):e859-e865.
30. Cohn R, Harwood K, Richards H, Schlumpf K. A case-based reasoning (CBR) model for the integration of insurance policy and regulations in professional physical therapist education. *J Phys Ther Educ.* 2015;29(2):13-20.
31. Kiehl D. Completely unreasonable: the "practice losses" theory as a basis for Stark violations in the era of value-based reimbursement. *J Health Care Finance.* 2016;43(1).
32. Berry S, Soltau E, Richmond NE, Kieltyka RL, Tran T, Williams A. Care coordination in a medical home in post-Katrina New Orleans: lessons learned. *Matern Child Health J.* 2011;15(6):782-793.
33. Griffin E, Coburn AF. Integrated care management in rural communities. (Working Paper #54). Portland, ME: University of Southern Maine, Muskie School of Public Service, Maine Rural Health Resource Center; 2014
34. Levinson DR. *The Medicare payment system for skilled nursing facilities needs to be reevaluated.* Washington, DC: Office of Inspector General, US Dept of Health & Human Services; 2015.
35. Levinson DR. *Inappropriate payments to skilled nursing facilities cost Medicare more than a billion dollars in 2009.* Washington, DC: Office of Inspector General, Dept of Health & Human Services; 2009
36. Carter C, Garrett AB, Wissoker D. Reforming Medicare payments to skilled nursing facilities to cut incentives for unneeded care and avoiding high-cost patients. *Hlth Affairs.* 2012;31(6):1303-1313.
37. DeBoer MJ. Medicare coverage policy and decision making, preventive services, and comparative effectiveness research before and after the Affordable Care Act. *Journal of Health & Biomedical Law.* 2012;7:493-572.
38. Simons G. Legal issues for physical therapists who provide fitness services. *Top Geriatr Rehabil.* 2010;26(4):324-334.
39. Ness P. *The Rest of Us Just Live Here.* New York, NY: HarperCollins Publishers; 2015.
40. American Physical Therapy Association. Guide to Physical Therapist Practice 3.0. *APTA.* http://guidetoptpractice.apta.org/. Published 2016. Accessed February 15, 2018.
41. BECK: Cognitive Behavior Therapy. https://www.beckinstitute.org/. *BECK: Cognitive Behavior Therapy.* Updated 2016. Accessed February 15, 2018.
42. Dobson KS, ed. *Handbook of Cognitive-Behavioral Therapies.* 3rd ed. New York, NY: Guilford Press; 2010.
43. Herning MM, Cook JH, Schneider JK. Cognitive behavioral therapy to promote exercise behavior in older adults: implications for physical therapists. *J Geriatr Phys Ther.* 2005;28(2):34-38.
44. Nezu AM, Nezu CM, D'Zurilla TJ. *Solving Life's Problems: A 5-Step Guide to Enhanced Well-Being.* New York, NY: Springer; 2007.
45. Visser MM, Heijenbrok-Kal MH, van 't Spijker A, Ribbers GM, Busschbach JJV. The effectiveness of problem solving therapy for stroke patients: study protocol for a pragmatic randomized controlled trial. *BMC Neurol.* 2013;13:67.
46. Lynch TR, Chapman AL, Rosenthal MZ, Kuo JR, Linehan MM. Mechanisms of change in dialectical behavior therapy: theoretical and empirical observations. *J Clin Psychol.* 2006;62(4):459-480.
47. Miller WR, Rollnick S. *Motivational Interviewing: Preparing People to Change Addictive Behavior.* New York, NY: Guilford;1991.
48. Nidecker M, DiClemente CC, Bennett ME, Bellack AS. Application of the transtheoretical model of change: psychometric properties of leading measures in patients with co-occurring drug abuse and severe mental illness. *Addict Behav.* 2008;33(8):1021-1030.
49. Miller WR, Rollnick S. Ten things that motivational interviewing is not. *Behav Cogn Psychother.* 2009;37(2):129-140.
50. Sargeant JM, Mann KV, van der Vleuten CP, Metsemakers JF. Reflection: a link between receiving and using assessment feedback. *Adv Health Sci Educ Theory Pract.* 2009;14(3):399-410.

51. Davis CM. *Patient Practitioner Interaction: An Experiential Manual for Developing the Art of Health Care*. 4th ed. Thorofare, NJ: SLACK Incorporated; 2006.
52. Rosenzweig S. Emergency rapport. *J Emerg Med*. 1993;11(6):775-776.
53. Jepson C. Neurolinguistic programming in dentistry. *CDA Journal*. 1992;20(3):28-32.
54. Konefal J. Chronic Disease and Stress Management. Paper presented at: NLP Comprehensive International Conference; 1992; Denver, CO.
55. Sturt J, Ali S, Robertson W, et al. Neurolinguistic programming: a systematic review of the effects on health outcomes. *Br J Gen Pract*. 2012;62(604):e757-e764.
56. Roderique-Davies G. Neuro-linguistic programming: cargo cult psychology? *JARHE*. 2009;1(2):58-63.
57. Nazarko L. People living with dementia: components of communication. *British Journal of Healthcare Assistants*. 2014;8(11):554-558.
58. Nazarko L. Top-quality communication skills remove obstacles to communicating with people with dementia. *British Journal of Healthcare Assistants*. 2015;9(2):60-65.
59. Carmona RH, Giannini M, Bergmark B, Cabe J. The Surgeon General's call to action to improve the health and wellness of persons with disabilities: historical review, rationale, and implications 5 years after publication. *Disabil Health Journal*. 2010;3(4):229-232.
60. Iezzoni LI, Frakt AB, Pizer SD. Uninsured persons with disability confront substantial barriers to health care services. *Disabil Health J*. 2011;4(4):238-244
61. Reschly DJ. Change dynamics in special education assessment: historical and contemporary patterns. *Peabody J Educ*. 2002;77(2):117-136.
62. Hallam RA, Rous B, Grove J, LoBianco T. Level and intensity of early intervention services for infants and toddlers with disabilities: the impact of child, family, system, and community-level factors in service provision. *J Early Interv*. 2009;31(2):179-196.
63. National Alliance on Mental Illness. *NAMI*. https://www.nami.org/. Updated 2017. Accessed February 15, 2018.
64. Personal stories: a letter to someone who doesn't understand. *National Alliance on Mental Illness*. https://www.nami.org/Personal-Stories/A-Letter-to-Someone-Who-Doesn-t-Understand#. Accessed April 17, 2018.
65. National Council for Behavioral Health. *Mental Health First Aid*. https://www.mentalhealthfirstaid.org/cs/. Updated 2018. Accessed February 15, 2018.
66. Academy of Geriatric Physical Therapy. *AGPT*. http://geriatricspt.org/. Updated 2016. Accessed February 15, 2018.
67. Lewis CB. Our future selves: unprecedented opportunities. *Phys Ther*. 2016;96(10):1493-1502.
68. International Organization of Physical Therapists in Mental Health. *World Confederation for Physical Therapy*. http://www.wcpt.org/ioptmh. Updated June 21, 2017. Accessed February 15, 2018.
69. Probst M. The international organization of physical therapists working in mental health (IOPTMH). *Mental Health and Physical Activity*. 2012;5(1):20-21.
70. PL Detail-Document. Potentially harmful drugs in the elderly: Beers list. *Therapeutic Research Center*. http://www.ngna.org/_resources/documentation/chapter/carolina_mountain/Beers%20Criteria%20Literature.pdf. June 2012. Accessed October 11, 2016
71. News Now Staff. APTA launches #ChoosePT campaign to battle opioid epidemic. *PT in Motion*. http://www.apta.org/PTinMotion/News/2016/6/7/ChoosePTCampaignLaunch/. Published June 7, 2016. Accessed February 15, 2018.

Background Information on Mental Illness

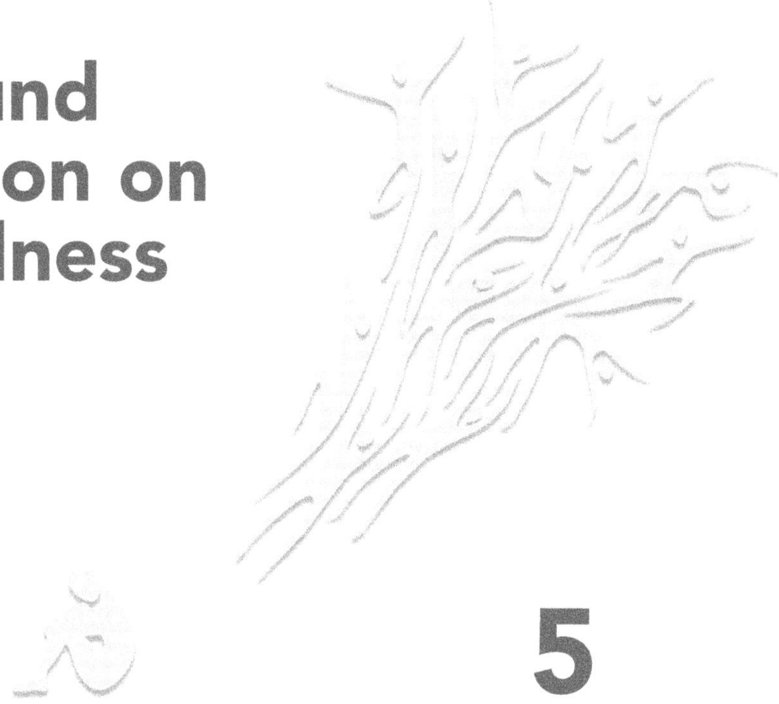

5

Outline

Johnson H.
Psychosocial Elements of Physical Therapy: The Connection of Body to Mind (pp 87-109).

Learning Objectives

- Acquire basic vocabulary related to interprofessional management of persons with psychological conditions
- Incorporate demographic and risk factor information for major mental health issues into the physical therapy patient management model (ie, a cycle of processes physical therapists follow in decision making)
- Justify skilled physical therapy intervention for persons with mental illness, based on the concept of the human movement system (ie, all parts of the body related to production and control of movement, including brain, mind, spinal cord/nerves, skin, muscles, tendons, bones, etc)
- Reflect on past and current management of patients with complex conditions

Why Physical Therapists Should Care About Mental Health Issues and Medical Complexity

Mental illness turns people inwards. That's what I reckon. It keeps us forever trapped by the pain of our own minds, in the same way that the pain of a broken leg or a cut thumb will grab your attention, holding it so tightly that your good leg or your good thumb seem to cease to exist.

—Nathan Filer[1]

As physical therapists, we specialize in human movement and the structures and functions that allow and control it (ie, the human movement system).[2] Thus, most therapists' training is mainly in the movement sciences, which span musculoskeletal, neuromuscular, cardiopulmonary, and other systems. Curricula and continuing-education offerings also examine psychosocial aspects of health care, since each patient's and therapist's attitudes, beliefs, values, and his or her individual circumstances are increasingly recognized as contributing to the success or failure of treatment.[3,4] The relationship of psychosocial aspects and treatment programs goes both ways; evidence suggests that, as the population ages, regular physical activity can prevent many mental health "conditions that affect cognition, emotion, and behavior,"[5] such as anxiety and depression.[6] The physical therapist is in a key position to influence how a patient becomes more consistently physically active.

This section uses a mental-illness lens to look briefly at psychosocial aspects of patient management, including cognition, stigma, and social support structure, because mental wellness is related to physical and social wellness[5] Indeed, a worldwide survey found that mental illnesses—especially posttraumatic stress disorder, bipolar disorders, and major depressive disorders (MDDs)—cause significant partial disability, which is comparable to the number of sick days taken by persons with chronic physical conditions.[7] Throughout this introductory section and the whole text, the reader should bear in mind that while mental health issues and multiple comorbidities can be obstacles to delivering the best quality physical therapy to the patient, **the psychosocially informed provision of physical therapy to these patients can positively impact their lives and the course of diseases.**

Although many doctor of physical therapy (DPT) programs include classes in psychosocial aspects, differential diagnosis, and patient management, the cognitive component may not be adequately addressed due to constraints on time, despite its demonstrated importance. For example, the function of community-dwelling elderly and restraint reduction in inpatient psychiatric settings depend on the patient's cognitive status and abilities.[8,9] Furthermore, clinical practice guidelines recommend non-pharmacological interventions (eg, physical therapy) for psychiatric disorders, including cognitive behavioral therapy to reduce depressive symptoms and the promotion of exercise behavior in older adults.[10,11]

Internationally, an organization of physical therapists has begun to describe the intersection of mental health with physical therapy,[12] yet the United States has not done so at this time. Several studies describe this lack of clear evidential guidance.[13-15] In order to facilitate translation of research knowledge to clinical practice that treats both body and mind, this book seeks to review current literature related to that intersection. Discussed in various chapters are the 3 aspects of the mind-body intersection, which are health promotion, stigma, and the human movement system (discussed later in this chapter).

Discussing health promotion, an integral part of physical therapist practice, Drench et al[4] notes that the population of persons with psychological conditions has a higher prevalence of chronic medical conditions and poor health behaviors, which increases the burden of care and likelihood of early death. Of persons over age 65 (this text's standard for geriatric), approximately 15% to 20% have a mental health diagnosis, according to the Surgeon General's Report on Mental Health.[16] Bipolar disorder, depression, personality disorders, anxiety disorders, and schizophrenia are among the top 10 most costly mental health disorders for large companies in the United States.[17]

Unfortunately, health care providers and members of the public may show harmful stigma when interacting with persons with mental illness. Due to limited general knowledge about causes and treatments for psychiatric conditions, stigma can be addressed via self-reflection about one's personal biases or lack of knowledge about psychological conditions (addressed in later chapters). If health care providers do not address stigma, it can cause the patient to have "shame ... fear, apprehension, and worry."[4] Because of this perceived stigma in others, the patient will delay seeking help (by an average of 8 to 9 years for mood disorders), which can entrench the disorder and thus decrease treatment efficacy. This is a significant barrier for wellness, which requires the individual to address his or her physical, emotional, intellectual, vocational, social, environmental, and spiritual needs with a health care team, ideally including a physical therapist, in a supportive setting.[16]

To combat stigma and the comparative lack of research literature related to physical therapy interventions for persons with mental health issues, one way for the clinician to help such patients is by giving social support:

> **Even a walking program is [effective] to provide mild exercise to improve mood symptoms. People with mental illness benefit more from group exercise than individual programs. Groups that provide support and motivation are significant factors for people whose symptoms include loss of interest and initiative.**[4]

As experts in the human movement system, physical therapists are in a unique position to prescribe physical activity interventions that will be most effective in each patient's specific context, including this need for interaction.

Scope of the Text

The distinction between diseases of "brain" and "mind," between "neurological" problems and "psychological" or "psychiatric" ones, is an unfortunate cultural inheritance that permeates society and medicine. It reflects a basic ignorance of the relation between brain and mind. Diseases of the brain are seen as tragedies visited on people who cannot be blamed for their condition, while diseases of the mind, especially those that affect conduct or emotion, are seen as social inconveniences for which sufferers have much to answer. Individuals are to be blamed for their character flaws, defective emotional modulation, and so on; lack of willpower is supposed to be the primary problem.

—António R. Damásio[18]

Within a psychosocial context, this text will set forth essential facts about and physical therapy effects on common mental illnesses. The *Diagnostic and Statistical Manual of Mental Disorders, 5th Edition* (DSM-5) classification of psychiatric illnesses and conditions is very broad.

Its categories span neurodevelopmental, obsessive-compulsive, trauma- and stressor-related, dissociative, somatic, feeding- and eating-related, elimination, sleep-wake, sexual, gender dysphoria, conduct, addictive, paraphilic, and medication-induced movement disorders.[19]

While students and physical therapists may see patients with many of the previously mentioned conditions in any clinical setting, this book intentionally limits its discussion to a few categories because:

- Anxiety, depressive, bipolar, schizophrenia spectrum, neurocognitive, personality, substance use, and domestic trauma-related disorders arguably have the greatest impacts on the plan of care.
- Many secondary effects of these included illnesses fall within a physical therapist's scope of practice. Such effects include metabolic syndrome due to sedentary behavior in depression and schizophrenia, falls due to decreased safety awareness in manic states or dementia, and increased muscle tension due to repeated panic attacks and fear of the next attack.
- The author wished to create a text of manageable length and structure for the student clinician working in settings with many patients over age 65, who have complex medical histories and have diagnosed or suspected mental illness. Given the information on selected conditions, as well as treatment approaches applicable to any condition (see Chapter 4), the practitioner will have a solid knowledge base for gaining knowledge and experience for expert clinical practice.

Background Terminology for the Physical Therapist

When had I stopped being a person with Paranoid Schizophrenia, and become a Paranoid Schizophrenic; defined by my illness?

—Michaela Haze[20]

Whether physical therapists work in an interdisciplinary team/interprofessional team (IDT/IPT; see Chapter 2) or in isolation during patient care, all practitioners need a common working vocabulary for effective communication. The following terms, also included in Appendix B, are a starting point. The practitioner may refer also to Figure 5-1 of the physical therapist's patient management model to guide his or her thought process in learning the terminology. One important point is that in any communication, person-first language is the profession's norm, never labeling the person by his or her condition, as the earlier quote by Michaela Haze illustrates.

General Terms

- Evidence-based practice: "the conscientious, explicit, and judicious use of the best evidence from systematic research to make decisions about the care of individual patients."[21]
- Human movement system: "the anatomic structures and physiologic functions that interact to move the body or its component parts."[22]
- Psychoneuroimmunology: "a field that explores the interactions among the central nervous system, the endocrine system, and the immune system; the impact of behavior or stress on these interactions; and how psychological and pharmacological interventions may modulate these interactions."[21]
- Judgment: "making decisions that are constructive and adaptive."[21]
- Insight: a "patient's understanding of the nature of the illness."[21]

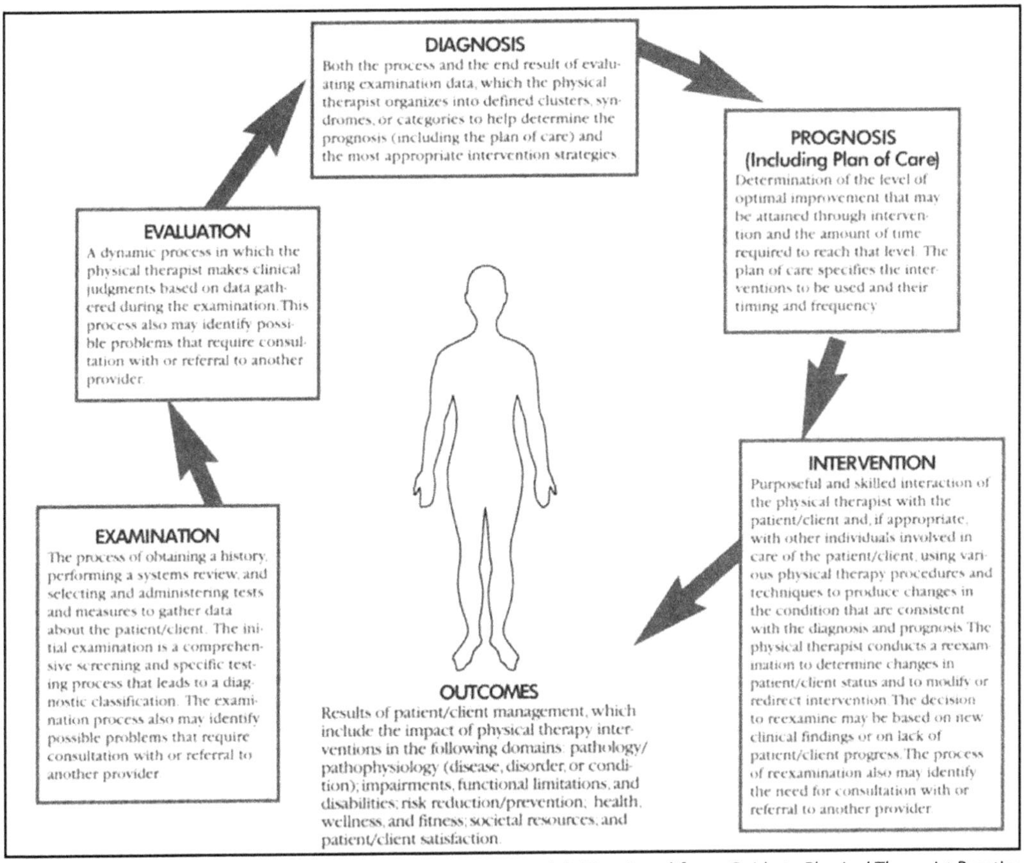

Figure 5-1. The physical therapist's patient management model. (Reprinted from *Guide to Physical Therapist Practice 3.0*, [http://www.apta.org/Guide/], with permission of the American Physical Therapy Association. © 2014 American Physical Therapy Association.)

- Social cognition or intelligence: "a theory of personality that refers to the expertise people bring to their experience of life tasks."[23]
- Executive function: a set of organizational and regulatory cognitive functions that allow goal-directed behavior. These include attention, abstract thinking, self-control, and stimulus monitoring.[24]
- Severe mental illness (SMI): defined legally, and in several articles throughout the text, as including schizophrenia, paranoia, bipolar spectrum disorders, and MDDs.

Diagnostic Terms

- Mood disorder: "a mood disturbance such as severe depression or depression alternating with mania."[23]
    - Mood: "the patient's self-report of the prevailing emotional state and reflects the patient's life situation."[21]
    - Affect: "the patient's prevailing emotional tone as observed by the [clinician] during the interview."[21]
    - Depression: "an abnormal extension or overelaboration of sadness and grief."[21]
    - Mania: "characterized by an elevated, expansive, or irritable mood."[21]

  - Anxiety: "a diffuse, vague apprehension associated with feelings of uncertainty and helplessness. This emotion has no specific object."[21]
  - Panic attack: "a discrete period of intense fear or discomfort in which at least four of the following symptoms develop abruptly and reach a peak within 10 minutes": tachycardia, sweating, trembling, shortness of breath, 'choking', angina, nausea, light-headedness, feelings of unreality or detachment from self, fear of losing control or going crazy, fear of dying, paresthesias, chills or hot flashes.[21]
  - Phobia: "a persistent and irrational fear of a specific object, activity, or situation that is excessive and unreasonable, given the reality of the threat."[23]
- Somatoform disorder: a group of symptoms without any somatic impairment.[21]
  - Somatization disorder: wherein "the person has many physical complaints."[21]
  - Conversion disorder: a disorder "in which a loss or alteration of physical functioning occurs."[21]
  - Hypochondriasis: "somatic over-concern with … details of body functioning."[21]
  - Body dysmorphic disorder: "a person with a normal appearance is concerned about having a physical defect."[21]
  - Pain disorder: where "psychological factors play an important role in the onset, severity, or maintenance of the pain."[21]
- Schizophrenia: "a serious, persistent brain disease that results in psychotic behaviors, concrete thinking, and difficulties in information processing, interpersonal relationships, and problem solving."[21]
- Schizoaffective disorder: including "both affective and schizophrenic symptoms" such that the condition qualifies as a separate condition from schizophrenia, depression, and mania.[25]
- Dementia (neurocognitive disorder): a typically chronic, slowly progressive collection of symptoms demonstrating impaired "memory, thinking, orientation, comprehension, calculation, learning capacity, language, and judgment" with frequent "deterioration in emotional control, social behaviour [sic], or motivation."[25]
- Delirium: a "nonspecific cerebral organic syndrome," including simultaneous impairments in "consciousness and attention, perception, thinking, memory, psychomotor behaviour [sic], emotion, and the sleep-wake schedule" that fluctuate over hours to days.[25]
- Personality disorder: "enduring, inflexible, and maladaptive patterns of behavior that are severe enough to cause either dysfunctional behavior or profound distress."[21]
  - Paranoid: marked by an "excessive sensitivity to setbacks, unforgiveness of insults, suspiciousness, a tendency to distort experience … and a combative and tenacious sense of personal rights."[25]
  - Schizoid: marked by a "withdrawal from affectional, social, and other contacts, with preference for fantasy, solitary activities, and [introspection]."[25] The person is unable to express feelings (alexithymia) or experience joy (anhedonia).
  - Schizotypal: marked by a lack of schizophrenic disturbances, but with "eccentric behaviour [sic] and anomalies of thinking and affect which resemble those seen in schizophrenia."[25]
  - Antisocial: marked by a "disregard for social obligations … a low tolerance to frustration and a low threshold for discharge of aggression, including violence [and] a tendency to blame others."[25]
  - Borderline: marked by impulsive actions, as well as "disturbances in self-image, aims, and internal preferences, by intense and unstable interpersonal relationships, and by a tendency to self-destructive behavior."[25]

- Histrionic: marked by "self-dramatization, theatricality, exaggerated expression of emotions, suggestibility, egocentricity, self-indulgence, [and] lack of consideration for others."[25] The person will also crave "appreciation, excitement, and attention."
- Narcissistic: marked by "an exaggerated sense of self-importance, an exhibitionistic need for attention and admiration, feelings of entitlement [and] envy, lack of empathy, and exploitation of others while disregarding their rights and feelings."[25]
- Avoidant: marked by "tension and apprehension, insecurity, and inferiority ... [and] a hypersensitivity to rejection and criticism."[25]
- Dependent: marked by "pervasive passive reliance on other people to make major and minor life decisions, great fear of abandonment, feelings of helplessness ... [and] passive compliance with the wishes of elders and others."[25]
- Obsessive-compulsive: marked by "personal insecurity and doubt leading to excessive conscientiousness, stubbornness, caution, and rigidity," but not severe enough to be diagnosed as obsessive-compulsive disorder.[25]

Signs and Symptoms

- Hallucination: "false sensory impressions or experiences."[21]
- Illusions: "false perceptions or false responses to a sensory stimulus."[21]
- Thought content: "the specific meaning expressed in the patient's communication,"[21] including:
    - Delusion: a "false belief that is firmly maintained even though it is not shared by others and is contradicted by social reality."[21] The categories of delusions are listed as follows:
        - Grandiose: with "exaggerated notions of capacities, possessions, and esteem which in delusional form are associated with mania, schizophrenia, and cerebral organic psychoses."[25]
        - Paranoid: where the patient is consumed by themes including "persecution, love, hate, envy, jealousy, honour [sic], litigation, grandeur, and the supernatural."[25]
        - Thought broadcasting: "the experience that one's thoughts are somehow immediately shared with other people or otherwise made public knowledge."[25]
        - Thought insertion or withdrawal: "the individual's experience of (1) thoughts recognized as alien intruding into his or her mental processes; (2) his or her own thoughts being taken away or otherwise appropriated by an external agency."[25]
    - Depersonalization: a "feeling of having lost self-identity."[21]
    - Ideas of reference: "incorrect interpretation of casual incidents ... as having direct personal references."[21]
    - Magical thinking: "belief that thinking equates with doing."[21]
    - Nihilistic ideas: "thoughts of nonexistence and hopelessness."[21]
    - Obsession: especially in anxiety disorders, an "idea, emotion, or impulse that repetitively and insistently forces itself into consciousness, although it is unwelcome."[21]
    - Phobia: especially in anxiety disorders, a "morbid fear associated with extreme anxiety."[21]
- Thought process: "the 'how' of the patient's self-expression ... observed through speech."[21]
    - Circumstantial: with "excessive and unnecessary detail that is usually relevant to a question."[21]
    - Flight of ideas: a "rapid shifting from one topic to another and fragmented ideas."[21]
    - Loose associations: "lack of a logical relationship between thoughts and ideas."[21]
    - Neologisms: "new word or words created by [the] patient, often a blend of other words."[21]
    - Perseveration: "involuntary, excessive continuation or repetition of a single response, idea, or activity."[21]

- Tangential: "similar to circumstantial, but [the] patient never returns to [the] central point and never answers [the] original question."[21]
- Thought blocking: a "sudden stopping in the train of thought or in the midst of a sentence."[21]
- Word salad: a "series of words that seem completely unrelated."[21]

- Negative symptoms of schizophrenia
  - Alexithymia: "difficulty naming and describing emotions."[21]
  - Apathy: "lack of feelings, emotions, interest, or concern."[21]
  - Anhedonia: also in depression, the "inability or decreased ability to experience pleasure, joy, intimacy, and closeness."[21]
  - Avolition: lack of motivation, initiative, interest, and engagement in goal-oriented behaviors
  - Alogia: lack of normal flow and quantity of speech during conversation
- Movement symptoms of schizophrenia
  - Tardive dyskinesia: a side effect of many antipsychotic drugs after prolonged use, marked by "abnormal, involuntary, slow, irregular movements of the tongue, lips, mouth, and trunk, and by choreoathetoid movements of the extremities.[25] Remission ranges from 5% to 90% depending on the severity of the initial dyskinesia.
  - Catatonia: A range of abnormal movement patterns including stereotypic movements, echopraxia, and impulsive movements. Movement may be increased (hyperkinesia), decreased (hypokinesia), or absent altogether (akinesia).[25]
  - Stereotypic movement disorder: marked by "voluntary, repetitive, stereotyped, non-functional (and often rhythmic) movements that do not form part of any recognized psychiatric or neurologic condition [including] body-rocking, head-rocking, hair-plucking ... and hand-flapping [if non–self-injurious] and head-banging, face-slapping, [or] eye-poking" if self-injurious.[25]
  - Waxy flexibility: in schizophrenia with catatonia, the tendency of a person to stay in the posture placed by another, without initiating movement him- or herself.
  - Echopraxia: a "pathologic imitation of the movements or gestures of another, usually semi-automatic in nature."[25]

While it is impossible to cover all the terms the clinician may need in working with persons with mental health conditions, the above serve as a framework, especially for the student or therapist with limited or no background in abnormal psychology. Finally, although many health care systems and facilities have transitioned to the current DSM-5 classification system, it is worthwhile to be aware of the earlier 5-axis system for classification of psychiatric disorders[21]:

1. Axis I: clinical disorders, the primary mental-health diagnosis (eg, flare-up of panic disorder)
2. Axis II: personality disorders and developmental disorders, including borderline personality disorder
3. Axis III: general medical conditions, the person's potentially relevant medical comorbidities
4. Axis IV: psychosocial and environmental problems, recently encountered stressors
5. Axis V: global assessment and functioning, rated on a 0 to 100 scale and higher scores indicating better function psychosocially

Demographics of Selected Mental Illnesses

The *Diagnostic and Statistical Manual of Mental Disorders, Fourth Edition* describes approximately 400 psychiatric conditions, with 22% of patients in the United States being annually diagnosed with a psychological condition, usually a mood disorder. Of these disorders, approximately

6% are classified as SMI. SMI may raise the risk for being admitted to a skilled nursing facility at an earlier age (62 years old) than persons without SMI.[26] This section examines the prevalence, or percent of people with current diagnoses, of the major mental health issues described in later chapters. The updated DSM-5 was the primary source for statistics, risk factors, and principal symptoms. As reiterated later, cultural factors influence diagnosis; for example, "for Native Americans, it is considered normal to hear and speak to dead ancestors."[4]

Anxiety disorders are an excessive duration or intensity of fear or anxiety. Not only are females diagnosed at twice the rate of males, but also anxiety may present differently in males, who approach a health care provider less often for diagnosis. In skilled nursing facilities, SMI that includes anxiety disorder occurs in 27.4% of residents.[26] Several types of anxiety disorders have distinct prevalence in the general population:

- Separation anxiety: 4% in children, while 0.9% to 1.9% in adults
- Selective mutism (choosing not to speak to or around certain people): less than 1% of adults and children
- Specific phobia: 7% to 9% in adults and children
    - Social phobia (related to social interaction situations): 7%
    - Agoraphobia (fear of being in public or open places, with any risk of embarrassment): 1.7%
- Generalized anxiety disorder: 0.9% in adolescents, while 2.9% in adults
    - Panic disorder: 2% to 3% with increased suicide risk
    - Panic attacks (isolated): 11.2% in adults

Depressive disorders, defined in DSM-5 as the "presence of sad, empty, or irritable mood, accompanied by somatic and cognitive changes that significantly affect the individual's capacity to function," can be categorized by "duration, timing, or presumed etiology."[19] Typically, a clinically diagnosed depressive disorder will last more than 2 weeks per episode. Prevalence for various types of depressive disorders include:

- Disruptive mood dysregulation disorder: 2% to 5% in children, with personality and genetic factors increasing the risk. This newly described disorder is marked by a persistent angry or irritable mood beyond what parents or teachers see as typical child moodiness.
- Major depressive disorder (intense and prolonged depressive symptoms without a manic phase): 7% influenced by personality, environmental, and genetic risk factors
- Dysthymia (chronic depressed mood over several years, not severe enough to be classified as major depression): 0.5%
- Medication-induced depression: 0.26%. Chapter 4 discusses side effects of potentially inappropriate medications for geriatric patients; several types of medications that can cause depression include anticonvulsants, barbiturates (for anxiety and seizure prevention), benzodiazepines, beta blockers, calcium channel blockers, opioids, and statins.
- Premenstrual dysphoric disorder (characterized by extreme mood shifts including depressive moods for several days prior to each menstrual period): 1.8% to 5.8% of menstruating women

Bipolar spectrum disorders, marked by alternating episodes of mania and depression, carry a greatly increased suicide risk across age groups. Prevalence and risks are noted as follows:

- Bipolar I disorder (including a manic episode): 0.6% with a 15-fold increased risk of suicide
- Bipolar II disorder (including a hypomanic episode, not severe enough to be classified as bipolar I): 0.8% in the United States vs 0.3% worldwide. In this population, 33% attempt suicide, and 15% have impaired psychosocial and physical functioning between episodes.
- Cyclothymic disorder (alternating hypomanic and hypodepressive episodes): 0.4% to 1%

Schizophrenia spectrum disorders include key features of at least one of delusions, hallucinations, disorganized thinking, disorganized or abnormal motor behavior (eg, catatonia), and negative symptoms (see earlier definitions). As with depressive disorders, these disorders are classified by duration and cause, considering cultural factors for diagnosis, differential diagnosis, and psychosocial functional impact. Prevalence is as follows:

- Delusional disorder: 0.2% characterized primarily by delusions
- Brief psychotic disorder: 9% with short duration of symptoms, with risk increased by personality traits
- Schizophrenia: 0.3% to 0.7%, with risk factors including a birthday during winter months and genetic traits
- Schizoaffective disorder: 0.3%, with increased risk if a family member has schizophrenia. This condition carries a 5% suicide risk.
- Substance-induced: 0.5%. Prescription or illicit drug abuse (cannabis, cocaine, LSD, or amphetamines) may increase schizophrenia symptoms in susceptible individuals.

Personality disorders have been briefly defined in the terminology section (see also Chapter 10). Gender and culture are important factors in diagnosis, as one's personality can vary widely depending on societal and familial expectations of the individual. For example, females display higher prevalence of histrionic personality disorder, while males may display more antisocial personality disorder. Prevalence of subtypes is as follows:

- Paranoid: 2.3% to 4.4%
- Schizoid: 3.1% to 4.9%
- Schizotypal: 0.6% to 4.6%, depending on geographic area and diagnostic methods
- Antisocial: 0.2% to 3.3%, with risk factors including alcohol use and male sex
- Borderline: 1.6% to 5.9%
- Histrionic: 1.84%
- Narcissistic: 6.2% or less
- Avoidant: 2.4%
- Dependent: 0.6%
- Obsessive-compulsive: 2.1% to 7.9%

Finally, dementias (classified as neurocognitive disorders in DSM-5), involve domains of complex attention, executive function, learning and memory, language skills, perceptual-motor skills, and social cognition. In total, severe forms of dementias affect approximately 1% of persons at 65 years old and 30% at 85 years old, while minor forms affect 2% to 10% at 65 years old and 5% to 25% at 85 years old. In long-term care facilities in developed countries, dementia is present in 58% of residents, and 78% of residents with dementia displayed behavioral and psychological symptoms of dementia.[27] Risk factors known to date include increased age and female sex (related to increased longevity). Prevalence of subtypes includes:

- Delirium (often confused with dementia): 1% to 2% in all ages, but 14% of persons over 85 years old
- Alzheimer's disease (AD): 5% to 25%
- Frontotemporal dementia (earlier onset than AD): 2 to 10 persons out of every 100,000
- Dementia with Lewy bodies/Lewy body dementia: 20% to 35% of all dementias, but 0.1% to 5% of the geriatric population
- Vascular dementia: 20% to 35% of persons poststroke, but 0.2% to 16% of the geriatric population
- Dementia due to HIV-AIDS infection: 33% to 50%; dementia is often an early sign of AIDS.

- Dementia due to Parkinson disease (PD): 75% of persons with PD, but 0.5% to 3% of the general population. Approximately 27% of persons with PD develop a minor form of dementia.
- Huntington disease: inevitably ends in dementia due to the progression of the illness

The Human Movement System

The American Physical Therapy Association (APTA) has integrated the concept of the human movement system into its vision for the profession of physical therapy since 2013: "Transforming society by optimizing movement to improve the human experience."[28] In subsequent publications, it continues to urge members of the profession to investigate research and interventions in terms of the movement system (ie, what structures and functions of the human body allow or hinder the particular movement we are investigating?). This section surveys current literature on the human movement system and its general changes associated with poor mental health; research is ongoing.

Exploration of the Human Movement System

Prominent physical therapists argue that clinicians should be identified by who they are, not what they do,[2] hence the push toward movement system expertise. However, other health care providers do deal with the movement system as part of their scopes of practice, as we deal with body systems in our scope of practice; for example, the cardiovascular system's impact on endurance-based activities such as running. To emphasize our unique contribution to human function, then, we individualize plans of care to each patient's goals and social contexts, analyze movement critically to identify and address defective components, and look at the person as a whole vs isolating the patient in terms of one body system. For example, an orthopedic specialist physical therapist and a neurologic specialist should integrate aspects of the nervous system and relevant aspects of the musculoskeletal system into plans of care.

Since the movement system is our specialty, the question has arisen of how to define and communicate to other professionals the problems that we treat. Patients may have medical diagnoses such as cardiovascular disease, osteoarthritis, and hypertension; our diagnostic labels need to clearly define underlying physical impairments to better coordinate care. The APTA House of Delegates formally advised the development of such movement system diagnostic labels starting in 2015.[2] Conference programming (Combined Sections Meeting 2012 and 2013) has offered seminars on developing specialty-specific diagnostic labels and processes, for such physical therapy specialties as oncology, women's health, and cardiovascular/pulmonary. Generally, diagnosis is becoming based more on validated physical tests and less on vague observation, influenced by legislative bodies, payment regulations (eg, denial of payment for services for a particular diagnostic code submitted in billing claims), and interprofessional communication.[29]

One current obstacle to adoption of movement system diagnoses is their awkwardness. For example, a patient diagnosed medically with adhesive capsulitis of the shoulder may have a movement system diagnosis of "global loss of both active and passive shoulder range of motion."[30] The physical therapist can use this phrase as it accurately captures the underlying abnormal movement features to be corrected by physical therapy. Although the labels are long, the orthopedics section of APTA recommends them as they specify the best physical therapy treatments, describe the movement deficits underlying the patient's problems, enable effective interprofessional communication, keep the treatment diagnosis within the therapist's scope of practice, and facilitate better diagnostic accuracy by well-designed clinical assessment tools. Other advantages include preservation of accurate biomedical terminology, focus on the patient's function within society, and facilitation of direct access to therapists without requiring an initial medical referral or specialist appointment.

The clinician must weigh these factors while seeking expertise in practice to continually facilitate better outcomes for patients. The label development process is ongoing and involves lively dialogue and debate among professionals in the APTA and others.[31] While on the research end, the analysis of the complexity of human movement is difficult, but on the practice end, this analysis and translation of knowledge to the clinic will benefit patients and therapists immensely.[32]

General Movement System Differences in Persons With Mental Illness

As noted in this chapter's terminology section, the human movement system comprises both structures and functions: microscopic, as well as at the system or organism level. Related to psychological conditions, literature continues to explore areas of change in movement system components. This text introduces general changes first, followed by specific differences as explored in the literature. As a nod to physical activity prescribers, such as physical therapists, Fox et al studied older adults in the Better Ageing Project and concluded that **even low-level "physical activity can prevent some aspects of mental illness in older people such as depression, dementia, and Alzheimer's disease."**[33] Though the study did not show quantitatively that increased exercise prevented mental illness, several interviews with participants and exercise facilitators "suggested that important improvements in perceived function and social benefits had been experienced."[33] The bottom line for physical therapist services is quality of life via better movement.

Common comorbidities across mental health issues are often related to secondary impairments from decreased physical activity. Microscopically, this may be caused by altered neurotransmitter function and levels; Lundy-Ekman[34] notes that glutamate transmission is abnormal in conditions affecting the central nervous system, including depression and schizophrenia. At the organ system level, metabolic syndrome is common in several mental illnesses as well. Metabolic syndrome is defined as "a cluster of risk factors (abdominal obesity, hypertension, dyslipidemia, glucose and insulin dysregulation)" and is a potential cause of "cardiovascular disease, diabetes, and dementia."[35] Several articles also note that it is common in schizophrenia.[12] Interestingly, cognitive performance seems to be improved in persons with early AD but who also have multiple risk factors in metabolic syndrome.

Obesity and diabetes mellitus type 2, as comorbidities in mental illness, have been studied extensively in the literature. Bartels et al[36] describe a coaching technique to promote healthy behaviors in persons with serious psychological conditions, noting sustained and significant improvements in weight and aerobic endurance as measured by the 6-Minute Walk Test. Brown et al[37] included coronary artery disease in their study of a nutrition management and instruction program combined with exercise; this was tailored to specific cognitive impairments in SMI and also facilitated slight weight loss. Finally, McBain et al,[38] in a recent article, examined a randomized controlled trial promoting a self-management program for type 2 diabetes in adults with schizophrenia. Though the evidence base for this type of intervention is currently limited to a single trial, weight and body mass index remained slightly improved at a 1-year follow-up.[38] As type 2 diabetes is twice as common in persons with vs without SMI, this is a critical area for high-quality research and translation into clinical practice.

Pain is another area of interest in populations with mental illness. Since many psychological conditions, especially dementias, may decrease a patient's cognitive and verbal abilities, standard scales, such as the Numeric Pain Rating Scale, may not accurately indicate pain quality, intensity, sites, or impact. This can impair correct diagnosis and an effective treatment plan. Defrin et al[39] explore how persons with cognitive impairment process pain. Since processing differs depending on the type of cognitive impairment, underlying clinical condition, or noxious stimulus, Defrin et al[39] note that "patients do feel noxious stimuli, with more evidence for hypersensitivity than hyposensitivity to these stimuli compared with cognitively unimpaired individuals." Currently, experimental models have not revealed specific neurobiological pathways or chemical changes that underlie this difference. Given the tendency toward hypersensitivity to pain, then, and the secondary effects of pain (and self-protective inactivity) on function (eg, contractures, weakness, fractures, and falls), it is imperative for physical therapists to learn how to accurately assess pain in persons with mental health issues and substance use disorders. This is discussed in greater detail in Chapters 6 through 12.

A final general difference in persons with vs without mental illness relates to lack of beneficial behaviors. Patients may demonstrate more aggression, less self-worth, poorer interpersonal relationships, and inability to hold a steady job. Stubbs and Hollins[40] focus on the geriatric population with cognitive impairment of varying etiology, including dementia. How health care providers control aggression that is common in this population can impact secondary impairments, including fracture, subluxation, and other injury. They recommend use of restraint as a last resort, and adapting restraint techniques, should aggressive behavior arise.[40] Examples include mid-range shoulder movements; holding of the patient's arms above vs at the wrists; and avoiding bringing the patient down to the floor, whenever possible, to avoid hip or spine fracture.

Due to less self-worth, patients with psychological conditions may avoid helpful behaviors, such as physical fitness, social interaction, and maintaining a job. Cairney et al[41] studied social and cognitive factors influencing the relationship between regular physical activity and improved mental health in older adults. They concluded that **"physical activity interventions focused on improving mastery or self-worth, as well as physical fitness, may yield the greatest benefit in alleviating psychological distress."**[41] This may also be related to the rapport developed by therapy providers with their patients. Hall et al[42] explore impacts of the therapist-patient relationship on treatment outcomes. Outcomes of interest to this text, measured via the Working Alliance Inventory, included adherence to treatment in patients with medically complex histories, "depressive symptoms in patients with cardiac conditions and those with brain injury," and "physical function in geriatric patients."[42] Finally, Van Til et al[43] note that SMI, including anxiety, depression, posttraumatic stress disorder, and substance abuse disorders, is common in veterans and causes difficulties in work reintegration. However, scholarly literature about reintegrating veterans into the workforce is limited at this time.

Beyond movement system differences associated with mental illness in general, literature describes correlations and causations between specific disorders, as well as treatments. Anxiety is influenced by pain and disability associated with osteoarthritis; this combination may be addressed by cognitive behavioral therapy (see Chapter 4) with targeted therapeutic exercise and manual therapy. This combination can "improve self-efficacy and reduce learned helplessness."[44] Kessler et al[45] and Ravindran and da Silva[46] note that patients with anxiety are using complementary and alternative medicine more widely, with potential interactions and side effects of herbs and supplements often recommended by non-medical doctors. Additional anxiety-related differences are addressed in Chapter 6.

Depression, especially MDD, causes more challenges in treatment of the movement system. Risk factors associated with severe depression in persons seeking outpatient physical therapy for musculoskeletal pain included being female, being seen in an industrial or pain clinic setting, having a history of chronic pain (especially neck or back), and history of surgery for this pain. This study concluded that "depressive symptoms had consistent detrimental influence on outcomes" of an episode of care, and "had a moderate to large effect on pain ratings and a small to large effect on functional status."[47] In geriatric patients specifically, pain, but not physical dependence, strongly correlated to level of depressive symptoms.[48]

Investigating the effects of exercise on depressive symptoms, several authors also hypothesized that underlying mechanisms and structures changed in the human movement system. At the system level (ie, cognition), Carta et al[49] investigated a 32-week addition of physical activity habits to treat women who had not responded to prior treatment for major depression. They noted that "subjective quality of life in bipolar and unipolar severe depression patients may not accurately reflect objective functional status, potentially due to diminished insight, demoralization, or altered life expectations over time."[49] Trivedi et al[50] examine this adjunctive effect of exercise at a microscopic level, again examining depression resistant to treatment with a selective serotonin reuptake inhibitor. They note that:

> [There] are also plausible neurobiological mechanisms for the efficacy of exercise as a treatment for depression, such as changes in serotonergic and noradrenergic neuromodulatory function similar to those observed with antidepressant treatments and increased hippocampal neurogenesis.[50]

Though dementias are explored more in Chapter 11, a few general movement system changes are worth noting here. Tangen et al[51] examined the spectrum of cognitive impairment from that which is subjective (ie, noticed by the patient but not an observer) to AD. They found that the level of executive function directly correlates to the patient's balance control, as measured by the sensitive Balance Evaluation Systems Test.[52] Venema et al assessed dual-task performance, a subset of executive function, where an individual has "to divide one's attention between motor and secondary tasks."[53] Clinically measurable cognitive impairment directly relates to dual-task cost, which impairs energy conservation and safety of physical function when the person is attempting to dual task. However, Venema et al "suggest that patients with [cognitive impairment] may be able to engage in more challenging tasks than might be assumed" due to demonstrated ability to perform dual tasks including backward counting, even with a Mini-Mental State Exam score as low as 7, indicating severe impairment.[53]

Management of the Medically or Psychiatrically Complex Patient

Since people are generally living longer, they have more likelihood of accumulating multiple short- or long-term medical conditions. For the rehabilitation professional, this means that a higher percentage of patients seen will be medically and psychosocially complex. However, a standard definition of complexity is difficult to find. Grant et al[54] explored how primary care physicians define complexity in their patients, and compared the definition and classification to 3 established algorithms that include chronic diseases and other factors. The physicians classified approximately one-quarter of their patients as complex. Younger complex patients tended to have mental health and substance use issues, while older complex patients required more clinical decision making and care coordination. These doctors' assessments, however, did not strongly agree with the algorithms, which accounted for patient age, number of chronic or dangerous conditions, and history of recent or recurrent hospitalization.

Rehabilitation literature describes how to work with a complex patient in many treatment settings, but again without defining well what complex means. Many might agree, however, that the greater the number of medical or psychiatric conditions the person has, the more complex the care. Nelson et al[55] note that clinical practice guidelines, which direct best practice for certain conditions, do not often mention concepts of complexity or comorbidity, and even less often provide specific guidance for management. Thus, this section will set forth principles with case examples based on the author's experience and that of others, to help the reader improve his or her approach to patients with multiple medical and psychiatric issues. Most chapters of this text contain additional diagnosis-specific case studies with graded complexity.

Strategies for Patient Management

Ideally, complex patient management practice begins in the entry-level physical therapist's education. One example is a dedicated geriatrics course within a DPT program, aimed at helping students to become more confident and capable in the management of the complex population over 65 years old. This type of course can incorporate "principles of adult learning, experiential learning theory, reflective practice, and active learning strategies" guided by a public list of essential competencies for the geriatric practitioner.[56] Such principles have been linked to development of expert practice in clinicians after graduation.

Before and after graduation from a DPT program, one tool to advance clinical reasoning skills and promote reflective practice that addresses the whole patient is the Physical Therapy Clinical Reasoning and Reflection Tool (PT-CRT). Developed by Atkinson and Nixon-Cave,[57] this tool integrates the *International Classification of Functioning, Disability and Health* (ICF) framework and the patient management model (see Figure 5-1). The ICF is taught in all DPT curricula and guides the user to tie a patient's movement problems to his or her ability to participate in society. When used with complex and simple patient cases, the PT-CRT can pinpoint strengths and weaknesses in clinical reasoning skills and facilitate pattern recognition, a key to expert practice.

Foster and Delitto[58] address complexity within the management of a common problem seen by physical therapists: low back pain. In low back pain, "there are complex, interdependent relationships between the physical and biomedical features ... and the psychological and social factors that are present concomitantly."[58] Challenges to adopting a biopsychosocial approach to patients with low back pain include:

- Education of DPT students that starts with the biomedical model, only later adding psychosocial concepts, after thought patterns are already set
- Clinical education experiences of DPT students that do not consistently and coherently reinforce the importance of psychosocial aspects of care
- Current physical therapist practice and continuing education courses that are heavily based on the biomedical model
- Patients who come with expectations about low back pain and therapy, and payor source regulations that do not reflect psychosocial factors because of lack of disseminated literature on this topic

These challenges often combine to disincentivize the clinician from sufficiently addressing the psychosocial needs. However, alternative payment models are being developed and tested to increase the financial incentive for the physical therapist to use complex decision-making processes, reflecting the patient's environmental needs and participation roles in the community (ie, how much functional impairment the medical conditions cause). Also, intensity of services required under such a model will vary depending on the clinician's judgment of the most effective dose. This is a difficult but worthy task to pursue across treatment settings.[59]

A treatment setting where complex patients are frequently seen is the acute care hospital, specifically the intensive care unit (ICU) and rehabilitation units. In the ICU itself, early initiation of physical therapy is generally accepted as safe and helpful if the therapists have training to handle complex decision making and care. Such training involves knowledge of mechanical ventilation; teams to coordinate care; and equipment, including custom walkers and neuromuscular electrical stimulation units for the very weak.[60]

Persons with critical illness (medical conditions requiring a stay in the ICU) survive more often now due to better medical care but may need continued physical therapy due to long-lasting impairments, "including muscle weakness and decreased functional ability and neuropsychiatric dysfunction [causing] decreased quality of life."[61] In these cases, keys for effective physical therapy include early rehabilitation, which requires smooth care-transition coordination between rehabilitation professionals; each team member's contributions; education of postacute care professionals, including outpatient therapists; and protocols for using high-quality interventions.

Practically, the author of this text has found that **managing the complex patient becomes easier with a broad knowledge base, reflection and discussion with self and colleagues, care coordination with other members of the patient's care team, and a commitment to lifelong learning.** Whether the patient's conditions are common or rare, the clinician can learn something new about the specific presentation, causes, or treatment. Reflecting and discussing can sharpen one's clinical reasoning skills, and coordinating care can ensure that all bases are covered for less risk of further complications to the patient. Finally, committing to lifelong learning helps the clinician stay more current in best evidence.

Counseling for Complex Patients: Opportunities and Challenges

The patient or client with multiple medical and psychiatric conditions, or even just a complicated family situation, presents challenges for the seasoned, as well as the novice, clinician. Given the relative simplicity of "paper patients" used in clinical reasoning exercises in DPT programs, it is hard to make the knowledge and skill connections to meet the complex patient's therapy goals. However, past APTA President R. Scott Ward reminds us that, as physical therapists helping people recover, we need to honor the possibilities that they (or we) see, and not prematurely limit them in therapy based on anybody's preconceptions, including our own.[62]

Counseling can bring another interpersonal piece to the table in such difficult situations, since by it the student or clinician can show compassion and empathy, model good health behaviors, facilitate communication within the IDT/IPT (see Chapter 2), and refer to other professionals as needed if the patient's needs fall outside the physical therapist's scope of practice. Compassion can be demonstrated by neurolinguistic psychology and other techniques, as discussed in Chapter 4, fueled by the physical therapist's desire and ability to care for others. Health behavior modeling also comes naturally to most clinicians, since they have higher adherence (beyond the *Healthy People 2010* targets) to the American College of Sports Medicine physical activity recommendations than do adults and non-therapist health professionals in the United States.[63]

Challenges for the clinician counseling a patient with complex medical and psychosocial issues are well documented. One challenge is the high percentage of unmet needs expressed by certain subgroups of patients. In an international example, a study of Norwegian adults with common cancers indicated that 40% of patients did not have their needs met related to therapy services, counseling, group support, subacute rehabilitation stay, and social worker consultation.[64] Another challenge is the limited efficacy of health promotion for common but complex conditions. Adding physical therapist counseling to supervised exercise for persons with type 2 diabetes in a college town did not significantly increase muscle strength and aerobic capacity, which are frequently impaired in the disease.[65]

A third challenge to counseling encountered by clinicians is the chance that certain groups of patients will not be receptive to medically necessary counseling. Skolasky et al[66] documented the following barriers to patient engagement in therapy after lumbar spine surgery and health behavior change counseling: less self-efficacy due to deficits in knowledge and support, more worry about how pain would be managed, and kinesiophobia (ie, fear of movement). Additional psychosocial factors (eg, patient personality, sense of entitlement, prior living setting, and history of frequent rehabilitation episodes) predict poor therapy outcomes, non-compliance with recommendations, and therapist burnout (L. Stevens, oral communication, April 17, 2017).

Despite the challenges, counseling does help patients and should be trialed and documented to show the therapist's knowledge and skill. When counseling alleviates a patient's psychosocial distress, that in turn can decrease disability for conditions such as low back pain.[67] In populations with low back pain complicated by fear-avoidance beliefs, education combined with physical therapy techniques can reduce days off of work while promoting general health.[68] Finally, if a person with myofascial chronic pain is referred via counseling to the appropriate professionals for management of depression and anxiety symptoms, multidisciplinary management of this pain has a higher chance of succeeding.[69] Literature related to other conditions is discussed in specific chapters.

The Patient's Social Support

Many students and therapists know intuitively how vital social support is in maintaining balance in life and regulating mood for optimal productivity. This section explores the benefits of social support from a mental-illness perspective. After all, to integrate the biopsychosocial model properly in patient-centered physical therapist practice requires us to master at least 3 tasks: (1) understand the patient's support system, (2) model good health behaviors professionally and interpersonally, and (3) support those patients who otherwise are alone. And to master these tasks, the therapist needs to have and use social support well.

Social support encompasses emotional, instrumental, and informational domains. That is, individuals can receive a sense of being cared for from others; actual assistance with daily or occasional tasks, such as transportation for work; and useful information from people they know or meet.[70] For many patients, a significant other provides a great deal of support; however, as the patient ages, this significant other may become ill or die. Family may range from extensive and closely involved to minimal and absent from health crises, when patients need the support most. Friends and acquaintances can also provide variable help to the patient, so it is important to ask questions about how patients receive social support in the 3 main domains.

Literature has shown many benefits to having and using positive social support, especially for people with SMI. One benefit is a person's improvement in coping strategies to allow him or her to function better within his or her life roles.[71] How one handles tough situations affects stress management, and by extension all potential consequences of stress. Additionally, strong social support "may help persons with SMI initiate and maintain lifestyle change," including improved eating and exercise habits.[72] Conversely, negative health behaviors may cause or worsen poor mental health. Thus, social workers may be a critical part of the IDT/IPT to specifically promote health behaviors related to cardiovascular risk in persons with mental illness; they can accomplish this by involving the person's relatives and by training other health care providers how to engage the person actively during fitness-related interventions.[73]

Practically, social support also improves meeting of temporal needs in persons with SMI. Gabrielian et al[74] explored how clients of the Veterans Affairs in Greater Los Angeles utilize various forms of support for obtaining permanent housing, with health care providers, case managers, family, or friends as options, depending on whether housing was stable or sheltered. The more stable and deep the patterns of social support, the better the housing status was, regardless of interpersonal conflicts.

Relative to emotional needs met or unmet by social support, Chronister et al note that persons with SMI typically have less support, which correlates to "higher levels of internalized stigma [relative to the disease] and lower levels of recovery and quality of life."[75] However, increasing the level of support, something physical therapists and the IDT/IPT influence, can improve the patient's recovery and quality of life. Outside of the IDT/IPT, social media can be a source of support, as explored by Naslund et al[76] looking at YouTube and other social media platforms. Naslund et al discovered peer support over 4 themes:

> [M]inimizing a sense of isolation and providing hope; finding support through peer exchange and reciprocity; sharing strategies for coping with day-to-day challenges of SMI; and learning from shared experiences of medication use and seeking mental health care.[76]

This is worth exploring, as many larger health care providers already maintain a social media presence: how can providers use social media to influence persons with SMI?

Summary

This chapter has laid the framework for evidence-based physical therapy for persons with psychological conditions and medical complexity. This framework includes a common vocabulary for the team of health care providers, as well as foundational concepts for effective care within the physical therapist's scope of practice. Statistics, known risk factors, and general differences related to aspects of the human movement system, especially related to complex patient cases, flesh out the framework. With this background, the reader can build a mental scaffold to deepen knowledge of specific mental illnesses and treatment techniques or modifications that are the focus of subsequent chapters.

Key Points

- Psychosocially informed physical therapy positively impacts life and disease in persons with complex medical and psychiatric histories.
- Persons with mental health issues often need the motivation and support of group exercise, even a walking program.
- Even low-level "physical activity can prevent some aspects of mental illness in older people such as depression, dementia, and Alzheimer's disease."[33]
- "Physical activity interventions focused on improving mastery or self-worth, as well as physical fitness, may yield the greatest benefit in alleviating psychological distress."[41]
- Complex patient management improves with a broad knowledge base, reflective discussion, care coordination, and lifelong learning.

Review Questions

- Based on the topics discussed in this chapter, what might be some reasons that cause you, as a physical therapist, to want or need to learn about persons with psychological conditions?
- Complete the following activities, then discuss with one or more classmates, if possible:
  - In your own words, define psychoneuroimmunology. How does that connect the study of mental health and illness to the scope of practice of a physical therapist?
  - Compare, contrast, and connect mood and affect. Does your clinical documentation (eg, paper patient cases, simulation labs, and clinical rotations) reflect distinctions between the 2?
- Review, for your own recall, the risk factors and prevalence of depressive and neurocognitive disorders.
- Define the human movement system in your own words. How does the contribution of various body systems to this system, including mental health and illness, define the physical therapist's scope of practice?
- Refer to Figure 5-1. Given a common example of a patient with comorbid depression and dementia, how might you use information from the text about risk factors, demographics, and medical comorbidities in each of the following aspects of patient management?
  - Examination
  - Evaluation
  - Diagnosis

  - Prognosis (including plan of care)
  - Intervention
  - Outcomes assessment
- How might you communicate the need for skilled physical therapy intervention to the primary medical care provider for a patient with mental health issues? Recall specific clinical examples, as applicable.
- Reflect on the case of a medically or psychosocially complex patient you have treated.
  - Why did you classify this patient as complex?
  - In what ways did you incorporate the skills of other professionals in patient care?
  - What do you feel you did most effectively to improve the outcome?
  - What might you do differently next time, and why?

Case Studies: First Impressions

As you review the following case studies, you may want to consider these questions for thought or discussion:

- What standardized tests and measures (including psychiatric, for example, a depression screen) would you select for this patient? Why?
- Based on available data, what short- and long-term goals would you write for your plan of care? Consider using the acronyms SMART (specific, measurable, attainable, realistic, and timely) or ABCDE (actor, behavior, conditions, degree, and expected time frame) to guide your goal writing.
- What elements (procedures, psychosocial aspects, communication aspects, etc) would you make sure to include or omit in your plan of care for this patient? Why?
- What are your anticipated needs, if any, for consultation and referral for this patient?
- How will you transition this patient toward lasting health behavior change following discharge (eg, recommending a YMCA membership trial)?

Case 1

A 46-year-old male was referred to outpatient physical therapy by his primary medical doctor, 1 week after a right partial anterior cruciate ligament tear, which was sustained while playing basketball with coworkers. His goals are to return to work full time and engage in leisure activities.

- Social history: he is employed full time in an office position with a 45-minute commute. He is married with 2 children; his wife cares for the children at home and is a freelance photographer. The family lives in a 2-story house with a basement; the patient's bedroom is on the second floor. He describes himself as a hard worker who likes to keep busy at all times.
- Medical/psychiatric history: hypercholesterolemia, hypertension, and situational depression postinjury
- Impairments, activity limitations, and participation restrictions found on initial interview and examination
  - Subjective right knee instability and pain rated 6/10 with weightbearing
  - Mild right knee inflammation causing functional weakness in knee extensors and hip abductors
  - Standing tolerance limited to 5 minutes
  - Unable to carry objects in both hands due to fear of falling (using single axillary crutch currently)

  - Unable to carry items up and down stairs
  - Unable to drive (must now carpool)

Case 2

A 27-year-old female was hospitalized for 3 days after the birth of her first child. She self-referred to outpatient women's health physical therapy 1 week after returning home, due to pelvic pain and increased episodes of incontinence. Her goals are to return to work and to care for her infant without pain and bothersome clothing changes.

- Social history: she works full time as an occupational therapist in an acute care setting but has 1 month of maternity leave remaining. Her husband works second shift and assists with laundry and childcare. They live in a ranch house with laundry in the basement, and her mother lives near enough to visit every 1 to 2 weeks to help with cooking and freezing meals.
- Medical/psychiatric history: type 1 diabetes mellitus, stress urinary incontinence, postpartum depression that started on hospital discharge, and a family history of postpartum depression
- Impairments, activity limitations, and participation restrictions found on initial interview and examination
  - Pain rated 5/10 in pelvis and occasionally radiating to upper thighs
  - Mild unsteadiness during gait, especially while carrying her infant (brought infant to clinic)
  - Several episodes of mild urinary incontinence daily, especially while transitioning sit to stand
  - Difficulty in walking more than household distances, especially while carrying her infant

Case 3

A 64-year-old female was referred to outpatient physical therapy 2 weeks after a left total hip replacement with anterior approach, thus avoiding posterior hip precautions of flexion over 90 degrees, adduction past neutral, and internal rotation past neutral. She completed inpatient and home health physical therapy prior to this. Her goal is to resume full household duties and at least 75% of her tutoring caseload.

- Social history: she works in the home as a piano teacher and reading tutor for children with learning disabilities; her husband assists with outdoor and light indoor household chores. They live in a 2-story house with her bedroom on the second floor and laundry in the basement. Their children no longer live at home but visit occasionally.
- Medical/psychiatric history: hyperlipidemia, hypertension, anxiety symptoms 50% of time, and depressive symptoms 75% of time
- Impairments, activity limitations, and participation restrictions found on initial interview and examination
  - Pain rated 4/10 in left hip and right knee with prolonged weightbearing activities
  - Generalized stiffness in large joints
  - Decreased left hip extensor and abductor strength
  - Standing tolerance limited to 10 minutes
  - Unable to walk continuously for greater than 5 minutes (progressing from 2-wheeled walker to single-point cane and previously required no device)
  - Difficulty in cooking, cleaning, and sitting for more than one consecutive student
  - Subjectively poor sleep quality

References

1. Filer N. *The Shock of the Fall.* New York, NY: St. Martin's Griffin; 2015.
2. APTA Staff. The movement system brings it all together. *PT In Motion.* http://www.apta.org/PTinMotion/2016/5/Feature/MovementSystem/. Published May 2016. Accessed February 19, 2018.
3. Overmeer T, Boersma K, Denison E, Linton S. Does teaching physical therapists to deliver a biopsychosocial treatment program result in better patient outcomes? A randomized controlled trial. *Phys Ther.* 2011;91(5):804-819.
4. Drench ME, Noonan AC, Sharby N, Ventura SH. *Psychosocial Aspects of Health Care.* 3rd ed. Upper Saddle River, NJ: Pearson; 2012.
5. Manderscheid R, Ryff C, Freeman E, McKnight-Eily L, Dhingra S, Strine, T. Evolving definitions of mental illness and wellness. *Prev Chronic Dis.* 2010;7(1):A19.
6. Mortazavi S, Mohammad K, Eftekhar Ardebili H, Dorali Beni R, Mahmoodi M, Keshteli AH. Mental disorder prevention and physical activity in Iranian elderly. *Int J Prev Med.* 2012;3(suppl 1):S64-S72.
7. Bruffaerts R, Vilagut G, Demyttenaere K, et al. Role of common mental and physical disorders in partial disability around the world. *Br J Psychiatry.* 2012;200(6):454-461.
8. Morala DT, Shiomi T, Maruyama H. Factors associated with the functional status of community-dwelling elderly. *J Geriatr Phys Ther.* 2006;29(3):101-106.
9. Stubbs B. Physical intervention in older adult psychiatry: an audit of physical ailments identified by physiotherapists and the implications for managing aggressive behavior. *Int Psychogeriatr.* 2009;21(6):1196-1197.
10. Qaseem A, Barry MJ, Kansagara D. Nonpharmacologic versus pharmacologic treatment of adult patients with major depressive disorder: a clinical practice guideline from the American College of Physicians. *Ann Intern Med.* 2016;164(5):350-359.
11. Herning MM, Cook JH, Schneider JK. Cognitive behavioral therapy to promote exercise behavior in older adults: implications for physical therapists. *J Geriatr Phys Ther.* 2005;28(2):34-38.
12. International Organization of Physical Therapists in Mental Health. *World Confederation for Physical Therapy.* http://www.wcpt.org/ioptmh. Updated June 21, 2017. Accessed February 19, 2018.
13. Morgan AJ, Jorm AF. Self-help interventions for depressive disorders and depressive symptoms: a systematic review. *Ann Gen Psychiatry.* 2008;7:13.
14. Stanton R, Happell B. Exercise for mental illness: a systematic review of inpatient studies. *Int J Ment Health Nurs.* 2014;23(3):232-242.
15. Tosh G, Clifton AV, Xia J, White MM. General physical health advice for people with serious mental illness. *Cochrane Database Syst Rev.* 2014;(3):CD 008567.
16. Haber D. *Health Promotion and Aging: Practical Applications for Health Professionals.* 4th ed. New York, NY: Springer; 2007.
17. Goetzel RZ, Hawkins K, Ozminkowski RJ, Wang S. The health and productivity cost burden of the "Top 10" physical and mental health conditions affecting six large US employers in 1999. *J Occup Environ Med.* 2003;45(1):5-14.
18. Damásio AR. *Descartes' Error: Emotion, Reason, and the Human Brain.* New York, NY: Penguin Books; 1994.
19. American Psychiatric Association. *Diagnostic and Statistical Manual of Mental Disorders.* 5th ed. Washington, DC: American Psychiatric Association; 2013.
20. Haze M. *The Bleeders.* United States: Dirty Jeans Publishing; 2010.
21. Stuart GW. *Handbook of Psychiatric Nursing.* 6th ed. St. Louis, MO: Elsevier Mosby; 2005.
22. American Physical Therapy Association. APTA white paper—the movement system. http://www.apta.org/MovementSystem/WhitePaper/. Published August 2015. Accessed February 19, 2018.
23. American Psychological Association. Glossary of psychological terms. *American Psychological Association.* http://www.apa.org/research/action/glossary.aspx. Published 2002. Accessed February 19, 2018.
24. Regents of UCSF. Executive functions. *UCSF Memory and Aging Center.* http://memory.ucsf.edu/ftd/overview/biology/executive/single. Updated 2018. Accessed February 19, 2018.
25. World Health Organization. Lexicon of psychiatric and mental health terms. 2nd ed. *World Health Organization.* http://apps.who.int/iris/bitstream/10665/39342/1/924154466X.pdf. 1994. Accessed February 19, 2018.
26. Grabowski D, Aschbrenner K, Feng Z, Mor V. Mental illness in nursing homes: variations across states. *Health Aff (Millwood).* 2009;28(3):689-700.
27. Seitz D, Purandare N, Conn D. Prevalence of psychiatric disorders among older adults in long-term care homes: a systematic review. *Int Psychogeriatr.* 2010;22(7):1025-1039.
28. American Physical Therapy Association. "Movement System" is our professional identity. *NEXT.* http://www.apta.org/NEXT/News/2015/6/6/MovementSystem/. Published June 8, 2015. Accessed February 19, 2018.
29. Delaune MF. Moving from mystery diagnosis to diagnosis in physical therapist practice. *PT In Motion.* 2009;10. http://www.apta.org/PTinMotion/2009/10/MysteryDiagnosis/. Accessed February 19, 2018.
30. Ludewig PM, Lawrence RL, Braman JP. What's in a name? Using movement system diagnoses versus pathoanatomic diagnoses. *J Orthop Sports Phys Ther.* 2013;43(5):280-283.

31. Hunter SJ, Norton BJ, Powers CM, Saladin LK, Delitto A. Rothstein Roundtable Podcast - "Putting all our of our eggs in one basket: human movement system." *Phys Ther.* 2015;95(11):1466.
32. Bumann RL, Valero-Cuevas FJ, Riener R. *Using load-cells to unveil limitations to the human movement system* [master's thesis]. Switzerland: ETH Zurich.
33. Fox KR, Stathi A, McKenna J, Davis MG. Physical activity and mental well-being in older people participating in the Better Ageing Project. *Eur J Appl Physiol.* 2007;100(5):591-602. DOI 10.1007/s00421-007-0392-0
34. Lundy-Ekman L. *Neuroscience: Fundamentals for Rehabilitation.* 3rd ed. St. Louis, MO: Saunders; 2007.
35. Watts AS, Loskutova N, Burns JM, Johnson DK. Metabolic syndrome and cognitive decline in early Alzheimer's disease and healthy older adults. *J Alzheimers Dis.* 2013;35(2):253-265.
36. Bartels SJ, Pratt SI, Aschbrenner KA, et al. Pragmatic replication trial of health promotion coaching for obesity in SMI and maintenance of outcomes. *Am J Psychiatry.* 2015;172(4):344-352.
37. Brown C, Goetz J, Hamera E. Weight loss intervention for people with SMI: a randomized controlled trial of the RENEW program. *Psychiatr Serv.* 2011;62(7):800-802.
38. McBain H, Mulligan K, Haddad M, Flood C, Jones J, Simpson A. Self management interventions for type 2 diabetes in adult people with severe mental illness. *Cochrane Database Syst Rev.* 2016;(4):CD011361.
39. Defrin R, Amanzio M, de Tommaso M, et al. Experimental pain processing in individuals with cognitive impairment: current state of the science. *Pain.* 2015;156(8):1396-1408.
40. Stubbs B, Hollins L. The safe application of physical interventions in aggressive older adults: considerations from the physiotherapy profession. *Int Psychogeriatr.* 2011;23(4):672-674.
41. Cairney J, Faulkner G, Veldhuizen S, Wade TJ. Changes over time in physical activity and psychological distress among older adults. *Can J Psychiatry.* 2009;54(3):160-169.
42. Hall AM, Ferreira PH, Maher CG, et al. The influence of the therapist-patient relationship on treatment outcome in physical rehabilitation: a systematic review. *Phys Ther.* 2010;90(8):1099-1110.
43. Van Til L, Fikretoglu D, Pranger T, et al. Work reintegration for veterans with mental disorders: a systematic literature review to inform research. *Phys Ther.* 2013;93(9):1163-1174.
44. Karp JF, Dew MA, Wahed AS, et al. Challenges and solutions for depression prevention research: methodology for a depression prevention trial for older adults with knee arthritis and emotional distress. *Am J Geriatr Psychiatry.* 2016;24(6):433-443.
45. Kessler RC, Soukup J, Davis RB, et al. The use of complementary and alternative therapies to treat anxiety and depression in the United States. *Am J Psychiatry.* 2001;158(2):289-294.
46. Ravindran AV, da Silva TL. Complementary and alternative therapies as add-on to pharmacotherapy for mood and anxiety disorders: a systematic review. *J Affect Disord.* 2013;150(3):707-719.
47. George SZ, Coronado RA, Beneciuk JM, et al. Depressive symptoms, anatomical region, and clinical outcomes for patients seeking outpatient physical therapy for musculoskeletal pain. *Phys Ther.* 2011;91(3):358-372.
48. Williams AK, Schulz R. Association of pain and physical dependency with depression in physically ill middle-aged and elderly persons. *Phys Ther.* 1988;68(8):1226-1230.
49. Carta MG, Hardoy MC, Pilu A, et al. Improving physical quality of life with group physical activity in the adjunctive treatment of major depressive disorder. *Clin Pract Epidemiol Ment Health.* 2008;4:1.
50. Trivedi MH, Greer TL, Church TS, et al. Exercise as an augmentation treatment for nonremitted major depressive disorder: a randomized, parallel dose comparison. *J Clin Psychiatry.* 2011;72(5):677-684.
51. Tangen GG, Engedal K, Bergland A, et al. Relationships between balance and cognition in patients with subjective cognitive impairment, mild cognitive impairment, and Alzheimer disease. *Phys Ther.* 2014;94(8):1123-1134.
52. Horak F. BESTest: balance evaluation—systems test. *BESTest.* http://www.bestest.us/files/4413/6358/0759/BESTest.pdf. 2008. Accessed February 19, 2018.
53. Venema DM, Bartels E, Siu KC. Tasks matter: a cross-sectional study of the relationship of cognition and dual-task performance in older adults. *J Geriatr Phys Ther.* 2013;36(3):115-122.
54. Grant RW, Ashburner JM, Hong CS, et al. Defining patient complexity from the primary care physician's perspective. *Ann Intern Med.* 2011;155(12):797-804.
55. Nelson MLA, Grudniewicz A, Albadry S. Applying clinical practice guidelines to the complex patient: insights for practice and policy from stroke rehabilitation. *Healthc Q.* 2016;19(2):38-43.
56. Ruckert E, Plack MM, Maring J. A model for designing a geriatric physical therapy course grounded in educational principles and active learning strategies. *J Phys Ther Educ.* 2014;28(2):69-84.
57. Atkinson HL, Nixon-Cave K. A tool for clinical reasoning and reflection using the *International Classification of Functioning, Disability and Health* (ICF) framework and patient management model. *Phys Ther.* 2011;91(3);416-430.
58. Foster NE, Delitto A. Embedding psychosocial perspectives within clinical management of low back pain: integration of psychosocially informed management principles into physical therapist practice—challenges and opportunities. *Phys Ther.* 2011;91(5):790-803.
59. Guccione AA, Harwood KJ, Goldstein MS, Miller SC. Can "severity-intensity" be the conceptual basis of an alternative payment model for therapy services provided under Medicare? *Phys Ther.* 2011;91(10):1564-1569.
60. Hodgson CL, Berney S, Harrold M, Saxena M, Bellomo R. Clinical review: early patient mobilization in the ICU. *Crit Care.* 2013;17:207.

61. Ohtake PJ, Strasser DC, Needham DM. Rehabilitation for people with critical illness: taking the next steps. *Phys Ther.* 2012:92(12):1484-1488.
62. Ward RS. 2009 APTA Presidential Address: We must see the possibilities. *Phys Ther.* 2009;89(11):1250-1252.
63. Chevan J, Haskvitz EM. Do as I do: exercise habits of physical therapists, physical therapist assistants, and student physical therapists. *Phys Ther.* 2010;90(5):726-734.
64. Thorsen L, Gjerset GM, Loge JH, et al. Cancer patients' needs for rehabilitation services. *Acta Oncol.* 2011;50(2):212-222.
65. Taylor JD, Fletcher JP, Tiarks J. Impact of physical therapist-directed exercise counseling combined with fitness center-based exercise training on muscular strength and exercise capacity in people with type 2 diabetes: a randomized clinical trial. *Phys Ther.* 2009;89(9):884-892.
66. Skolasky RL, Maggard AM, Li D, Riley LH, Wegener ST. Health behavior change counseling in surgery for degenerative lumbar spinal stenosis. Part II: patient activation mediates the effects of health behavior change counseling on rehabilitation engagement. *Arch Phys Med Rehabil.* 2015;96(7):1208-1214.
67. Nisenzon AN, George SZ, Beneciuk JM, et al. The role of anger in psychosocial subgrouping for patients with low back pain. *Clin J Pain.* 2014;30(5):501-509.
68. Godges JJ, Anger MA, Zimmerman G, Delitto A. Effects of education on return-to-work status for people with fear-avoidance beliefs and acute low back pain. *Phys Ther.* 2008;88(2):231-239.
69. Sorrell MR, Flanagan W, McCall JL. The effect of depression and anxiety on the success of multidisciplinary treatment of chronic resistant myofascial pain. *J Musculoskel Pain.* 2003;11(1):17-21.
70. Seeman T. Support and social conflict: section one - social support [definition and background]. *MacArthur Research Network on SES & Health.* http://www.macses.ucsf.edu/research/psychosocial/socsupp.php. Updated April 2008. Accessed February 19, 2018.
71. Davis L, Brekke J. Social support and functional outcome in severe mental illness: the mediating role of proactive coping. *Psychiatry Res.* 2014;215(1):39-45.
72. Aschbrenner KA, Mueser KT, Bartels SJ, Pratt SI. Perceived social support for diet and exercise among persons with serious mental illness enrolled in a healthy lifestyle intervention. *Psychiatr Rehabil J.* 2013;36(2):65-71.
73. Aschbrenner KA, Mueser KT, Bartels SJ, et al. The other 23 hours: a qualitative study of fitness provider perspectives on social support for health promotion for adults with mental illness. *Health Soc Work.* 2015;40(2):91-99.
74. Gabrielian S, Young AS, Greenberg JM, Bromley E. Social support and housing transitions among homeless adults with serious mental illness and substance use disorders [published online ahead of print August 22, 2016]. *Psychiatr Rehabil J.* DOI: 10.1037/prj0000213.
75. Chronister J, Chou CC, Liao HY. The role of stigma coping and social support in mediating the effect of societal stigma on internalized stigma, mental health recovery, and quality of life among people with serious mental illness. *J Community Psychol.* 2013;41(5):582-600.
76. Naslund JA, Grande SW, Aschbrenner KA, Elwyn G. Naturally occurring peer support through social media: the experiences of individuals with severe mental illness using YouTube. *PLoS One.* 2014;9(10):e110171. DOI: 10.1371/journal.pone.0110171

Anxiety Disorders

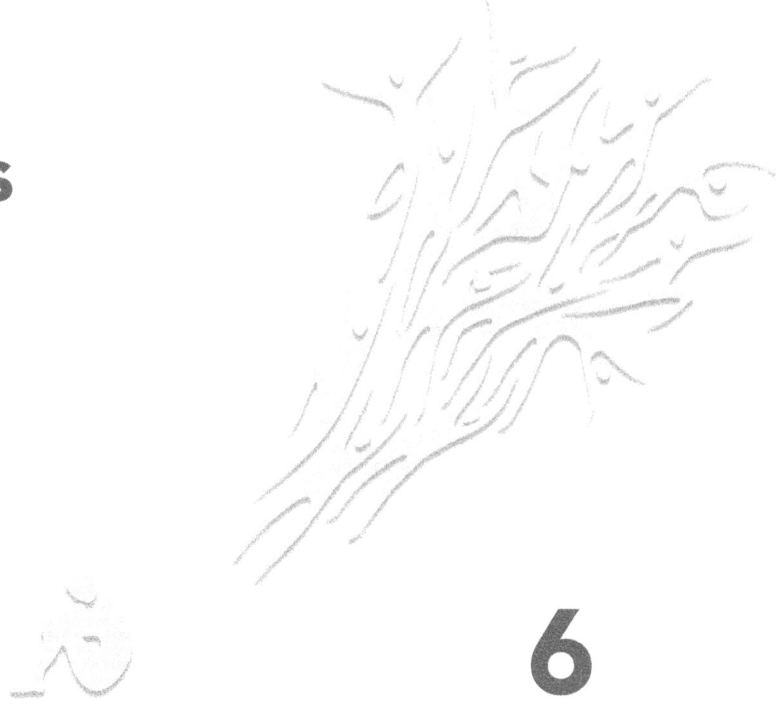

6

Outline

- Scope and Classification of Anxiety Disorders
- Neurophysiological Background, Etiology, and Risk Factors
- Comorbid Medical and Psychosocial Issues
- Specific Clinical Approaches to Improve Outcomes of Physical Therapy
    - Body-Focused Therapies
    - Mind-Focused Therapies
- Summary
- Key Points
- Review Questions
- Case Studies: First Impressions
- Quick Reference

Learning Objectives

- Demonstrate awareness of anxiety disorders per the *Diagnostic and Statistical Manual of Mental Disorders, Fifth Edition* (DSM-5) classification
- Summarize research related to alterations in the human movement system for anxiety disorders
- Incorporate risk factor assessment for anxiety disorders into the patient/client interview

Johnson H.
Psychosocial Elements of Physical Therapy: The Connection of Body to Mind (pp 111-122).

- Delineate impact of common comorbidities into patient care, being aware of the patient management model
- Propose changes to the physical therapist's approach, based on a diagnosis of an anxiety disorder, into assessments, exercise prescription, home exercise programs, building/maintaining rapport, and clinical documentation to improve outcomes

Anxiety disorders, a common mental health issue especially in the United States, encompass multiple distinct clinical conditions. They predispose the individual to other health conditions and potentially suicide. Thus, it is vital for the physical therapist to be aware of each disorder, as well as specific ways to adapt the plan of care to better serve these patients.

Scope and Classification of Anxiety Disorders

Anxiety isn't an attack that explodes out of me; it's not a volcano that lies dormant until it's triggered by an earth-shattering event. It's a constant companion. Like a blowfly that gets into the house in the middle of summer, flying around and around. You can hear it buzzing, but you can't see it, can't capture it, can't let it out. My anxiety is invisible to others, but often it's the focal point on my mind. Everything that happens on a day-to-day basis is filtered through a lens colored by anxiety.

—Jen Wilde[1]

As noted in Chapter 5, anxiety is "a diffuse, vague apprehension associated with feelings of uncertainty and helplessness. This emotion has no specific object."[2] An anxiety disorder, per the DSM-5,[3] involves at least 6 months of persistent, excessively intense anxiety. This anxiety may occur due to a specific situation, or it may be due to the individual trying to decrease other somatic symptoms; for example, the sensation of one's heart pounding may make the person more anxious in a vicious cycle. The outworking of this anxiety affects mind, behavior, and body, producing worry, panic, avoidance of anxiety triggers, and the fight-or-flight response.[4]

Several disorders fall under the umbrella of anxiety. These include generalized anxiety disorder (GAD), panic disorder, posttraumatic stress disorder (PTSD), obsessive-compulsive disorder (OCD), and phobias including social phobia and agoraphobia. Statistics for several of these are included in Chapter 5. The following is a list of brief descriptions from the DSM-5 for different types of anxiety disorders.

- GAD: excessive, ongoing, and uncontrollable worry about day-to-day matters. These patients may have insomnia, headaches, irritability, and fatigue.
- Panic disorder: typically occurring with agoraphobia (fear of open or public spaces), this includes 5 to 10 minute panic attacks involving intense fear and sympathetic nervous system arousal. Patients may have fear of panic attacks themselves, elevated heart rate, dizziness, and shortness of breath.
- PTSD: hypervigilance, nightmares, and unwanted flashbacks after a traumatic event
- OCD: uncontrollable thoughts causing repetitive actions (hoarding, hand-washing, arranging objects) to decrease the thought-induced anxiety. Patients usually recognize the irrationality of their obsessions, but this may make them feel more helpless.
- Phobia: persistent, excessive fear and subsequent avoidance of an object or situation regardless of actual danger level

Physical activity, especially aerobic exercise per the American College of Sports Medicine guidelines, is shown to be one of several helpful interventions for several anxiety disorders in adults.[5] However, limited research focuses on persons over age 65.[6] It is still an important issue for health care providers and especially physical therapists, because geriatric anxiety increases "risk of comorbid depression, falls, physical and functional disability, and loneliness."[7] This is complicated by the fact that anxiety in this age group is both difficult to diagnose (due to under-recognition and patients' reticence in talking about their own mental health) and frequently resistant to medication (up to half of individuals do not experience resolved anxiety symptoms after a first-line intervention such as medication).[8]

Lewis and Bottomley, in their hallmark text on geriatric rehabilitation, note that symptoms seen more frequently by physical and occupational therapists "include tremor, headaches, chest pain, weakness and fatigue, neck and back pain, dry mouth, dizziness, paresthesia, and a nonproductive cough."[9] Because these symptoms may have other potential causes including "[excessive] caffeine [intake], hypoglycemia, or thyroid disease," asking follow-up questions about a patient's background may help tease out the underlying anxiety disorder and its potential etiology.[9]

Neurophysiological Background, Etiology, and Risk Factors

Research has explored molecular and systemic causes of anxiety disorders across the lifespan, as well as potential treatment mechanisms. Per the biopsychosocial model of health care, health care providers should look at the person as a whole; this includes biological, psychological, and social aspects contributing to the person's makeup. Research literature, discussed next, is starting to scratch the surface in this domain.

At the microscopic level, potential changes in the locus ceruleus, oxygen sensors, autonomic nervous system hypersensitivity and arousal, and the individual's genetic makeup may contribute to anxiety or panic symptoms.[4] The locus ceruleus is in the brainstem and is the primary region that produces norepinephrine (noradrenaline); thus, it contributes to physiological symptoms of stress or panic. Faulty oxygen sensors in the central and peripheral nervous systems can also contribute to shortness of breath, chest tightness, and hyperventilation seen in panic attacks.

At the system level, the self-referential brain network (made up of the ventromedial prefrontal cortex, dorsomedial prefrontal cortex, and posterior cingulate cortex) has become implicated in anxiety disorders because "self-views can powerfully influence how a person thinks, feels, and behaves, particularly in social contexts."[10] In turn, this network relates especially to social anxiety disorder, where the person has an inaccurate and negative view of him- or herself. In a randomized controlled trial, mindfulness-based stress reduction (see Chapter 4) was shown to be superior to aerobic exercise as an isolated treatment for social anxiety disorder, by enabling uncued "recruitment of cognitive and attention regulation neural networks" to decrease unwanted impairments in the patient's self-image and self-assessment.[10] However, both mindfulness and aerobic exercise were better than no treatment. The study did not address the effects of combined mindfulness and aerobic exercise, but did show brain changes that occur in anxiety disorders.[10]

Finally, several authors have investigated anxiety sensitivity. Broman-Fulks and Storey define anxiety sensitivity as "the belief that anxiety-related sensations [eg, shortness of breath] can have negative consequences."[11] This can cause and prolong anxiety disorders. As few as 6 20-minute sessions of aerobic exercise can significantly decrease sensitivity, potentially because aerobic activity is a safe way to induce anxiety-like, but safe, sensations (eg, sweating, rapid heart rate, and shortness of breath). Smits et al[12] investigated exercise combined with a "cognitive restructuring intervention" incorporating education on anxiety sensitivity, for 2 weeks with a 3-week follow-up. They hypothesized that **physical activity could be "an additional psychosocial intervention for conditions such as panic disorder, where anxiety sensitivity is a prominent component of pathology."**[12] Thus, even very brief exercise can reduce anxiety symptoms.

Comorbid Medical and Psychosocial Issues

Anxiety disorders are associated with biopsychosocial abnormalities that affect function, health, and use of the health care system. Medically, the repeated cardiovascular stress associated with an anxiety disorder, along with the person's beliefs about the symptoms that will influence seeking treatment, can increase the risk of sudden death, blood clots, atherosclerosis, and cardiac dysrhythmias.[4] The proposed mechanism by which psychological disorders, such as anxiety, affect medical conditions is that neurohormones and neurotransmitters change immune system parameters, and that symptoms can directly or indirectly change health behaviors. For example, shortness of breath may cause the person to avoid exercise for fear of not being able to breathe at all. Anxiety, along with catastrophizing (ie, thinking the worst about a situation's potential outcome), depression, and low expectations for treatment, can predict a poor outcome for physical therapy for neck pain.[13]

Due to comorbid medical conditions and their treatments, of which people with anxiety may try many different kinds to manage symptoms, anxiety disorders rank as one of the most expensive psychological conditions. According to Olesen et al,[14] anxiety disorders incur a 74.4-billion euro cost ($79.3 billion in 2017) to treat as of 2010. For comparison, general mood disorders conservatively cost 113.4 billion euros ($120.9 billion in 2017), while dementias cost at least 105.2 billion euros ($112.1 billion in 2017). Olesen et al[14] note that limited data prevent a more accurate, and likely higher, cost estimate.

Specific Clinical Approaches to Improve Outcomes of Physical Therapy

Current literature on treatment for anxiety disorders, adult and geriatric, may be classified into 2 major domains pertinent to this text. These domains span mind and body, with overlap often more effective than either one in isolation. Throughout this section, one caution for the reader is the current paucity of research on geriatric second-line treatments. Barton et al[7] noted that, as of 2014, no high-level research (a randomized controlled trial or systematic review) existed to support a specific intervention for older people with anxiety that has not responded to a first-line medication.

Body-Focused Therapies

Of primary interest to the clinician is exercise effectiveness for anxiety disorders and the best exercise choice; ample evidence shows that physical activity is effective. While trials investigating the best dosage or type of exercise have yet to be completed, **current literature supports the use of both strength training (progressive resistance exercise [PRE]) and moderate- to vigorous-intensity aerobic training (barring medical contraindications) to manage primary and secondary impairments and symptoms of anxiety disorders.** Several studies are summarized in Table 6-1.

Table 6-1

Exercise Interventions for Anxiety Disorders

STUDY	DISORDER(S) STUDIED	INTERVENTION	FINDINGS
Bartley et al[15]	Varied anxiety disorders	Aerobic exercise	Works significantly better as adjunct therapy than alone
Broocks et al[5]	Panic disorder	Running program	Effective, but less effective alone than medication
Herring et al[16]	GAD	6 weeks of lower-body PRE or aerobic exercise	Worry reduced, 40% to 60% remission rates (30% remission for medication alone)
Jazaieri et al[10]	Social anxiety disorder	Aerobic exercise	Equally effective to mindfulness-based stress reduction
Meyer et al[17]	Varied anxiety disorders	10-week running program	Improves endurance, but did not correlate to anxiety scores

Other investigated body-related interventions include body awareness and yoga. Breitve et al[18] examined Norwegian psychomotor physical therapy for management of depression and anxiety symptoms. This technique, performed for at least 6 to 12 months in the study, is based on facilitating awareness of one's own body. Combining "movement exercises and massage," practicing clinicians also seek to validate their patients' experiences of the subjective or "hidden" aspects of mood disorders, including those symptoms without an apparent organic cause. This validation can influence the "visible" aspects by extension, to improve a patient's posture, muscle strength, balance, and movement patterns.[18]

Related to breath awareness, which is lacking in many conditions including anxiety or panic disorder, Sureka et al[19] found that Sudarshan Kriya improved anxiety, depression, global functioning, positive well-being, and general health in incarcerated adult males who were diagnosed with anxiety or depression. Sudarshan Kriya was described as a 6-week practice of each subject sitting daily "in an armchair with his eyes closed and [paying] gentle attention to [his] breath."[19] Compared to no intervention, this technique significantly improved anxiety symptoms. Finally, Kirkwood et al[20] found in a systematic review of studies that yoga shows promise for certain anxiety conditions including OCD.

Mind-Focused Therapies

Bridging the gap between mind and body, several studies also examined the effects of exercise as an adjunct to specific psychological therapies. Gaudlitz et al[21] found that aerobic exercise improves the effectiveness of cognitive behavioral therapy (CBT) for persons with a panic disorder. With 1 month of CBT intervention for all participants, an additional 8 weeks of aerobic exercise significantly improved subjects' scores on the Hamilton Anxiety Scale. This exercise was prescribed at 30 minutes, 3 times per week, at 70% of each subject's VO_2max, thus qualifying as moderate intensity. This supports the use of multifaceted and multidisciplinary interventions for anxiety disorders, since treatment resistance to medications may potentially be lessened by adding psychological and physical therapies, including CBT and aerobic exercise or PRE.

Psychological therapy is the first choice for many individuals for treatment of their anxiety disorders. Categories include CBT, humor therapy, and specific social support. CBT and its subtypes are discussed in more depth in Chapter 4, as this area applies to many different psychological conditions. Sue et al[4] also recommend modeling; restructuring irrational thoughts; and controlling exposure to an anxiety, or obsession-producing stimulus, while the therapist prevents the patient from responding as he or she typically would. For OCD, this technique is called *flooding*; by using it, the individual can be desensitized to what would normally trigger compulsive behavior. For example, one person's obsession might be a fear of germs, causing compulsive, repeated hand-washing far beyond what is necessary. A flooding intervention would include perceived high exposure to germs (handshake with a stranger), without allowing handwashing for a time.

Although it is common knowledge that humor and producing a happy mood can relieve anxiety and depression symptoms, limited scholarly evidence has studied this for the geriatric population specifically. Ganz and Jacobs[22] analyzed a humor therapy workshop for Israeli community-dwelling elders participating at senior centers. These workshops included one 2- to 3-hour session per week for 5 months, where a humorist and social worker worked to integrate humorous situations into daily activities, maintain a "supportive and mirthful environment," and preserve each participant's humorous anecdotes on video for group viewing.[22] Ganz and Jacobs[22] found that, while well-being improved and symptoms of anxiety and depression decreased significantly, psychological stress did not decrease, nor did general health increase. Thus, further research in this area is needed, especially in giving the clinician tools to work evidence-based humor interventions into the plan of care for better outcomes.

An impressive example of combining multiple treatments into an interprofessional program for anxiety and depression is found in a pair of studies.[8,23] These studies investigated the effects of an intensive short-term dynamic residential treatment on people with anxiety, depression, and occasional comorbid personality disorders, that did not respond to initial treatment (half of patients seeking treatment). Components of this 8-week intervention included individual psychotherapy for 90 minutes once per week, group psychotherapy for 90 minutes twice per week, art therapy groups, education, a walking program twice per week, and training in body awareness. Dramatic outcomes included:

- Rapid improvement (sustained at 14 months) in symptom distress and functioning in interpersonal relationships. Many depressive and personality disorders make relationships especially difficult.
- Clinical recovery rates of 46.26% for mood disorders and 63.93% for personality disorders
- Return-to-work rate of 71.18%, psychotropic drug use decrease of 28.62%, and health care utilization reduction of 65.55%

Thus, therapist facilitation of social support and relationships is key to the treatment of anxiety and other psychiatric disorders, since individuals diagnosed often cannot easily develop or maintain these requirements for function in today's world. In a study of the residents of assisted living or long-term care facilities in Malta and Australia, "mobility was found to foster an active life, which appeared to help residents to control their anxiety and depression. Rehabilitation programmes [sic] and facilitation of strategies were recommended to strengthen relationships" with social support.[24] Chapter 1 more thoroughly discusses social support for the therapist and patient.

The clinician may well encounter a patient in the early or middle stages of a panic attack. Strategies to mitigate this situation include addressing the trigger (if known), helping the patient to ground, and having the patient take a fast-acting anxiolytic medication, if available and appropriate. Grounding involves as many senses as possible: while talking softly and calmly to the patient, the therapist may use gentle hand contact and direct the patient to look at something, listen to something, hold on to something, and smell something in the environment. Since the physiological aspects of a panic attack (muscle tension, rapid pulse and respiratory rate) will self-limit after a few minutes, the therapist can guide the patient to distract him- or herself until those symptoms pass.

Finally, since non-pharmaceutical, complementary and alternative medicine (CAM) techniques for anxiety disorders are increasing, with or without evidence basis, providers need to know the state of the evidence. Joyce and Herbison conducted a Cochrane systematic review of Reiki, "a 2500 year old treatment described as vibrational or subtle energy therapy [which] is most commonly facilitated by light touch on or above the body,"[25] with very limited evidence on benefits or harms. Other techniques, specific to relaxation and easily applicable by the clinician, include diaphragmatic breathing, progressive muscle relaxation, visualization of a pleasant or relaxing scene, meditation, acupuncture, massage, chiropractic referral, hypnosis referral, biofeedback, aromatherapy, and laughter.[26]

More broadly, Ventegodt et al[27] examined major classes of CAM for effects, side effects, and adverse effects. Principles of any non-pharmaceutical therapy include:

- Salutogenesis: heal the whole person
- Similarity: trauma is said to reside in the subconscious mind.
- Hering's Law of Cure: "you will get well in the opposite order of the way you got ill."[27]
- Resources: replenish what was absent when the illness occurred
- Use "as little force as possible" to avoid doing harm[27]

Ventegodt et al[27] identified the major classes of CAM as:

- Chemicals, including herbs or "mildly bioactive often nontoxic drugs" with dietary changes[27]
- Physical therapy without high-velocity, low-amplitude joint manipulation
- Psychotherapy, including CBT
- Spiritual therapy, including prayer and spiritual healing, depending on the person's background
- Mind-body medicine, including homeopathy, the Alexander technique, and acupuncture
- Holistic medicine, focused on the whole person
- Shamanism, with hallucinogenic drugs

Impressively, **Ventegodt et al noted that CAM is demonstrably more efficient than medication for treating and curing conditions including:**

> **[S]ubjectively poor physical health … chronic pain, subjectively poor mental health, schizophrenia, major depression, anxiety, social phobia … subjectively poor quality of life, sense of coherence, suicidal prevention, low self-esteem, [and] poor working ability.[27]**

While this review found various randomized controlled trials supporting the use of CAM for anxiety and other disorders, a needed research direction is to examine how such methods interact with physical therapy techniques.

Summary

Anxiety disorders, including GAD, OCD, and PTSD, are woven into the fabric of many people's lives in the United States and around the world. While symptoms may be invisible or nearly invisible to others, they can severely affect the individual's function, by causing avoidance of potential anxiety triggers, as well as secondary impairments in the cardiovascular, neurologic, and musculoskeletal systems. These put patients at risk of suicide or other premature death. While risk factors for anxiety disorders vary, comorbid medical conditions are often stress-related and can impact the physical therapy plan of care in many ways, including the therapist's selection of exercise modality or complementary techniques to address the mind along with the body. People with anxiety disorders can benefit from physical therapy, and it behooves clinicians to be aware of the underlying factors, as well as evidence-based recommendations for specific treatment techniques.

Key Points

- Physical activity is a valuable adjunctive treatment for conditions marked by anxiety sensitivity.
- Strength training and moderate- to vigorous-intensity aerobic training have strong literature support of being able to manage primary and secondary anxiety-related impairments.
- Interdisciplinary, comprehensive interventions can have dramatic outcomes for mood disorders.
- CAM has literature support for multiple medical and mental health issues, with limited known side effects to date.

Review Questions

- Briefly recall clinical cases where an anxiety disorder was in the patient's past medical history. How did you incorporate an awareness of that condition into the patient interview, establishment of rapport, and plan of care for that patient?
  - Based on what you learned in this chapter, what changes would you make for a similar patient presentation in the future?
  - How might you document specific adjunct interventions aimed at the patient's anxiety symptoms to demonstrate an awareness of the patient as a whole person?
- What are some potential barriers to a person with an anxiety disorder participating in aerobic exercise to reduce symptoms? How might you address these barriers? Consult classmates or colleagues as needed.
- How might you incorporate psychosocial techniques such as humor and mindfulness into your intervention plans for persons with anxiety disorders?
- Develop a personal list of organizations in your area to which you could refer a patient after discharge from the physical therapy episode of care, to enable the person to maintain his or her gains related to anxiety symptoms (eg, aerobic fitness group).
- Identify at least 3 potential research or literature review questions you might explore to improve your clinical skills related to persons with anxiety disorders in your current or anticipated practice setting.

Case Studies: First Impressions

As you review the following case studies, you may want to consider these questions for thought or discussion:

- What standardized tests and measures (including psychiatric, for example, a depression screen) would you select for this patient? Why?
- Based on available data, what short- and long-term goals would you write for your plan of care? Consider using the acronyms SMART (specific, measurable, attainable, realistic, and timely) or ABCDE (actor, behavior, conditions, degree, and expected time frame) to guide your goal writing.
- What elements (procedures, psychosocial aspects, communication aspects, etc) would you make sure to include or omit in your plan of care for this patient? Why?
- What are your anticipated needs, if any, for consultation and referral for this patient?
- How will you transition this patient toward lasting health behavior change following discharge (eg, recommending a YMCA membership trial)?

Case 1

A 23-year-old female college soccer player was referred to outpatient physical therapy 2 weeks after a left combined anterior and medial cruciate ligament tear. Her goal is to return to practice by the end of the semester, which is 4 weeks away.

- Social history: she lives on campus on the third floor of a dormitory without an elevator available. She is involved in extracurricular activities, including theater (backstage this semester), a student service club, and campus worship services.
- Medical/psychiatric history: GAD (diagnosed 4 years previously), attention-deficit hyperactivity disorder, and pain medication prescribed occasionally impairs concentration
- Impairments, activity limitations, and participation restrictions found on initial interview and examination
    - Pain rated 8/10 at times in left knee, especially after using crutches to walk between classes
    - Left knee joint inflammation that impairs positioning while sitting
    - Left quadriceps weakness (able to hold knee straight against gravity without resistance)
    - Difficulty managing stairs to dormitory with backpack due to shortness of breath
    - Slightly decreased grades in 2 classes due to sleepiness from pain medications
    - Unable to participate in soccer practice

Case 2

A 41-year-old male construction worker is starting rehabilitation through worker's compensation for a back injury sustained in a fall from a 10-foot height through roof beams to the floor below. His goal is to return to work.

- Social history: he lives in a 2-story house with his wife, who works as a schoolteacher. Her parents assist with caring for their 2 children while both are at work. He has counseling twice per month for PTSD; finally, he reports difficulty with obtaining transportation to 25% of scheduled therapy appointments.
- Past medical and psychiatric history: recurrent lumbar disc protrusions, obesity, partial rotator cuff tear (2 years prior to current injury), PTSD from serving overseas in the military in his 20s, and a long history of taking low-dose opioid pain medications as needed

- Impairments, activity limitations, and participation restrictions found on initial interview and examination
  - Radiating pain throughout middle and lower back, especially in sitting and supine
  - Impaired single-limb balance and balance with eyes closed
  - Stiffness during postural transitions (supine/prone to quadruped and to standing)
  - Difficulty in accessing second story of house
  - Increased subjective anxiety and respiratory rate when in an open treatment area
  - Increased time and instruction needed to understand home exercise program handouts

Case 3

A 67-year-old male was admitted to subacute rehabilitation following a 3-week hospitalization for a right below-knee amputation. His goal is to get his prosthesis and return home.

- Social history: he lives alone in a ranch house with stoop step to enter. He is retired and widowed, but has adult children who live nearby.
- Medical/psychiatric history: panic disorder with agoraphobia, type 2 diabetes, obesity, hypertension, nicotine dependence, and coronary artery disease. He is on medications for all these conditions, as well as for pain and paresthesia due to amputation and diabetic neuropathy.
- Impairments, activity limitations, and participation restrictions found on initial interview and examination
  - Pain rated 9/10 with activity reported in residual limb
  - Phantom pain during the night, resulting in sleep disturbances and occasional falls due to trying to get out of bed unassisted
  - Difficulty complying with a diabetic diet as shown by a HbA1c value of 8.8 (a goal value for good glycemic control over the past 3 months is 7.0 or below)
  - Mild weakness in bilateral lower extremities
  - Slowly healing surgical wound
  - Good motivation to participate in therapies
  - Intermittent confusion when blood sugars are low

Quick Reference

- Possible diagnoses and their signs/symptoms:
  - GAD: constant worry, restlessness, fatigue, poor concentration, headache, nausea, or trouble falling asleep
  - Panic disorder: panic attacks in response to seemingly innocuous stimuli or situations; may include hyperventilation, heart racing, sense of impending doom, feeling of choking or smothering
  - PTSD: irritability, hypervigilance, insomnia, loneliness, anhedonia, intrusive thoughts, emotional detachment, hostility, or flashbacks
  - OCD: anxiety, depression, repetitive behavior (usually related to germs), impulsivity, hoarding, hypervigilance, compulsive behavior
  - Phobia: anxiety or panic symptoms related to a particular situation or object
- Questions to ask the patient (or friend/family member):
  - Do you often feel any of the symptoms (listed previously)?
  - Have you ever been diagnosed with one of the conditions (listed previously)? What was going on in your life around the time of that diagnosis?
  - How do you deal with your anxiety? How well does that work for you?
  - What should I know about what triggers your anxiety (or PTSD, OCD, phobia)?
- Referral options:
  - Psychiatrist for diagnosis, behavioral and pharmacological therapy
  - Support group for persons with similar conditions
  - Exercise group to capture benefits of aerobic exercise on anxiety sensitivity (after primary physician clearance for medical safety to exercise)

References

1. Wilde J. *Queens of Geek: Two Love Stories*. New York, NY: Swoon Reads; 2017.
2. Stuart GW. *Handbook of Psychiatric Nursing*. 6th ed. St. Louis, MO: Elsevier Mosby; 2005.
3. American Psychiatric Association. *Diagnostic and Statistical Manual of Mental Disorders*. 5th ed. Arlington, VA: American Psychiatric Association; 2013.
4. Sue D, Sue DW, Sue S. *Understanding Abnormal Behaviors*. 6th ed. Boston, MA: Houghton Mifflin; 2000.
5. Broocks A, Bandelow B, Pekrun G, et al. Comparison of aerobic exercise, clomipramine, and placebo in the treatment of panic disorder. *Am J Psychiatry*. 1998;155(5):603-609.
6. Byrne GH, Pachana NA. Anxiety and depression in the elderly: do we know any more? *Curr Opin Psychiatry*. 2010;23(6):504-509.
7. Barton S, Karner C, Salih F, Baldwin DS, Edwards SJ. Clinical effectiveness of interventions for treatment-resistant anxiety in older people: a systematic review. *Health Technol Assess*. 2014;18(50):1-59.
8. Solbakken OA, Abbass A. Intensive short-term dynamic residential treatment program for patients with treatment-resistant disorders. *J Affect Disord*. 2015;181:67-77.
9. Lewis CB, Bottomley JM. *Geriatric Rehabilitation: A Clinical Approach*. 3rd ed. Upper Saddle River, NJ: Pearson; 2008.
10. Jazaieri H, Goldin PR, Werner K, Ziv M, Gross JJ. A randomized trial of MBSR versus aerobic exercise for social anxiety disorder. *J Clin Psychol*. 2012;68(7):715-731.
11. Broman-Fulks JJ, Storey KM. Evaluation of a brief aerobic exercise intervention for high anxiety sensitivity. *Anxiety Stress Coping*. 2008;21(2):117-128.
12. Smits JAJ, Berry AC, Rosenfield D, et al. Reducing anxiety sensitivity with exercise. *Depress Anxiety*. 2008;25(8):689-699.

13. Hill JC, Lewis M, Sim J, Hay EM, Dziedzic K. Predictors of poor outcome in patients with neck pain treated by physical therapy. *Clin J Pain.* 2007;23(8):683-690.
14. Olesen J, Gustavsson A, Svensson M, Wittchen HU, Jönsson B. The economic cost of brain disorders in Europe. *Eur J Neurology.* 2012;19(1):155-162.
15. Bartley CA, Hay M, Bloch MH. Meta-analysis: aerobic exercise for the treatment of anxiety disorders. *Prog Neuropsychopharmacol Biol Psychiatry.* 2013;45:34-30.
16. Herring MP, Jacob ML, Suveg C, Dishman RK, O'Connor PJ. Feasibility of exercise training for the short-term treatment of generalized anxiety disorder: a randomized controlled trial. *Psychother Psychosom.* 2012;81(1):21-28.
17. Meyer T, Broocks A, Bandelow B, Hillmer-Vogel U, Rüther E. Endurance training in panic patients: spiroergometric and clinical effects. *Int J Sports Med.* 1998;19(7):496-502.
18. Breitve MH, Hynninen MJ, Kvåle A. The effect of psychomotor physical therapy on subjective health complaints and psychological symptoms. *Physiother Res Int.* 2010;15(4):212-221.
19. Sureka P, Govil S, Dash D, Dash C, Kumar M, Singhal V. Effect of Sudarshan Kriya on male prisoners with non psychotic psychiatric disorders: a randomized control trial. *Asian J Psychiatr.* 2014;12:43-49.
20. Kirkwood G, Rampes H, Tuffrey V, Richardson J, Pilkington K. Yoga for anxiety: a systematic review of the research evidence. *Br J Sports Med.* 2005;39(12):884-891.
21. Gaudlitz K, Plag J, Dimeo F, Ströhle A. Aerobic exercise training facilitates the effectiveness of cognitive behavioral therapy in panic disorder. *Depress Anxiety.* 2015;32(3):221-228.
22. Ganz FD, Jacobs JM. The effect of humor on elder mental and physical health. *Geriatr Nurs.* 2014;35(3):205-211.
23. Solbakken OA, Abbass A. Symptom and personality disorder changes in intensive short-term dynamic residential treatment for treatment-resistant anxiety and depressive disorder. *Acta Neuropsychiatr.* 2016;28(5):257-271. DOI: 10.1017/neu.2016.5
24. Baldacchino DR, Bonello L. Anxiety and depression in care homes in Malta and Australia: part 2. *Br J Nurs.* 2013;22(13):780-785.
25. Joyce J, Herbison GP. Reiki for depression and anxiety. *Cochrane Database Syst Rev.* 2015;(4):CD006833.
26. Haber D. *Health Promotion and Aging: Practical Applications for Health Professionals.* 4th ed. New York, NY: Springer; 2007.
27. Ventegodt S, Andersen NJ, Kandel I, Merrick J. Effect, side effects and adverse effects of non-pharmaceutical medicine. A review. *Int J Disabil Hum Dev.* 2009;8(3):227-235.

Depressive Disorders

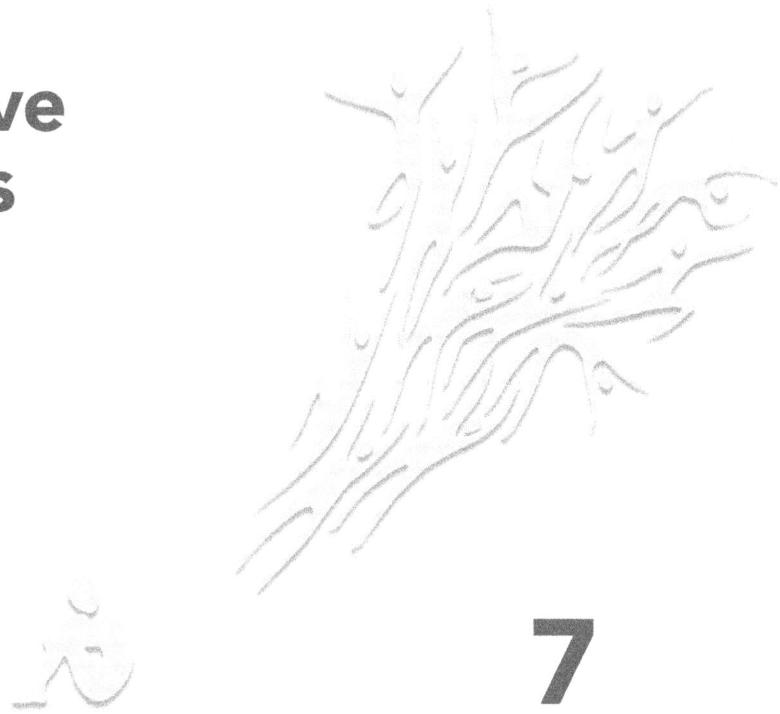

7

OUTLINE

- Scope and Classification of Depressive Disorders
- Neurophysiological Background, Etiology, and Risk Factors
- Comorbid Medical and Psychosocial Issues
  - Screening
  - Medication Concerns
  - Comorbidities
- Specific Clinical Approaches to Improve Physical Therapy Outcomes
  - Examination, Evaluation, and Diagnosis
  - Prognosis
  - Intervention
- Summary
- Key Points
- Review Questions
- Case Studies: First Impressions
- Quick Reference

Johnson H.
Psychosocial Elements of Physical Therapy: The Connection of Body to Mind (pp 123-138).

Learning Objectives

- Demonstrate awareness of depressive disorder diagnoses per the *Diagnostic and Statistical Manual of Mental Disorders, 5th edition* classification
- Summarize research related to changes in the human movement system for depressive disorders
- Incorporate risk factor assessment for a depressive disorder diagnosis into the patient interview
- Delineate impact of common comorbidities into patient care, per the patient management model
- Propose changes to the physical therapist's approach, based on each depressive disorder diagnosis, into assessments, exercise prescription, home exercise programs, building/maintaining rapport, and clinical documentation to increase successful outcomes

A physical therapist working in acute care reflects on the challenging case of a patient with comorbid depression, schizophrenia, and a failed suicide attempt by gunshot to the mouth:

> He came to us for surgery (total joint replacement). This was actually his second replacement, but he was not recovering as anticipated (compared to the other side); [he] ended up going to subacute and unfortunately fell so [he] had to come back for a pinning. With the frequent surgeries, anesthesia and changing environment, the patient had acute delirium. It was a challenge to redirect the patient, keep him focused on one task and to educate him on the importance of consistent therapy for recovery. No subacute facility would take him because of his history and recent fall plus acute delirium, so he stayed in our hospital for months. We got him to a point where he could safely be wheelchair level and returned home with caregiver support that he already had. The interesting part is when he came back to visit ... [he] walked in with his walker and told us about his experience: that he knew he was mentally off but could not control it and, even though he was delirious, he still remembered hearing what people said. Thankfully it was positive and no one said anything inappropriate (thinking he wouldn't understand or remember). He was very thankful and continues to complete therapy. (M. Hunter, PT, DPT, written communication, October 28, 2016)

Depressive disorders are common in patients seen by physical therapists, more common than anxiety or mania.[1] While the most common diagnosed depressive disorder is major depression, others include dysthymia (persistent mild depression), medication-induced depression, and disruptive mood dysregulation disorder. Additionally, depression occurs frequently with other medical conditions relevant to our scope of practice. This chapter discusses current literature related to physical therapy for various depressive disorders.

Scope and Classification of Depressive Disorders

Most people associate depression with a sad mood. However, this "is not an essential feature of the diagnosis."[2] Rather, a "triad of cognitive signs is a hallmark of depression ... the depressed person feels helpless, hopeless, and worthless."[2] Brünger and Spyra[3] examined the prevalence of depressive symptoms in German adults in rehabilitation settings. Depression rates (measured by the 2-question version of the Patient Health Questionnaire) were 4 times higher in persons in rehabilitation than in the general population (33.1% vs 7.8%), mostly in neurological and orthopedic settings, but least in cancer rehabilitation. "Depressive symptoms were significantly associated with higher comorbidity and impairment due to pain, with lower social support and self-efficacy and with specific work-related problems."[3] As noted in Chapter 5, depressive disorders include:

- Major depressive disorder (MDD): marked by intense and prolonged depressive symptoms without a manic phase
- Dysthymia: marked by chronic depressed mood over several years, but not severe enough to be classified as major depression
- Medication-induced depression: caused by anticonvulsants, barbiturates, benzodiazepines, beta blockers, calcium channel blockers, opioids, and statins, among others
- Disruptive mood dysregulation disorder: marked by persistent angry or irritable mood beyond what parents or teachers see as typical child moodiness
- Premenstrual dysphoric disorder (PMDD): marked by extreme mood shifts including depressive moods for several days prior to each menstrual period

Clinical depression appears different depending on the patient's age. While adolescents and children may withdraw from previously enjoyable activities, senior citizens may tend to have somatic symptoms including fatigue and insomnia.[3] This changing presentation, depending on age group, influences underdiagnosis and undertreatment, especially in geriatric clients. Only 50% of depressive diagnoses are treated in persons over 65 years old.[4]

Common symptoms and signs of depression in the elderly occur in the cognitive, somatic, and affective domains. Cognitive symptoms include "poor concentration, low self-esteem, indecisiveness, guilt, hopelessness, inability to concentrate, [and] suicidal ideations."[5] Somatic symptoms may include "fatigue, altered sleep patterns, weight gain or loss, tearfulness, agitation, heart palpitations, [and] overall weakness."[5] Finally, affective symptoms encompass "sadness, anxiety, irritability, fear, anger, depersonalization, [and] feelings of isolation (loneliness)."[5] The Geriatric Depression Scale (GDS) is a 30-question, publicly accessible yes/no questionnaire assessing these symptoms. The questionnaire has also been validated in a 15-question version for older adults. Web links for each screen and outcome measure are available in Appendix C.

More factors in geriatric depression include treatment setting, spousal or caregiver support, and the presence of physical disability. In persons over 65 years old living in the community, clinical depression affects 26% and major depression affects 6%. However, in long-term care settings, 35% have clinically significant depression, and 12% major depressive disorders.[4] As the population ages (over half of caregivers are over 50 years old), spousal depression risk increases significantly, especially if the spouse is the caregiver. If a spouse or other social support disappears or passes away, and if the person's perceived health status becomes poorer, suicide risk increases; age is directly proportional to suicide risk.

Certain aspects of the patient's past medical history are directly relevant to depression. Diseases that can cause depression include Parkinson's disease, stroke, dementias, coronary artery disease, cerebrovascular disease, and multiple sclerosis.[4] This can be due to the disease process itself or to increased disability related to secondary impairments from the diseases. "Some of the dangers of not treating depression [in geriatrics] are increased risk of suicide and mortality, increased physical disability, and increased risk for complications of other medical conditions."[4] However, "overall, depression has long been considered to be the most treatable psychiatric disorder affecting older adults."[4] This involves an interdisciplinary team/interprofessional team including the physical therapist.

Presentation of depression may be compared to that of bipolar disorder (see Chapter 8) and borderline personality disorder (see Chapter 10) as shown by a table from Malhi et al[6] in their comprehensive, publicly accessible clinical practice guidelines for multidisciplinary management of mood disorders.

Neurophysiological Background, Etiology, and Risk Factors

At the microscopic level, depression is related to several abnormalities in brain chemistry and structure. As noted in Chapter 5, glutamate transmission changes are associated with depression; additionally, "low levels of serotonin are associated with depression and suicidal behaviors" due to effects on mood and pain perception.[7] Common classes of antidepressants (monoamine oxidase inhibitors, tricyclic antidepressants, and selective serotonin reuptake inhibitors [SSRIs]) act to increase alpha-1 and serotonin receptors in the brain while decreasing abnormal activity in beta receptors. Brain-derived neurotrophic factor (BDNF) is related, if sometimes unclearly, to multiple disorders, including MDD. In a study examining aerobic treadmill exercise vs electroconvulsive therapy or a combination of the 2 for treating MDD, the combined intervention decreased depressive symptoms and increased plasma BDNF levels the most; however, "BDNF levels were not associated with symptoms of depression,"[8] thus leaving the question open as to the molecule's reliability as a biomarker.

Structurally, left prefrontal cortex damage is also associated with depression.[7] Consequently, areas of cognitive dysfunction in MDD include "attention, verbal and nonverbal learning and memory, and executive functioning."[9] Greer et al[9] found a dose-response relationship between exercise (as an adjunct to antidepressant medication) and cognitive dysfunction areas of "psychomotor speed, attention, visual memory and spatial planning." Also, a recent bout of exercise, in persons with current or past depression, can desensitize or habituate the person to stimuli that would otherwise induce a sad mood; the mechanism of action is still unknown.[10]

Risk factors for depression, especially in the elderly, include pain, level of disability, number of comorbidities, and nutritional deficits including failure to thrive.[11] Like all mental health conditions, depression's etiology is multifactorial, including biological differences, neurochemical differences, genetic predisposition, and hormonal changes. Since depression often begins in one's third or fourth decade, specific risk factors in the younger to middle-aged adult population include low self-esteem, pessimism, history of stressful or traumatic events or circumstances, personal history of mental health issues or chronic disease, substance abuse, certain medications, and first-degree relatives with a mood disorder.[12]

Comorbid Medical and Psychosocial Issues

That's the thing about depression: A human being can survive almost anything, as long as she sees the end in sight. But depression is so insidious, and it compounds daily, that it's impossible to ever see the end.

—Elizabeth Wurtzel[13]

Across the lifespan, depressive disorders increase the risk of medical comorbidities, functional decline, and inability to remain living independently. These risks may be due to primary symptoms, as well as medications for depression. Thus, it is important for the clinician to know how to screen for depression, what risk factors may be present, and when to refer to a specialist for more effective patient care.

Screening

Physical therapists do not rate or notice depression accurately when using subjective information or decision-making processes. To increase objectivity, therapists can use "a 2-item screening test for depression taken from the Primary Care Evaluation of Mental Disorders Procedure (PRIME-MD)," which is accessible at www.emich.edu/psychology/forms/prime-md_adult_only.pdf.[14] These questions are:

- "During the past month, have you often been bothered by feeling down, depressed, or hopeless?"
- "During the past month, have you often been bothered by little interest or pleasure in doing things?"

A "yes" answer to one or both of these questions prompts follow-up questions about secondary symptoms, such as impaired sleep, impaired appetite, loss of energy, impaired concentration, feelings of worthlessness, psychomotor retardation (slower movement or speech than normal), and suicidal thoughts or plans.

While the PRIME-MD may be used to screen any patient for depression, Williams[11] notes that geriatric or cognitively impaired individuals, especially in long-term care, need adapted screening procedures. While dementia is the most common psychiatric pathology in a skilled nursing facility, depression is the second. Many residents have comorbid depression and dementia. For geriatric depression, clinicians should know that commonly prescribed SSRIs increase fall risk. Thus, the therapist may need to select strength training over aerobic training to manage this fall risk, and potentially increase patient adherence, per recommendations for geriatric rehabilitation.[11]

In residents with comorbid cognitive impairment or dementia, the GDS is best for mild to moderate dementia because the Hamilton Depression Rating Scale (commonly used in research studies) is inappropriate. When a resident is non-verbal, the Apparent Emotions Rating is preferred:

> Actions signifying anxiety include furrowed brow, motor restlessness, repeated motions, sighing, hand wringing, crying, hyperventilation, and clinging. Signals of depression include crying, sad facial expression, slowness to respond, turning away, slow motor activity, and downcast eyes.[11]

If it is not clear whether a patient with depression also has dementia, screening tools need to guide clinical reasoning. Vieira et al notes that it is within the physical therapist's scope of practice, and indeed an essential **competency area, to administer outcome measures for cognition and depression; refer as needed; adapt communication style; and "differentiate between depression, delirium, and dementia on the basis of symptoms and comorbidities"** (see also Chapter 11).[15] However, screening in older adult populations can be "complicated by coexisting medical illness, pain, cognitive impairment, anxiety, and disability."[15] Thus, besides the PRIME-MD questions about anhedonia and depressed mood, and follow-up questions about secondary symptoms, the 15-question version of the GDS is useful in patients who can accurately report emotional symptoms. Since caregivers may "be unaware of behavioral symptoms associated with depression,"[15] the clinician can use the semi-structured patient interview format of the Cornell Scale for Depression in Dementia, which also assesses cognitive impairment. Refer to Table 1 in Vieira et al[15] and Appendix C of this book for online resources for therapists, families, and patients with depressive disorders.

Medication Concerns

In older adults, SSRI antidepressants can increase fall risk and subsequent injury. On the other end of the lifespan, a case report described antidepressant-induced mania and behavioral activation, or "increased activity, aggression, sleep disturbance, disinhibition, and subjective feelings of increased energy."[16] Risk factors for these serious side effects include "mental retardation, anxiety disorders, autism spectrum disorders, and tic disorders" in children, hence a black-box warning for antidepressants including sertraline.

In adults, antidepressants are associated with acute or chronic side effects in 63% of users. Benign, acute side effects include "diarrhea, dizziness, dry mouth, headaches, nausea, sweating, [and] tremors," while more dangerous effects include "drowsiness or confusion, feelings of panic or dread, increased thoughts of suicide, insomnia … nervousness and agitation, [and] weight gain."[17] Chronic diseases associated with use include type 2 diabetes mellitus, increased fracture risk, and gastrointestinal bleeding.

Also, psychotropic medications or anxiety may change blood pressure; hypothyroidism, co-occurring with depression, may decrease heart rate; and anxiety symptoms may cause sinus tachycardia. Antidepressant medications vary in tolerability and efficacy; the most efficacious classes are SSRIs, serotonin/norepinephrine reuptake inhibitors, tricyclic antidepressants, and monoamine oxidase inhibitors. Adults using most antidepressants (except SSRIs) may have severe and irritating side effects, such as weight gain, anticholinergic effects, and central nervous system sedation or agitation.[6]

Comorbidities

In a patient with depression, pain is an important comorbidity for the clinician to consider. Since depression decreases recovery from low back pain,[14] lumbar stenosis surgery,[18] fusion surgery for chronic low back pain,[19] and neck pain (especially in older individuals),[20] therapists need to pay attention to assessing and managing pain. **If possible, the plan of care needs to be lengthened**, to allow time for mood effects of exercise,[21] rapport, motivational interviewing and other techniques (see Chapter 4), and combating the psychomotor retardation that is common in depression.

Sedentary behavior due to depressive symptoms leads to other medical conditions, which can delay functional recovery in the acute hospital setting and cascade into earlier placement into long-term care.[2,22] Depression strongly predicts traumatic brain injury in adults over age 65.[23] This may be due to deconditioning that increases fall risk as the individual becomes weaker and less flexible. Metabolic syndrome, type 2 diabetes, and cardiovascular disease are so-called "sitting diseases," which are more common in persons with depression; Knapen et al[24] strongly advocate motivational strategies with exercise-focused physical therapy plans of care to combat these conditions. Malhi et al[6] note that these comorbidities, as well as chronic obstructive pulmonary disease, obstructive sleep apnea, and obesity, are related to inactivity.

Physical therapists can target depression-related metabolic symptoms. In persons with moderate to severe depression, a 6-week, thrice-weekly adjunctive exercise program significantly improved aerobic capacity, waist circumference, and high-density lipoprotein cholesterol levels.[25] Alosaimi and Baker[26] examining cognitive behavioral therapy, principles of which many clinicians use, found superior effects of cognitive behavioral therapy over medication. To facilitate antidepressant medication review in persons with comorbid depression and cardiac disease, they noted that:

> [S]ertraline, citalopram, and mirtazapine were safe from a cardiac perspective, but only sertraline and citalopram were clearly more effective than placebo in [coronary heart disease] patients with moderate-to-severe type, recurrent MDD, or MDD episode onset before the [coronary heart disease] event.[26]

Besides addressing pain and metabolic changes, clinicians should be aware of risk factors for relapse into depression. Several risk factors can be changed: stress level, poor management of medical comorbidities, non-compliance with treatment regimens, substance use, and poor social support. Factors that are difficult or impossible to change include female gender, severe or prolonged depression, presence of psychosis, and residual symptoms.[6] Taken together, these comorbidities, risk factors, and associated psychosocial issues have a high cost; Olesen et al[27] conservatively estimate the cost of mood disorders (including depression and anxiety) as at least 113.4 billion euros ($122.2 billion in 2017) in Europe in 2010.

Specific Clinical Approaches to Improve Physical Therapy Outcomes

Listen to the people who love you. Believe that they are worth living for even when you don't believe it. Seek out the memories depression takes away and project them into the future. Be brave; be strong; take your pills. Exercise because it's good for you even if every step weighs a thousand pounds. Eat when food itself disgusts you. Reason with yourself when you have lost your reason.

—Andrew Solomon[28]

This section is organized according to the patient management model from the *Guide to Physical Therapist Practice 3.0*.[29] Throughout, the benefits of clinicians providing and facilitating social support can be seen, especially in the geriatric population.[30]

Examination, Evaluation, and Diagnosis

For a patient with depression, the clinician can alter the examination and evaluation process in the following ways. Interpersonally, the clinician should practice patience and rapport skills (see Chapter 4) and assess for risk factors (see previous section). For geriatric patients with depression, which commonly overlaps with delirium, mild cognitive impairment, or dementia, use additional outcome measures.[31] Documentation of tests and knowing risk factors, symptoms, and behaviors for each disorder is essential to geriatric care.

Beyond the PRIME-MD screen with follow-up (comprising the Patient Health Questionnaire-9) and GDS, clinicians may confidently and quickly use the following accessible scales for depressive symptoms in cognitively intact individuals[31] (see Appendix C for links to these scales):

- Center for Epidemiologic Studies Depression Scale: a 20-question scale indicating likely depression with a score over 16.
- Beck Depression Inventory: a 21-item measure differentiating between borderline, mild, moderate, and severe depression.
- Zung Self-Rating Depression Scale: a 20-item Likert scale with a score over 50 indicating depression.

For coexisting depression and cognitive impairment, the Cornell Scale for Depression in Dementia, a 30-minute caregiver and patient interview, examines mood-related signs, behavioral disturbances, physical signs, cyclic functions (sleep-wake alterations), and ideational disturbance (pessimism or suicidal thoughts). The Delirium Rating Scale (accessible by request to its developer) can be used to differentiate delirium, dementia, schizophrenia, and depression. While the physical therapist may not make a medical diagnosis, this screening knowledge can guide the psychosocial aspects of the plan of care.

Prognosis

Insurance companies need to be aware (via physical therapist documentation) of research supporting longer episodes of care for better outcomes in people with depression; also, the clinician can rely on rapport and social support to increase patient participation for more successful treatment outcomes. For the geriatric practitioner, Wallace et al[32] note that older adults tend to use disengagement strategies more than engagement strategies to combat late-life depression. While younger adults may prefer engagement (ie, "the investment of cognitive and behavioral resources to achieve health goals"), **older adults usually use "the withdrawal of these resources from obsolete or unattainable health goals, combined with goal restructuring."**[32] This may be due to the increased energy cost for practically all activities, mental and physical, in the aging body.

Exercise supervision by a physical therapist affects participation in the episode of care. In exercise-related randomized controlled trials including people with depression, those with MDD drop out 17.2% of the time, while 18.1% of normal controls drop out prior to study completion. Since this meta-analysis did not specify the severity of depressive symptoms in each specific study, one cannot assign a "typical" severity (mild, moderate, or severe) to this slightly lower rate. However, drop-out rate increased with "higher baseline depressive symptoms" and decreased with more "supervised interventions delivered by physiotherapists and exercise physiologists."[33]

A home exercise program (HEP) is vital for carryover of progress after discharge from therapy. Picorelli et al[34] found that weighting the plan of care towards supervised vs unsupervised exercise programs improved adherence rates for geriatric patients, with fewer depressive symptoms and better cognitive levels also improving adherence. Finally, Forkan et al[35] found that older adults are less affected by motivators than by barriers to HEP adherence, with a non-adherence rate of 37%. Barriers to carry-through, over a 3-year follow-up, were "no interest, poor health, weather, depression, weakness, fear of falling, shortness of breath, and low outcomes expectation."[35] It is important, especially in geriatric patients with depression, for the clinician and each patient to talk through personal barriers for solutions.

Intervention

General or unspecified physical exercise is well-researched for depressive symptoms and secondary impairments. A meta-analysis controlling for heterogeneity of studies found that any exercise modality lessens depressive symptoms; supervised exercise showed a small additional benefit over unsupervised.[36] Focusing on neurologic disorders, including Alzheimer's disease, Parkinson's disease, and stroke, Adamson et al[37] found that any exercise modality meeting the American College of Sports Medicine (ACSM) guidelines produced a moderate effect size (0.38), improving depressive symptoms, while exercise not meeting ACSM guidelines produced a small positive effect size (0.19). However, a meta-analysis found no difference between physical activity interventions meeting ACSM guidelines or not; **all studies showed large positive impacts on depressive symptoms and moderate effects on aerobic capacity.**[38]

Methodological quality and sample size of trials affect applicability of research interventions; 3 papers critique the universal application of exercise as a sole treatment for depression. A large, individualized pragmatic trial with 12-month follow-up found that telephone-based facilitation of physical activity caused an increase in activity levels, but this increase may not have been large enough "to lead to a measurable influence" on depression or use of medications.[39] This intervention was also less cost-effective than medication alone.

Chalder et al noted that "only more vigorous activity might be of benefit [and] previous studies had only recruited individuals with a pre-existing commitment to physical activity."[39] In a Cochrane systematic review, Cooney et al[40] found only "a smaller effect in favour [sic] of exercise. When compared to psychological or pharmacological therapies [alone], exercise appears to be no more effective, though this conclusion is based on a few small trials." Finally, a study of patients over age 65, with physical disability and living in assisted-living or long-term care facilities, in a 3-month, high-intensity functional weightbearing exercise program improved depressive symptoms only in persons with dementia and only at 3-month follow-up.[41] Table 7-1 summarizes other studies.

Table 7-1

Aerobic Exercise Interventions for Depressive Disorders

STUDY	INTERVENTION	FINDINGS
Babyak et al[42]	6-month follow-up to a 4-month trial of sertraline vs aerobic exercise	"Exercising on one's own during the follow-up period was associated with a reduced probability of depression diagnosis at the end of that period"[42]
Crumbie et al[43]	Dance at moderate intensity for 1 hour, 1 to 2 times per week, for 10 to 15 weeks, individual or group	Improved depressive symptoms, well-being, balance, function, cognition, socialization, and psychological stress
Danielsson et al[44]	Physical therapist-guided aerobic exercise to fight symptoms of "numbness and stagnation"[44]; study used semi-structured interviews	Patient-perceived themes: "(1) struggling toward a healthy self, (2) challenging the resistance, (3) feeling active but not euphoric, and (4) needing someone to be there for you"[44]
Hoffman et al[45]	For adults over age 40 with mild depression: supervised aerobics 3 times per week at 70% to 85% of heart rate reserve vs HEP or sertraline x 4 months	Improved aerobic fitness, but no more cognitive improvement (verbal memory, working memory, and verbal fluency) than sertraline takers
Hoffman et al[46]	1-year follow-up to 4-month trial of sertraline vs aerobic exercise	"Exercise during the follow-up period seems to extend the short-term benefits of exercise [on depression] and may augment the benefits of antidepressant use"[46]
Legrand and Neff[47]	10-day adjunctive aerobics vs stretching for inpatients just started on antidepressant medication	Aerobics superior to stretching; both groups improved in Beck Depression Inventory scores significantly
Mota-Pereira et al[48]	For treatment-resistant depression: 30 to 45 minutes per day of walking, 5 times per week for 12 weeks, with 1 walk per week supervised	Depression scores improved, 21% response and 26% remission vs 0% for medication alone
Oertel-Knöchel et al[49]	45-minute aerobic exercise (vs mental relaxation training) 3 times per week for 4 weeks, combined with cognitive training in psychiatric inpatient setting	Depressive symptoms significantly improved, with moderate improvement in cognitive performance and subjective quality of life
Silveira et al[50]	Systematic review comparing progressive resistance exercise to aerobic exercise	Age and symptom severity influenced outcome; both types significantly effective

Other modes of physical exercise for depression have varied benefits. Mind-body interventions include yoga, Sudarshan Kriya, and Norwegian psychomotor physical therapy. In Chapter 6, each of these interventions showed promise for anxiety symptoms; the same results hold for depressive symptoms:

- Yoga: a systematic review recommends yoga for short-term improvement of depression.[51]
- Sudarshan Kriya: a 6-week, daily intervention of adults with mood disorders, instructed to sit comfortably in a supportive chair, while focusing on breathing with eyes closed significantly improved depressive symptoms and other health indicators.[52]
- Norwegian psychomotor physical therapy: a 6- to 12-month intervention of body awareness, therapist validation of the patient's "invisible" symptoms, therapeutic exercises to correct movement, and massage or manual therapy techniques significantly improved depressive symptoms.[53]

Weather and environment permitting, some patients may prefer still other modes of exercise. One 12-week intervention of Nordic walking, with handheld poles, 3 hourly sessions per week, improved depressive symptoms, lower extremity strength, and balance in cognitively intact but physically frail adults over age 70.[54] Meekums et al[55] and Verrusio et al[56] studied dance movement therapy in elderly subjects with depression. While the 2015 systematic review found only low-quality evidence supporting this therapy, the 2014 pilot study found a significant short- and long-term improvement in stress biomarkers and depressive symptoms in combined exercise and music therapy as compared to medication only. Refer to Chapter 6 for a discussion of complementary and alternative therapies.

Various other exercise modalities have been studied as well. Virtual reality dance exercise, 30 minutes per day at 5 times per week, combined with 30 minutes of neurodevelopmental treatment and 15 minutes of functional electrical stimulation for 6 weeks improved depressive symptoms in patients with Parkinson's disease, which commonly causes depression.[57] A 9-week telerehabilitation intervention of internet-delivered educational modules, with weekly guidance by a therapist, significantly improved depressive symptoms but not physical activity levels at 6-month follow-up.[58] This study did not specify the content of each module, thus opening a research direction into tailoring content to specific impairments or functional limitations by the physical therapist.

Since many exercise modalities adjunctively treat depression, how does the clinician choose the best one for a patient? **Given the 3 principles of evidence-based practice (patient preference, clinician expertise, and high-quality research), the bottom line is to select treatments using more social support to encourage more physical activity for a longer time**, while documenting the therapist's skill and judgment. Dunn et al[59] found a dose-response relationship between intensity of physical exercise and reduction in depressive symptoms over 12 weeks. Solbakken and Abbass[60,61] examined a multidisciplinary intervention for treatment-resistant psychological conditions (see Chapter 6). Mather et al[62] noted a modest short- and long-term response of 10 weeks of group exercise in treatment-resistant depression, where medications had failed to resolve the initial disorder. Nyström et al[63] summarize that **"individually customized [physical activity] for at least 30 minutes, preferably performed under supervision and with a frequency of at least three times per week is recommended when treating MDD."**

Summary

Depression is a multifactorial collection of disorders, influenced by genetic predisposition; environmental trauma; some medications; and other medical conditions, including neurological disorders such as Parkinson's disease, stroke, and multiple sclerosis. Any depressive disorder increases the risk for metabolic syndrome, cardiovascular and pulmonary conditions, cognitive impairment, and functional decline. Thus, effective physical therapist management of this population requires familiarity with the scope of the patient's physical and mental health impairments, side effects of antidepressants, and specific preferences for exercise mode to tailor the plan of care. Increasing social support for the patient is important for success, whether by the clinician alone or by an interdisciplinary team/interprofessional team.

Key Points

- The geriatric clinician should be able to differentiate delirium, depression, and dementia by their symptoms and signs.
- If possible, treat persons with depression over longer periods to allow exercise to improve mood.
- Due to decreased physical and mental resources, older adults may tend to revise their therapy goals and divert resources away from goals they perceive as unattainable.
- Aerobic exercise, regardless of meeting ACSM guidelines, has a large positive impact on depressive symptoms and a moderate impact on aerobic capacity.
- Use evidence-based practice (patient preference, clinician expertise, and published research) to choose treatments high in social support for promoting permanent physical activity habits.
- MDD best benefits from tailored physical activity, 30 or more minutes at least 3 times per week, under physical therapist supervision.

Review Questions

- Referring to Malhi et al,[6] in your own words, compare and contrast MDD, bipolar disorders, and borderline personality disorder.
- Why is a medication review for each patient (regardless of a diagnosis of depression) important?
- What are some ways you might incorporate a broader focus on aerobic conditioning into your plans of care, especially for persons with depressive disorders?
- Reflect on your preferred management of common comorbidities to depression. What factors related to the depressive disorder itself would prompt you to alter your approach? How?
- In your current or most recent clinical practice setting, what movement system impairments have you seen more commonly in patients with depression vs those without?
- Instead of prescribing a HEP at the middle or end of an episode of care, how might you customize your approach to benefit patients with depression on your current or past caseload?
- Recall, if applicable, a patient over 65 years old that you have worked with who has depression as well as cognitive impairment.
  - How did you screen for depressive symptoms, given the cognitive impairment?
  - Was your patient evaluation and case management effective?
  - How did you measure this effectiveness?
  - How might you become more effective in the future, based on new knowledge from this chapter?

Case Studies: First Impressions

As you review the following case studies, you may want to consider these questions for thought or discussion:

- What standardized tests and measures (including psychiatric, for example, a depression screen) would you select for this patient? Why?
- Based on available data, what short- and long-term goals would you write for your plan of care? Consider using the acronyms SMART (specific, measurable, attainable, realistic, and timely) or ABCDE (actor, behavior, conditions, degree, and expected time frame) to guide your goal writing.
- What elements (procedures, psychosocial aspects, communication aspects, etc) would you make sure to include or omit in your plan of care for this patient? Why?
- What are your anticipated needs, if any, for consultation and referral for this patient?
- How will you transition this patient toward lasting health behavior change following discharge (eg, recommending a YMCA membership trial)?

Case 1

A 30-year-old female was referred to outpatient physical therapy 1 week after surgery for a traumatic right hip labral tear. Her goals are to return to walking 2 miles daily and resuming normal activity as a high school teacher.

- Social history: she needs to carpool to work, and she lives alone in a first-floor apartment without family nearby.
- Medical/psychiatric history: PMDD, carpal tunnel syndrome, history of patellofemoral syndrome, and currently taking ibuprofen and prescribed oxycodone as needed for pain
- Impairments, activity limitations, and participation restrictions found on initial interview and examination
    - Intermittent dull pain and subjective weakness in right hip and knee musculature
    - Currently requires single-point cane for weightbearing-as-tolerated surgical restriction
    - Standing tolerance limited to 5 minutes by pain
    - Walking tolerance limited to one-quarter mile by pain and fatigue

Case 2

A 52-year-old male living in a group home was referred to home health physical therapy due to recent falls involving loss of balance or tripping over objects. His goal is to stay in the group home; his caregivers would like the incidence of falls to decrease by 75%.

- Social history: he lives in a single-story group home with 5 other residents and a ramp to enter. He receives limited assistance and cues as needed from caregivers to complete activities of daily living. Physically, he has a sedentary lifestyle.
- Medical/psychiatric history: MDD (single episode), developmental delay, coronary artery disease, obesity, osteopenia, and asthma. He refuses medications from staff approximately one-third of the time.
- Impairments, activity limitations, and participation restrictions found on initial interview and examination
  - Generalized joint stiffness, especially in large joints, noted from a young age
  - Shortness of breath with exertion
  - Hip and knee extensor weakness
  - Wide-based gait pattern without an assistive device
  - Difficulty standing unsupported when lights are dimmed or off

Case 3

A 73-year-old female in an assisted living setting was referred to home health physical therapy after a hospitalization for exacerbation of congestive heart failure. Her goal is to be able to transfer herself independently and easily, without staff assistance.

- Social history: she has been widowed for 6 years and has 2 adult children who, though local, do not often visit. The assisted living facility offers activities she occasionally participates in.
- Medical/psychiatric history: Currently seeing a speech therapist for difficulty in safely consuming regular-consistency foods and thin liquids. She has dysthymia, generalized anxiety disorder, chronic obstructive pulmonary disease, stage 2 chronic kidney disease, coronary artery disease, hyperlipidemia, and mild left hemiparesis from a stroke at age 70 (she is right-hand dominant). She is on medications for all conditions except dysthymia, as she had a medication interaction the last time she tried antidepressants.
- Impairments, activity limitations, and participation restrictions found on initial interview and examination
  - Shortness of breath at rest and increased with activity
  - Currently requires 50% assistance for transfers and ambulating within her room to the bathroom (previously was able to walk to and from meals independently with a 4-wheeled walker)
  - Currently on oxygen as needed via nasal cannula (previously on none)
  - Moderate weakness in trunk and lower extremity musculature grossly

Quick Reference

- Possible diagnoses and their signs/symptoms:
  - MDD: poor appetite, weight and sleep changes, slow activity, poor concentration, social isolation, guilt, anhedonia
  - Dysthymia: milder symptoms but of longer duration than MDD
  - Medication-induced depression: a side effect within a month of starting beta blockers, corticosteroids, benzodiazepines, stimulants, anti-Parkinson's medications, anticonvulsants, proton pump inhibitors, anticholinergic gastrointestinal medications, and statins
  - Disruptive mood disorder: severe tantrums, irritability, and anger
  - PMDD: mood swings, sleep changes, bloating, self-critical thoughts, pelvic or breast pain
- Questions to ask the patient (or friend/family member):
  - Do you often feel any of the symptoms (listed previously)?
  - Have you ever been diagnosed with a depressive disorder (listed previously)? What was going on in your life around the time of that diagnosis?
  - How do you deal with your depression? How well does that work for you?
  - What should I know about your depression?
- Referral options:
  - Psychiatrist for diagnosis, behavioral and pharmacological therapy
  - Support group for persons with similar conditions
  - Exercise group to capture benefits of aerobic exercise and socialization on depression (after primary physician clearance for medical safety to exercise)

References

1. Sue D, Sue DW, Sue S. *Understanding Abnormal Behaviors*. 6th ed. Boston, MA: Houghton Mifflin; 2000.
2. Drench ME, Noonan AC, Sharby N, Ventura SH. *Psychosocial Aspects of Health Care*. 3rd ed. Upper Saddle River, NJ: Pearson; 2012.
3. Brünger M, Spyra K. Prevalence of comorbid depressive symptoms in rehabilitation: a cross-indication, nationwide observational study. *J Rehabil Med*. 2016;48(10):70-75.
4. Blackburn JA, Dulmus CN. *Handbook of Gerontology: Evidence-Based Approaches to Theory, Practice, and Policy*. Hoboken, NJ: Wiley; 2007.
5. Lewis CB, Bottomley JM. *Geriatric Rehabilitation: A Clinical Approach*. 3rd ed. Upper Saddle River, NJ: Pearson; 2008.
6. Malhi GS, Bassett D, Boyce P, et al. Royal Australian and New Zealand College of Psychiatrists clinical practice guidelines for mood disorders. *Aust N Z J Psychiatry*. 2015;49(12):1087-1206.
7. Lundy-Ekman L. *Neuroscience: Fundamentals for Rehabilitation*. 3rd ed. St. Louis, MO: Saunders; 2007.
8. Salehi I, Hosseini SM, Haghighi M, et al. Electroconvulsive therapy (ECT) and aerobic exercise training (AET) increased plasma BDNF and ameliorated depressive symptoms in patients suffering from major depressive disorder. *J Psychiatr Res*. 2016;76:1-8.
9. Greer TL, Grannemann BD, Chansard M, Karim AI, Trivedi MH. Dose-dependent changes in cognitive function with exercise augmentation for major depression: results from the TREAD study. *Eur Neuropsychopharmacol*. 2015;25(2):248-256.
10. Mata J, Hogan CL, Joormann J, Waugh CE, Gotlib IH. Acute exercise attenuates negative affect following repeated sad mood inductions in persons who have recovered from depression. *J Abn Psychol*. 2013;122(1):45-50. DOI: 10.1037/a0029881
11. Williams AK. Psychosocial issues in long-term care. *Top Geriatr Rehabil*. 1999;15(2):14-21.

12. Mayo Clinic Staff. Depression (major depressive disorder). *Mayo Clinic*. http://www.mayoclinic.org/diseases-conditions/depression/basics/definition/con-20032977. Published February 3, 2018. Accessed February 21, 2018.
13. Wurtzel E. *Prozac Nation*. Boston, MA: Houghton Mifflin; 1994.
14. Haggman S, Maher CG, Refshauge KM. Screening for symptoms of depression by physical therapists managing low back pain. *Phys Ther*. 2004;84(12):1157-1166.
15. Vieira ER, Brown E, Raue P. Depression in older adults: screening and referral. *J Geriatr Phys Ther*. 2014;37(1):24-30.
16. Bradshaw DM, Young-Walker L. An 11-year-old girl with suicidal thoughts, hallucinations. *Psychiatr Ann*. 2011;41(8):386-389.
17. Consumer Reports. Using antidepressants to treat depression: comparing effectiveness, safety, and price. *Consumer Reports Best Buy Drugs*. https://www.consumerreports.org/cro/2013/09/best-treatments-for-depression/index.htm. Accessed May 2, 2018.
18. Sinikallio S, Lehto SM, Aalto T, Airaksinen O, Kröger H, Viinamäki H. Depressive symptoms during rehabilitation period predict poor outcome of lumbar spinal stenosis surgery: a two-year perspective. *BMC Musculoskelet Disord*. 2010;11:152.
19. Daubs MD, Norvell DC, McGuire R, et al. Fusion versus nonoperative care for chronic low back pain. *Spine*. 2011;36(suppl 21):S96-S109.
20. Hill JC, Lewis M, Sim J, Hay EM, Dziedzic K. Predictors of poor outcome in patients with neck pain treated by physical therapy. *Clin J Pain*. 2007;23(8):683-690.
21. Blumenthal JA, Babyak MA, Moore KA, et al. Effects of exercise training on older patients with major depression. *Arch Intern Med*. 1999;159(19):2349-2356.
22. Lohmann S, Strobl R, Mueller M, Huber EO, Grill E. Psychosocial factors associated with the effects of physiotherapy in the acute hospital. *Disabil Rehabil*. 2011;33(23-24):2311-2321.
23. Dams-O'Connor K, Gibbons LE, Landau A, Larson EB, Crane PK. Health problems precede traumatic brain injury in older adults. *J Am Geriatr Soc*. 2016;64(4):844-848.
24. Knapen J, Vancampfort D, Moriën Y, Marchal Y. Exercise therapy improves both mental and physical health in patients with major depression. *Disabil Rehabil*. 2015; 37(16):1490-1495.
25. Kerling A, Tegtbur U, Gützlaff E, et al. Effects of adjunctive exercise on physiological and psychological parameters in depression: a randomized pilot trial. *J Affect Disord*. 2015;177:1-6.
26. Alosaimi FD, Baker B. Clinical review of treatment options for major depressive disorder in patients with coronary heart disease. *Saudi Med J*. 2012;33(11):1159-1168.
27. Olesen J, Gustavsson A, Svensson M, Wittchen HU, Jönsson B; CDBE2010 Study Group; European Brain Council. The economic cost of brain disorders in Europe. *Eur J Neurology*. 2012;19(1):155-162.
28. Solomon A. *The Noonday Demon: An Atlas of Depression*. New York, NY: Scribner; 2001.
29. American Physical Therapy Association. Guide to Physical Therapist Practice 3.0. *APTA*. http://guidetoptpractice.apta.org/. Updated 2016. Accessed February 21, 2018.
30. Baldacchino DR, Bonello L. Anxiety and depression in care homes in Malta and Australia: part 2. *Br J Nurs*. 2013;22(13):780-785.
31. Francis NJ. Assessment tools for geriatric patients with delirium, mild cognitive impairment, dementia, and depression. *Top Geriatr Rehabil*. 2012;28(3):137-147.
32. Wallace ML, Dombrovski AY, Morse JQ, et al. Coping with health stresses and remission from late-life depression in primary care: a two-year prospective study. *Int J Geriatr Psychiatry*. 2012;27(2):178-186.
33. Stubbs B, Vancampfort D, Rosenbaum, et al. Dropout from exercise randomized controlled trials among people with depression: a meta-analysis and meta regression. *J Affect Disord*. 2016;190:457-466.
34. Picorelli AMA, Pereira LSM, Pereira DS, Felício D, Sherrington C. Adherence to exercise programs for older people is influenced by program characteristics and personal factors: a systematic review. *J Physiother*. 2014;60(3):151-156.
35. Forkan R, Pumper B, Smyth N, Wirkkala H, Ciol MA, Shumway-Cook A. Exercise adherence following physical therapy intervention in older adults with impaired balance. *Phys Ther*. 2006;86(3):401-410.
36. Schuch FB, Vancampfort D, Richards J, Rosenbaum S, Ward PB, Stubbs B. Exercise as a treatment for depression: a meta-analysis adjusting for publication bias. *J Psychiatr Res*. 2016;77:42-51.
37. Adamson BC, Ensari I, Motl RW. Effect of exercise on depressive symptoms in adults with neurologic disorders: a systematic review and meta-analysis. *Arch Phys Med Rehabil*. 2015;96(7):1329-1338.
38. Rosenbaum S, Tiedemann A, Sherrington C, Curtis J, Ward PB. Physical activity interventions for people with mental illness: a systematic review and meta-analysis. *J Sci Med Sport*. 2014;18(supple 1):e150.
39. Chalder M, Wiles NJ, Campbell J, et al. A pragmatic randomised controlled trial to evaluate the cost-effectiveness of a physical activity intervention as a treatment for depression: the treating depression with physical activity (TREAD) trial. *Health Technol Assess*. 2012;16(10):1-164.
40. Cooney GM, Dwan K, Greig CA, et al. Exercise for depression. *Cochrane Database Syst Rev*. 2013;(9):CD004366.
41. Conradsson M, Littbrand H, Lindelöf N, Gustafson Y, Rosendahl E. Effects of a high-intensity functional exercise programme on depressive symptoms and psychological well-being among older people living in residential care facilities: a cluster-randomized controlled trial. *Aging Ment Health*. 2010;14(5):565-576.

42. Babyak M, Blumenthal JA, Herman S, et al. Exercise treatment for major depression: maintenance of therapeutic benefit at 10 months. *Psychosom Med.* 2000;62(5):633-638.
43. Crumbie V, Olmos F, Watts C, Avery J, Nelson R. The impact of dance interventions on mood and depression in older adults. *Ther Recreation J.* 2015;49(2):187-190.
44. Danielsson L, Kihlbom B, Rosberg S. "Crawling out of the cocoon": patients' experiences of a physical therapy exercise intervention in the treatment of major depression. *Phys Ther.* 2016;96(8):1241-1250.
45. Hoffman BM, Blumenthal JA, Babyak MA, et al. Exercise fails to improve neurocognition in depressed middle-aged and older adults. *Med Sci Sports Exerc.* 2008;40(7):1344-1352.
46. Hoffman BM, Babyak MA, Craighead E, et al. Exercise and pharmacotherapy in patients with major depression: one-year follow-up of the SMILE study. *Psychosom Med.* 2011;73(2):127-133.
47. Legrand FD, Neff EM. Efficacy of exercise as an adjunct treatment for clinically depressed inpatients during the initial stages of antidepressant pharmacotherapy: an open randomized controlled trial. *J Affect Disord.* 2016;191:139-144.
48. Mota-Pereira J, Silverio J, Carvalho S, Ribeiro JC, Fonte D, Ramos J. Moderate exercise improves depression parameters in treatment-resistant patients with major depressive disorder. *J Psychiatr Res.* 2011;45(8):1005-1011.
49. Oertel-Knöchel V, Mehler P, Thiel C, et al. Effects of aerobic exercise on cognitive performance and individual psychopathology in depressive and schizophrenia patients. *Eur Arch Psychiatry Clin Neurosci.* 2014;264(7):589-604. DOI 10.1007/s00406-014-0485-9
50. Silveira H, Morales H, Oliveira N, Coutinho ESF, Laks J, Deslandes A. Physical exercise and clinically depressed patients: a systematic review and meta-analysis. *Neuropsychobiology.* 2013;67(2):61-68.
51. Balasubramaniam M, Telles S, Doraiswamy PM. Yoga on our minds: a systematic review of yoga for neuropsychiatric disorders. *Front Psychiatry.* 2013;3:117.
52. Sureka P, Govil S, Dash D, Dash C, Kumar M, Singhal V. Effect of Sudarshan Kriya on male prisoners with non psychotic psychiatric disorders: a randomized control trial. *Asian J Psychiatr.* 2014;12:43-49.
53. Breitve MH, Hynninen MJ, Kvåle A. The effect of psychomotor physical therapy on subjective health complaints and psychological symptoms. *Physiother Res Int.* 2010;15(4):212-221.
54. Lee HS, Park JH. Effects of Nordic walking on physical functions and depression in frail people aged 70 years and above. *J Phys Ther Sci.* 2015;27(8):2453-2456.
55. Meekums B, Karkou V, Nelson EA. Dance movement therapy for depression. *Cochrane Database Syst Rev.* 2015;(2):CD009895.
56. Verrusio W, Andreozzi P, Marigliano B, et al. Exercise training and music therapy in elderly with depressive syndrome: a pilot study. *Complement Ther Med.* 2014;22(4):614-620.
57. Lee NY, Lee DK, Song HS. Effect of virtual reality dance exercise on the balance, activities of daily living, and depressive disorder status of Parkinson's disease patients. *J Phys Ther Sci.* 2015;27(1):145-147.
58. Ström M, Uckelstam CJ, Andersson G, Hassmén P, Umefjord G, Carlbring P. Internet-delivered therapist-guided physical activity for mild to moderate depression: a randomized controlled trial. *PeerJ.* 2013;1:178.
59. Dunn AL, Trivedi MH, Kampert JB, Clark CG, Chambliss HO. The DOSE study: a clinical trial to examine efficacy and dose response of exercise as treatment for depression. *Control Clin Trials.* 2002;23(5):584-603.
60. Solbakken OA, Abbass A. Intensive short-term dynamic residential treatment program for patients with treatment-resistant disorders. *J Affect Disord.* 2015;181:67-77.
61. Solbakken OA, Abbass A. Symptom- and personality disorder changes in intensive short-term dynamic residential treatment for treatment-resistant anxiety and depressive disorder. *Acta Neuropsychiatrica.* 2016;28(5):257-271. DOI: 10.1017/neu.2016.5
62. Mather AS, Rodriguez C, Guthrie MF, McHarg AM, Reid IC, McMurdo MET. Effects of exercise on depressive symptoms in older adults with poorly responsive depressive disorder. *Br J Psychiatr.* 2002;180(5):411-415.
63. Nyström MBT, Neely G, Hassmén P, Carlbring P. Treating major depression with physical activity: a systematic overview with recommendations. *Cogn Behav Ther.* 2015;44(4):341-352.

Bipolar Disorders

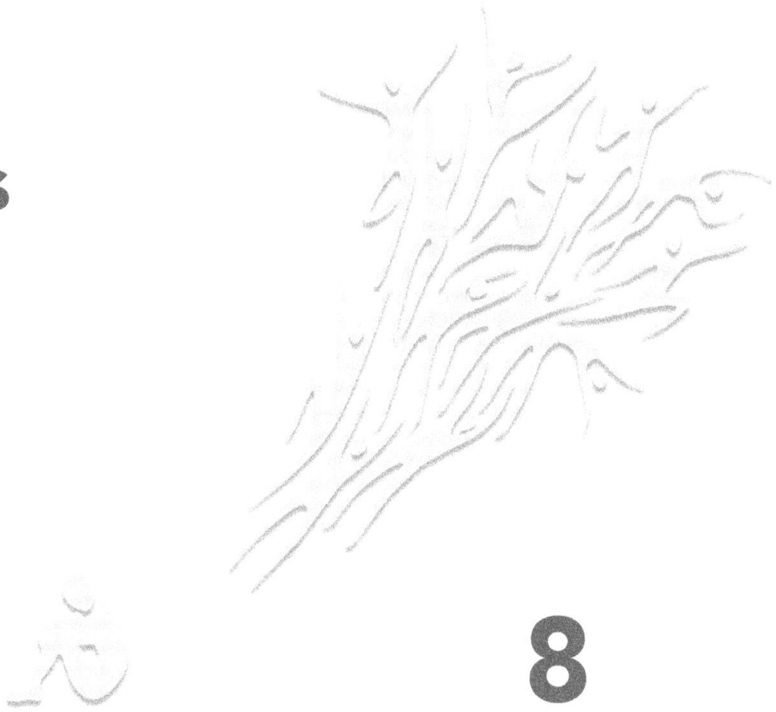

8

Outline

- Scope and Classification of Bipolar Disorders
- Neurophysiological Background, Etiology, and Risk Factors
- Comorbid Medical and Psychosocial Issues
- Specific Clinical Approaches to Improve Physical Therapy Outcomes
- Summary
- Key Points
- Review Questions
- Case Studies: First Impressions
- Quick Reference

Learning Objectives

- Demonstrate awareness of bipolar disorder diagnoses per the *Diagnostic and Statistical Manual of Mental Disorders, 5th Edition* (DSM-5) classification, including bipolar I, antidepressant-induced mania, bipolar II, and cyclothymic disorder
- Summarize research related to alterations in the human movement system for bipolar disorders
- Incorporate risk factor assessment for bipolar disorder diagnoses into the patient/client interview
- Delineate impact of common comorbidities into patient care for persons with bipolar disorders
- Propose changes to the physical therapist's approach, based on a bipolar disorder diagnosis, into assessments, exercise prescription, home exercise programs, building/maintaining rapport, and clinical documentation to increase successful outcomes

Johnson H.
Psychosocial Elements of Physical Therapy: The Connection of Body to Mind (pp 139-147).

Bipolar robs you of that which is you. It can take from you the very core of your being and replace it with something that is completely opposite of who and what you truly are. Because my bipolar went untreated for so long, I spent many years looking in a mirror and seeing a person I did not recognize or understand. Not only did bipolar rob me of my sanity, but it robbed me of my ability to see beyond the space it dictated me to look. I no longer could tell reality from fantasy, and I walked in a world no longer my own.

—Alyssa Reyans[1]

Bipolar spectrum disorders include mood disorders involving depression as well as mania (see definitions in Chapter 5). For the most part, physical therapist management of patients with bipolar disorders is similar to that for depressive disorders, unless the patient has frequent episodes of mania. As sports physical therapist Lacey McRoy relates (written communication, September 30, 2016):

> I have a patient with manic depressive [that is, bipolar I] disorder with neck and back pain who continually re-injured herself while in a manic state. It complicated her recovery a bit. To address it effectively, we acknowledged that it was a thing. She was working on strategies with her psychiatrist to manage, and we worked on symptom management. She is coming down from her manic state and is able to better control her activity level. Her pain has been a little better, but still only doing fair.

Mania, a medical emergency, demands an additional set of knowledge and interpersonal skills. This chapter will explore literature related specifically to bipolar disorder background and management. For information on managing the depressive aspect, the reader can refer to Chapter 7.

Scope and Classification of Bipolar Disorders

Bipolar disorders are characterized by alternating periods of depression and mania (Table 8-1). Belmaker[2] defines mania as characterized by excessive optimism and a low amount of sleep that impairs judgment. These periods of alternating mood symptoms vary in severity, lending a continuum-based classification.[2] The DSM-5 identifies the following several specific disorders[3]:

- Bipolar I disorder is clinically significant depression, plus at least one manic episode, and associated with a 15-fold increased risk of suicide.
- Bipolar II disorder is significant depression plus at least one hypomanic episode; hypomania is not as severe as mania (a medical emergency), but these patients typically have residual functional impairment between episodes.
- Cyclothymic disorder includes hypomania and hypodepression, which is less severe than major depression but still harmful to the person's function.

The reader may refer to Chapter 5 for statistics related to each bipolar spectrum disorder. For a comparison of major depressive disorder, bipolar disorders, and borderline personality disorder, refer to Malhi et al.[4]

Table 8-1

Symptoms of Depression and Mania

DOMAIN	DEPRESSION	MANIA
Affective	Sad, unhappy, anxious, apathetic, brooding	Elated, grandiose, irritable
Cognitive	Pessimistic, guilty, unable to concentrate, negative thoughts, decreased motivation and interest, suicidal	Flighty, pressured thoughts, decreased focus/attention, impaired judgment
Behavioral	Little energy and attention to appearance, crying, agitation, psychomotor retardation	Overactive, talkative, speech hard to understand
Physiological	Altered appetite, menses, and sleep; decreased libido; constipation	Increased arousal, decreased need for sleep

Reprinted with permission from Sue D, Sue DW, Sue S. *Understanding Abnormal Behaviors.* 6th ed. Boston, MA: Houghton Mifflin; 2000.

Neurophysiological Background, Etiology, and Risk Factors

As with other mood and psychotic disorders, bipolar disorders have multifactorial etiology and specific changes in the movement system. Magnetic resonance imaging studies of affected patients found that the brain's more external gray matter appears to be progressively lost, specifically in the "prefrontal and anterior cingulate cortex and the subgenual region," as well as possibly the temporal and subcortical areas over time in a person with a bipolar disorder.[5] These areas are important for judgment, perception, and information processing. Usher et al,[6] examining amygdala volume (impacting fear response and emotional regulation) related to age, found that change in volume is inconsistent across patients with bipolar disorders, indicating a weaker relationship between volume changes and disorder progression. Generally, however, they found that in children and most people with bipolar disorders, amygdala volume is smaller bilaterally but seems to increase with age, potentially enhancing its function.

Regarding the complex etiology of bipolar disorders, Belmaker noted that a genetic component is clearly present, but without details known at this time. In identical (monozygotic) twins, the concordance rate or chance of both twins having a diagnosis is 40% to 80%.[2] In fraternal (dizygotic) twins, however, this concordance rate is only 10% to 20%. Potential pathophysiological factors include:

- Abnormal intracellular regulation of calcium ions in B-lymphoblasts
- Increased neuronal sensitivity to serotonin
- Abnormalities in the brain extracellular matrix
- Decreased neuronal density or normalcy of function
- Decreased inositol-driven signaling within the brain
- Abnormal neurological development, with the neuroglia less dense in the cerebral cortex
- "Abnormal emotional responsiveness to social stimuli" related to "decreased gray matter and blood flow in the subgenual prefrontal cortex"[2]

A variety of other potential contributors to the symptoms and signs of bipolar disorders include:

- Emotional: self-anger; interpretation of experiences as unpleasant via faulty and imbalanced thought patterns, which include arbitrary inference (conclusions without an evidence base), selected abstraction (focus on one detail at random), over-generalization, and magnification or minimization of a thought
- Social: separation or loss, learned helplessness, and decreased social support
- Personal characteristics: female sex. Belmaker[2] also notes that many artists have bipolar disorder, due to the temporary increase in creativity just prior to the onset of full-blown mania. Personality traits do not, however, predict bipolar disorder.
- Health-related: elevated cortisol levels (relating to stress), altered neurotransmitter levels (termed the *catecholamine hypothesis*), and decreased sleep[7]

An example of a patient with many of these risk factors was an adult female treated by the author. This patient had generalized anxiety disorder, depression, bipolar disorder (type unspecified), posttraumatic stress disorder (PTSD), and tobacco dependence. She frequently had hallucinations and PTSD-related flashbacks during her therapy episode of care, as well as poor sleep due to anxiety symptoms. She had uncertain social support and high stress levels due to chronic unemployment and a disfiguring, debilitating skin condition. To address low back pain and balance deficits for a safe return home, the author collaborated with occupational therapy and nursing staff, attended a psychiatric evaluation with the patient, and used a rapport-focused approach with gentle manual therapy and consistent session structure. The author started the patient's home program with one exercise, adding one at a time as the patient showed mastery and verbalized criteria for progression.

Comorbid Medical and Psychosocial Issues

As with depressive disorders, bipolar disorders have comorbidities and challenges for the physical therapist in cognitive, metabolic, and participation-related domains. Research on promoting physical activity for persons with bipolar disorder is limited at this time; an international survey recommended examination of benefits, potential safety issues, optimal dosage and assessment, key barriers, translation of research to practice, makeup of the interdisciplinary team/interprofessional team, and prevention of sedentary behavior.[8] This section introduces recent articles addressing several related research questions.

A basic clinical question is this: what factors affect adherence to treatment by individuals with bipolar spectrum disorders? Murru et al[9] examined bipolar I and schizoaffective disorder (bipolar type) in an outpatient setting. Studying how well patients took psychiatric medication as scheduled, they found a non-adherence rate of 32% for persons with bipolar I and 44% for schizoaffective disorder (bipolar type). Predictive factors included "presence of psychotic symptoms, higher number of manic relapses, comorbidity with personality disorders, and lithium therapy."[9] As a side note, lithium can easily become toxic, especially to the kidneys, requiring monitoring of serum levels of the medication and potential side effects that include drowsiness, hand tremors, uneasiness, dry mouth, and gastrointestinal distress. While the physical therapist cannot necessarily address these symptoms directly, he or she should screen for and anticipate non-adherence, documenting accordingly.

To avoid medical emergencies, the patient with a history of mania should use antidepressants only with caution. If the patient currently has mania, very short-term use of neuroleptics (eg, dopamine blockers) is safe to avoid tardive dyskinesia and metabolic side effects that include "weight gain, changes in lipid levels, and abnormalities in glucose tolerance."[2] Poulin et al[10] found that an 18-month intervention consisting of **education on diet and physical activity, combined with structured, supervised exercise, produced significant improvements in body mass index, waist circumference, cholesterol levels, fasting glucose, and HbA1c levels**, indicating decreased risk or impact of metabolic syndrome. Interestingly, this active intervention had an 85% adherence rate and improved participants' mental health as measured by the Short Form, 36-question version.[10]

Integrating physical activity and education into a broader set of lifestyle interventions (psychosocial aspects and nutritional improvement) shows promise in bipolar disorder, as well. A systematic review identified "a beneficial role of lifestyle interventions on mood, weight, blood pressure, lipid profile, physical activity and overall well-being."[11] While significant methodological limitations exist in the studies, future high-quality trials may continue to uncover benefits related to specific tailored interventions, including patient preferences to increase adherence. As Malhi et al[4] state in their clinical practice guideline for mood disorders, psychological aspects of interventions should:

- Improve the patient's regulation and self-monitoring of stress, sleep quality, mood, and symptoms before mania
- Educate significant others; get patients back into their life roles
- Correct erroneous patterns of thoughts or beliefs
- "Reduce drug or alcohol misuse"[4] as a poor coping strategy

Since physical therapists are invaluable interdisciplinary team/interprofessional team members to promote physical activity and other interventions for persons with bipolar disorders, they need to **be aware of neurocognitive impairment in this disease.** Many people with bipolar disorders do not regain their true prior level of function after affective symptoms are treated; etiology of this progressive neurocognitive impairment is unknown. A significant proportion of immediate relatives without a diagnosed bipolar disorder do, however, also have impaired "verbal declarative memory and some facets of executive function," while in affected persons, the number of manic episodes predicts poor "verbal declarative memory performance."[12] Thus, it may be more difficult for the patient to give an accurate history during the initial therapy evaluation.

Wingo et al[13] agree that residual functional impairment is common, but that it "is far less likely than syndromal and even symptomatic recovery." However, high unemployment (55%) is one potentially devastating result of neurocognitive impairment, however severe. This may affect physical therapy plans of care due to payment issues and the need for volunteer (pro bono) services. Chapter 4 sets forth general principles related to payment issues for severe mental illness (SMI) in general.

Specific Clinical Approaches to Improve Physical Therapy Outcomes

The majority of strategies and information discussed in Chapter 7 (depressive disorders) also applies to persons with bipolar disorders because depression is a prominent feature between episodes of mania. While the literature related to physical therapy in this regard is limited, several authors recommend a focus on psychosocial interventions. Sue et al[7] imply that a background knowledge of interpersonal psychotherapy and cognitive behavioral therapy across the team helps patients to analyze and reframe their thoughts. Beynon et al[14] affirms the potential benefits of cognitive behavioral therapy, in individual or group sessions, to minimize risk of relapse. Finally, Drake et al[15] note that a variety of counseling and team-based interventions reduce functional and participation deficits in persons with comorbid SMI and substance use disorder.

SUMMARY

Bipolar spectrum disorders affect physical therapist management in several ways beyond the effects of the underlying depressive component. Primary distinctions lie in the management of manic symptoms, antipsychotic drug side effects, potential for comorbid substance use disorders, and increased suicide risk. As with other mood disorders and SMI, awareness of medical and psychosocial concerns is of great importance for patient management, especially in a team-based health care environment.

Key Points

- Supervised exercise and education on dietary and physical activity approaches to weight management improves metabolic indicators in persons with bipolar spectrum disorders.
- Be alert for neurocognitive impairment in examination of persons with bipolar spectrum disorders.

REVIEW QUESTIONS

- If you suspect a patient may have an undiagnosed bipolar disorder, how might you screen for the purpose of referral, per the list of risk factors and symptoms from Sue et al?[7]
- Why is prevention and management of metabolic abnormalities (including elevated cholesterol and decreased glucose tolerance) important in the population with bipolar disorders?
- Recall a patient recently on your caseload with a diagnosis of bipolar I, bipolar II, or cyclothymic disorder. How did this diagnosis and associated medications, if any, affect your examination, evaluation, and approach to your plan of care?
  - Are there any aspects of care coordination (eg, referral to specialist) that you would change if working with a similar patient in the future?
  - If possible, discuss this case in a small group of health care professionals or students you interact with. What aspects does each profession bring to the table for better outcomes?
- Given the common neurocognitive deficits present in individuals with bipolar disorders, how might you tailor your exercise program and discharge recommendations for more effective carryover?

CASE STUDIES: FIRST IMPRESSIONS

As you review the following case studies, you may want to consider these questions for thought or discussion:

- What standardized tests and measures (including psychiatric, for example, a depression screen) would you select for this patient? Why?
- Based on available data, what short- and long-term goals would you write for your plan of care? Consider using the acronyms SMART (specific, measurable, attainable, realistic, and timely) or ABCDE (actor, behavior, conditions, degree, and expected time frame) to guide your goal writing.

- What elements (procedures, psychosocial aspects, communication aspects, etc) would you make sure to include or omit in your plan of care for this patient? Why?
- What are your anticipated needs, if any, for consultation and referral for this patient?
- How will you transition this patient toward lasting health behavior change following discharge (eg, recommending a YMCA membership trial)?

Case 1

A 26-year-old male software engineer was referred to outpatient physical therapy for low back pain. His personal goals are to be able to work full days and start working out to gain physical fitness.

- Social history: he was referred to counseling for depression, as well as to physical therapy by his primary care provider. He lives in a 2-story house with a basement and a roommate who works third shift; his job requires frequent 10-hour days and is a 40-minute drive or train ride away.
- Medical/psychiatric history: prehypertension, mildly overweight, and cyclothymic disorder. He is currently on non-steroidal anti-inflammatory medications as needed and was issued a back brace.
- Impairments, activity limitations, and participation restrictions found on initial interview and examination
  - Central low back pain rated 5/10 with bending and lifting tasks
  - Mild trunk weakness
  - Impaired proprioceptive awareness related to spinal positioning
  - Shortness of breath after climbing a flight of stairs to his office or bedroom
  - Sitting tolerance limited to 10 minutes without medication or back brace
  - Standing tolerance limited by pain to 15 minutes
  - Unable to complete meal preparation and laundry without frequent breaks

Case 2

A 43-year-old female was sent to your subacute rehabilitation facility for intravenous antibiotics due to systemic infection, following a 1-week hospitalization for a brief psychiatric crisis. Her goals are to return to her apartment and care for her cat as she looks for part-time work.

- Social history: she lives alone in a second floor apartment with her cat; she has no significant other or family support, and has limited compliance with medications when in a hypomanic phase.
- Medical/psychiatric history: bipolar II disorder, premenstrual dysphoric disorder, and pemphigus (an autoimmune disease that produces blisters). The blisters that form tend to get infected.
- Impairments, activity limitations, and participation restrictions found on initial interview and examination
  - Moderate balance deficits on foam and in single-limb stance
  - Limited periods of daytime alertness
  - Exertion rated 8/10 (rating of perceived exertion) when walking 0.5 mph on level ground
  - Requires both rails to negotiate stairs to apartment

Case 3

A 68-year-old male has orders to be seen in acute care due to non-healing wounds that required bilateral below-knee amputations 1 day prior to your evaluation. His goal is to return home with his wife, who has limited ability to physically assist him.

- Social history: he is retired and lives in a ranch house with 2 stoop steps to enter. His wife is non-ambulatory and uses a wheelchair for mobility due to lower extremity osteoarthritis. Prior to amputations, he previously completed all heavy cleaning, cooking, shopping, and laundry tasks; they have 2 adult children that live in the area and have visited the patient in the hospital.
- Medical/psychiatric history: bipolar I disorder, PTSD from military service overseas (50 years ago), type 2 diabetes, early stage glaucoma, obesity, hypertension, nicotine dependence, and chronic obstructive pulmonary disease. He requests a female therapist due to PTSD symptoms.
- Impairments, activity limitations, and participation restrictions found on initial interview and examination
    - Decreased protective sensation in both hands
    - Phantom pain during periods of sitting
    - Shortness of breath at rest, with an order for oxygen as needed via nasal cannula
    - Severely limited trunk and lower extremity flexibility and strength
    - Frequent refusals of nursing care for various reasons
    - Difficulty in remembering safety precautions while setting up wheelchair for a slide board transfer

Quick Reference

- Possible diagnoses and their signs/symptoms:
    - Bipolar I: abrupt mood or sleep changes, euphoria or risk-taking behaviors, poor concentration, racing or slow thoughts, paranoia, abrupt activity level changes
    - Bipolar II: less severe symptoms than bipolar I
    - Cyclothymic disorder: irritability, mood swings, may increase over time
- Questions to ask the patient (or friend/family member):
    - Do you often feel any of the symptoms (listed previously)?
    - Have you ever been diagnosed with a bipolar disorder (listed previously)? What was going on in your life around the time of that diagnosis?
    - How do you deal with your bipolar disorder? How well does that work for you?
    - What should I know about your bipolar disorder?
- Referral options:
    - Psychiatrist for diagnosis, behavioral and pharmacological therapy
    - Inpatient psychiatric program or the person's psychiatrist if the patient appears to be entering or in a manic episode, which must be treated as a medical emergency
    - Support group for persons with bipolar disorders
    - Exercise group or facility, preferably where staff are trained to work sensitively with persons with bipolar and other psychological disorders

References

1. Reyans A. *Letters from a Bipolar Mother.* Alyreyans Press; 2012.
2. Belmaker RH. Medical progress: bipolar disorder. *N Engl J Med.* 2004;351:476-486.
3. American Psychiatric Association. *Diagnostic and Statistical Manual of Mental Disorders.* 5th ed. Washington, DC: American Psychiatric Association; 2013.
4. Malhi GS, Bassett D, Boyce P, et al. Royal Australian and New Zealand College of Psychiatrists clinical practice guidelines for mood disorders. *Aust N Z J Psychiatry.* 2015;49(12):1087-1206.
5. Lim CS, Baldessarini RJ, Vieta E, Yucel M, Bora E, Sim K. Longitudinal neuroimaging and neuropsychological changes in bipolar disorder patients: review of the evidence. *Neurosci Behav Rev.* 2013;37(3):418-435.
6. Usher J, Leucht S, Falkai P, Scherk H. Correlation between amygdala volume and age in bipolar disorder—a systematic review and meta-analysis of structural MRI studies. *Psychiat Res Neuroim.* 2010;182(1):1-8.
7. Sue D, Sue DW, Sue S. *Understanding Abnormal Behaviors.* 6th ed. Boston, MA: Houghton Mifflin; 2000.
8. Vancampfort D, Rosenbaum S, Probst M, et al. Top 10 research questions to promote physical activity in bipolar disorders: a consensus statement from the International Organization of Physical Therapists in Mental Health. *J Affect Disord.* 2016;195:82-87.
9. Murru A, Pacchiarotti I, Amann BL, Nivoli AMA, Vieta E, Colom F. Treatment adherence in bipolar I and schizoaffective disorder, bipolar type. *J Affect Disord.* 2013;151:1003-1008.
10. Poulin MJ, Chaput JP, Simard V, et al. Management of antipsychotic-induced weight gain: prospective naturalistic study of the effectiveness of a supervised exercise programme. *Aust N Z J Psychiatry.* 2007;41(12):980-989.
11. Bauer IE, Gálvez JF, Hamilton JE, et al. Lifestyle interventions targeting dietary habits and exercise in bipolar disorder: a systematic review. *J Psychiatr Res.* 2016;74:1-7.
12. Robinson LJ, Ferrier IN. Evolution of cognitive impairment in bipolar disorder: a systematic review of cross-sectional evidence. *Bipolar Disord.* 2006;8(2):103-116.
13. Wingo AP, Harvey PD, Baldessarini RJ. Neurocognitive impairment in bipolar disorder patients: functional implications. *Bipolar Disord.* 2009;11(2):113-125.
14. Beynon S, Soares-Weiser K, Woolacott N, Duffy S, Geddes JR. Psychosocial interventions for the prevention of relapse in bipolar disorder: systematic review of controlled trials. *Br J Psychiatry.* 2008;192(1):5-11.
15. Drake RE, O'Neal EL, Wallach MA. A systematic review of psychosocial research on psychosocial interventions for people with co-occurring severe mental and substance use disorder. *J Subst Abuse Treat.* 2008;34(1):123-138.

Schizophrenia Spectrum Disorders

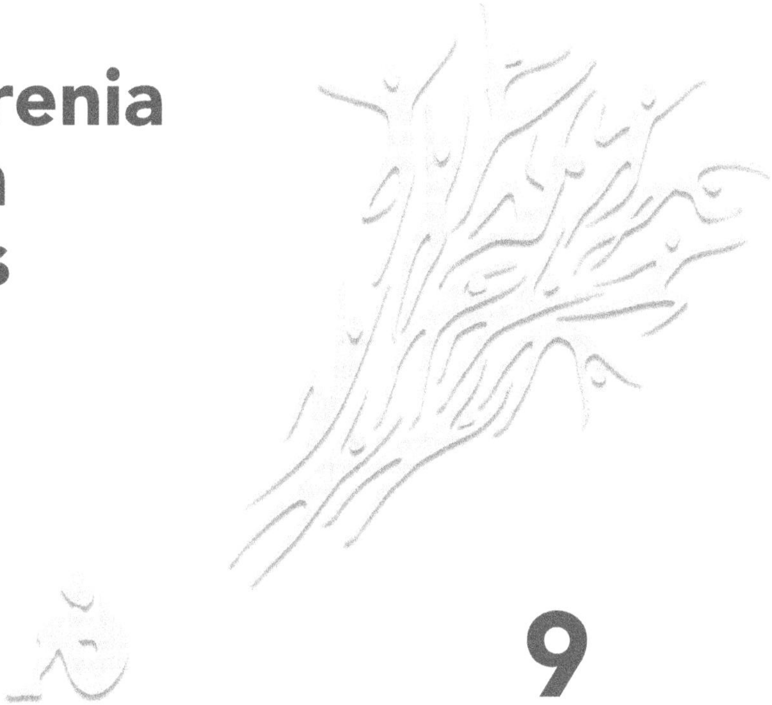

9

Outline

- Scope and Classification of Schizophrenia Spectrum Disorders
- Neurophysiological Background, Etiology, and Risk Factors
- Comorbid Medical and Psychosocial Issues
- Specific Clinical Approaches to Improve Physical Therapy Outcomes
    - Psychosocial Interventions
    - Physical Activity Interventions
- Summary
- Key Points
- Review Questions
- Case Studies: First Impressions
- Quick Reference

Learning Objectives

- Demonstrate awareness of schizophrenia spectrum disorder diagnoses per the *Diagnostic and Statistical Manual of Mental Disorders, 5th Edition* (DSM-5) classification, including paranoia, catatonia, schizophreniform, and schizoaffective disorder
- Summarize research related to changes in the human movement system for a schizophrenia spectrum disorder diagnosis

Johnson H.
Psychosocial Elements of Physical Therapy: The Connection of Body to Mind (pp 149-160).

- Incorporate risk factor assessment for schizophrenia spectrum disorders into the patient/client interview
- Delineate impact of common comorbidities into patient care, based on the patient management model
- Propose changes to the physical therapist's approach, based on a schizophrenia spectrum disorder diagnosis, into assessments, exercise prescription, home exercise programs, building/maintaining rapport, and clinical documentation to improve outcomes

A schizophrenia spectrum disorder, often starting in one's 20s or 30s, is a confusing and often frightening part of a patient's medical history, for the patient and the rehabilitation professional. However, research clearly shows a need for therapy services in this population. This chapter presents research about the disorder and its symptoms, medical management, and physical activity strategies to improve outcomes for this population in need of physical therapists' knowledge and skill.

Stubbs et al[1] surveyed members of the International Organization of Physical Therapists in Mental Health (IOPTMH) and found that persons with schizophrenia live about a decade less than unaffected persons, influenced by poor physical activity habits, despite the low cost and high effectiveness of physical activity prescription. Internationally based physical therapists specializing in mental health believe that physical activity clearly benefits schizophrenia, especially if clinicians supervise and prescribe it in the context of psychiatric intervention: it improves "mental health, socialization and quality of life."[1] A systematic review of physical therapy within a multidisciplinary care plan for persons with schizophrenia spectrum disorders found that many types of exercise can reduce psychiatric symptoms, baseline anxiety, short-term memory, and psychological distress.[2] Finally, Vera-Garcia et al[3] found additional evidence that aerobic exercise and yoga significantly impact psychiatric symptoms, while also addressing cardiometabolic risk factors.

Scope and Classification of Schizophrenia Spectrum Disorders

The only thing you have for measuring what's real is your mind ... so what happens when your mind becomes a pathological liar?

—Neal Shusterman[4]

Symptoms of schizophrenia spectrum disorders include at least 6 months' intermittent (and 1 month continuous) duration of delusions, hallucinations, disorganized speech (including neologisms, or nonsense words often based on existing words), disorganized or catatonic behaviors, flat affect, avolition, alogia, and anhedonia (see Chapter 5 for definitions). A person with schizophrenia will have at least 2 of these symptoms. For a diagnosis of schizophrenia, symptoms must negatively impact function and not be due to organic disorders or substance use.[5]

The spectrum of schizophrenia disorders includes paranoia; disorganized or catatonic behavior; schizophreniform; and schizoaffective disorder, which is an underlying mood disorder with isolated psychotic symptoms.[5,6] Under the fourth edition of the *Diagnostic and Statistical Manual of Mental Disorders*, these were classified as distinct subtypes; however, under DSM-5, schizophrenia is termed a *single spectrum disorder*, affecting the patient's sense of reality and named by its primary symptom in a patient.[7] Cultural interpretation of human behavior affects diagnosis and etiology. For example, "for Native Americans, it is considered normal to hear and speak to dead ancestors."[8]

For a diagnosis of schizophreniform disorder (which has a 33% spontaneous remission rate but otherwise progresses to schizophrenia), psychotic symptoms must last between 1 and 6 months total. On the other end of the spectrum, schizoaffective disorder will predominantly have symptoms of the underlying mood disorder (eg, depression or bipolar disorder), with weaker psychotic symptoms. Because schizoaffective disorder lacks many psychotic symptoms, it has a better prognosis than schizophrenia but is still a lifelong disorder.

Neurophysiological Background, Etiology, and Risk Factors

Schizophrenia spectrum disorders are still poorly understood in terms of specific etiology and causes, but literature does implicate multiple areas of the brain and central nervous system. Proposed risk factors include genetic abnormality or heredity, higher dopamine levels, ventricular enlargement, smaller cerebrum and thalamus, poor frontal lobe function, family influence, and lower social class.[5] Lundy-Ekman[9] connects these changes to alterations in the basal ganglia, dopamine receptors, and corpus callosum; in imaging studies, the frontal and temporal lobes, amygdala, and hippocampus show decreased function.

Exercise affects neurological changes in schizophrenia spectrum disorders. A systematic review showed correlation of hippocampal volume increase "with improvements in aerobic fitness and short-term memory."[10] Volume changes, however, had an unclear relationship to aerobic exercise, indicating a need for further focused research. In a pilot study, Vancampfort et al[11] examined the positive effects of "single sessions of yoga or aerobic exercise," for 20 to 30 minutes at each patient's self-selected intensity, on symptoms. The intervention, with a large effect size of 0.82 to 1.01, "significantly decreased state anxiety, decreased psychological stress, and increased subjective well-being compared to a no exercise control condition."[11]

Comorbid Medical and Psychosocial Issues

The medication given during mental-ill health makes you rather weaker in body, in soul and in spirit.

—Lailah Gifty Akita

Comorbid conditions related to schizophrenia spectrum disorders may be classified into several categories: social/functional, medical, and pharmacological. Each of these can contribute to the high costs of providing patient care. As Olesen et al[12] note, schizophrenia and other psychotic disorders impose a high economic cost, at least 93.9 million euros in 2010 ($101.1 billion in 2017) alone in Europe; the United States often has much higher health care costs due in part to differences in infrastructure and availability of specific services.

The course of a schizophrenia spectrum disorder usually takes a downward path. As with multiple sclerosis, individuals can experience single or multiple incidents of psychotic symptoms, with negligible, moderate, or severe residual impairment, and cognitive decline that stabilizes after about 5 years.[5] Due to this, clinicians may notice poor adherence to aspects of case management. Murru et al[13] found a 44% non-adherence rate in persons with schizoaffective disorder (bipolar type). Predictors of poor adherence included "presence of psychotic symptoms, higher number of manic relapses, comorbidity with personality disorders, and [oral] lithium therapy."[13]

Rastad et al[14] took a broader view of non-adherence in younger outpatients with a relatively longer duration of diagnosed schizophrenia. They identified barriers to physical activity as:

- Disease or illness symptoms, including fatigue, loneliness, and overweight/obesity
- Immediate negative outcomes, including pain and lack of positivity
- Negative expectations, including fear of failure and lack of time

- Misconceptions about physical activity, including that it required special equipment and environment
- Body perception, including wintry environments and difficulty finding exercise clothing
- Lack of resources, including money, equipment, and access to an exercise facility[14]

Corresponding motivators for physical activity included immediate positive outcomes (well-being, self-confidence, alertness, and feeling free) and positive expectations (reduced psychotic symptoms, improved appearance, and good memories of group exercise). Rastad et al[14] found that strategies to increase the likelihood of patient participation in physical activity included:

- Mental preparation: acknowledging one's own limits, improving self-talk, deciding firmly to exercise, and making mental images of the process and effects of exercise
- Personal support: recruiting someone to provide well-timed impetus and accountability, obtaining one-on-one instruction, and maximizing continuity of activity especially in groups
- Activity planning: stress reduction strategies, scheduled time for exercise, and self-selected enjoyable activity

Besides barriers associated with disease symptoms, long-term prescription and use of antipsychotic medications can cause issues for the physical therapist. Tardive dyskinesia, a distressing movement symptom, is caused by dopamine blockers, with the exception of clozapine.[9] Lynn and Plant[15] explored this and other dyskinesias in chronic schizophrenia from a psychiatric nurse's perspective, since these nurses often refer patients to physical therapy. In interviews by Lynn and Plant, the nurses thought that medications were a major cause of dyskinesia.[15] However, physical therapist intervention can address movement disorders caused by either medications or organic (related to brain function) factors. Abnormal movement patterns, besides the repetitive orofacial movements of tardive dyskinesia, include postural changes, gait deviations, and limb or hand tremors.

Because medications for schizophrenia and Parkinson's disease (PD) can each cause the other disorder, symptom monitoring and shorter duration of prescription are essential. Fujino et al[16] published a case study of a 71-year-old woman, with a 43-year history of schizophrenia with paranoia. This patient developed initial symptoms of PD following 13 years of taking thioridazine and sulpiride. However, treatment of this disease with levodopa and carbidopa worsened her psychosis for 2 years prior to admission to a psychiatric hospital with intact cognition but stage IV Hoehn and Yahr symptoms of PD. Physical function was initially low (Barthel Index 35 out of 100). On initiation of aripiprazole administration to minimize risk of sedation and orthostatic hypotension, the woman's psychosis, independent ambulation, and motivation to participate in physical therapy sessions improved. At discharge and 6-month follow-up, her PD symptoms had improved to stage III Hoehn and Yahr, and physical function had improved to a 65 on the Barthel Index, indicating potential for independent living.[16]

A pair of case studies highlights another potential adverse effect of antipsychotic medication use: contractures in neuroleptic malignant syndrome. Features of this syndrome include "sweating, pyrexia, muscular rigidity, fluctuating confusion, labile blood pressure, and grossly elevated creatine phosphokinase."[17] Following anti-schizophrenia medication administration, 2 younger adults developed the syndrome and subsequent resistance to mobilization and stretching, causing the need for surgical release of disabling upper-extremity contractures.

Finally, medical conditions associated with secondary impairments in schizophrenia spectrum disorders include "disease of the circulatory, digestive, endocrine, nervous and respiratory systems, suicide and undetermined death," as well as smoking-related mortality.[18] These conditions cause premature death and can be addressed by focusing on "patients' smoking and exposure to other environmental risk factors," as well as "improving the management of medical disease, mood disturbance and psychosis."[18] One condition involving digestive, endocrine, and cardiovascular dysfunction is metabolic syndrome, which is marked by at least 3 of the following risk factors: abdominal obesity (waist circumference over 35 to 40 inches); elevated triglyceride levels;

decreased high-density lipoprotein (HDL), or good cholesterol levels; elevated blood pressure; and fasting blood sugar levels over 100 mg/dL.[19] Metabolic syndrome is of high importance to the physical therapist.

Overweight and obesity, due to sedentary lifestyle and chronic antipsychotic medication use, contribute to metabolic syndrome. Littrell et al[20] tested the effects of a 4-month intervention, including "weekly psychoeducation classes focused on nutrition, exercise, and living a healthy lifestyle," in persons with schizophrenia spectrum disorders. This intervention, at 2-month follow-up, prevented weight gain in the group as a whole, vs an average 10-pound increase for each person in the control group. However, men still "gained significantly more weight than did women" in both groups.[20] An 18-month supervised exercise program combined with education on diet and physical activity had, besides an impressive 85% adherence rate, significant improvements in body mass index, waist circumference, body weight, cholesterol levels (both HDL and low-density lipoprotein), fasting glucose, hemoglobin A1c (HbA1c) levels (a measure of diabetes management), and physical and mental health.[21]

Type 2 diabetes mellitus specifically, and metabolic syndrome generally, are addressed in several studies, since the risk for both is far greater in patients with schizophrenia spectrum disorders.[22] Cimo et al[23] recommend "continuous metabolic monitoring" (including checks of HbA1c levels), as well as multifaceted diabetes education incorporating "diet and exercise components, while using a design that addresses challenges such as cognition, motivation, and weight gain." **Specific techniques include a slow pace of educational module presentation, gradual introduction of any new topic, use of memory aids, and simplification of messages by minimizing text in printed materials.**

Vancampfort et al[24] surveyed the IOPTMH (see Chapter 4) for consensus on physical activity recommendations within multidisciplinary rehabilitation to minimize cardiovascular and metabolic risk factors in patients with schizophrenia spectrum disorders. Combined "physical inactivity, unhealthy diet, substance abuse ... effects of antipsychotic treatment ... [and] limited access to physical health care" increased risk.[24] However, prescription of 150 minutes of moderate-intensity or 75 minutes of vigorous-intensity physical exercise is effective when patients can choose the type of activity. When addressing motivation, physical therapists "should consider illness symptoms, side-effects of antipsychotic medication, low self-efficacy and the lack of social support" faced by patients. Specific illness symptoms include "disembodiment, body image disturbances and deficits in the feeling of being an agent in their own bodies and lives."[24] Also, if a patient is on psychotropic medication, increasing gait speed can reduce medication-induced gait deviations.

Specific Clinical Approaches to Improve Physical Therapy Outcomes

To facilitate a focus on the whole person for the best health care, this section first examines psychosocial treatments for patients with schizophrenia spectrum disorders, and then physical activity interventions. Many such patients hear voices in their heads telling them to think, say, or do damaging things. Coping strategies include distracting oneself with a different activity, ignoring the voices (requiring presence of mind to realize that the voices are not real), selectively listening, and setting limits (telling the voice it will not be listened to after a certain time).[4] Within the interdisciplinary team/interprofessional team, more interventions can include individualized psychotherapy; community-focused hospitals; cognitive behavioral therapy, especially for social skills; and communication with and education of family members to help the patient maintain or improve function.

Psychosocial Interventions

The physical therapist can directly implement several psychosocial treatments for schizophrenia spectrum disorders and should be aware of them if the patient is receiving them elsewhere. Approaches from the literature include structured humor, social support, and mind-body integration; these and others fall under complementary and alternative medicine, which can be used by physical therapists and other health care providers. Ventegodt et al[25] reviewed classes of complementary and alternative medicine, including herbs, massage therapy, psychotherapy, mind-body medicine (eg, Alexander technique or acupuncture), and holistic medicine, any of which patients seen by physical therapists may be pursuing. While each technique is effective for decreasing symptoms of schizophrenia spectrum disorders, it is important for the clinician to ask about specific techniques to ensure minimal side effects and maximum efficacy of physical therapy.

Clinicians naturally use unstructured humor in their treatment sessions, but literature has also formally studied structured humor. Cai et al[26] investigated a 10-session humor intervention, which included increasing self-awareness of one's own sense of humor, practicing laughing, and learning how to use humor to reframe mistakes and stress. The authors noted that persons with schizophrenia can appreciate humor, but have difficulty recognizing it or laughing when they find something amusing; the more the subjects were able to laugh, the lower their stress levels and the higher their socialization skills became.[26]

Connecting with humor, social support can encourage patients to participate in physical activity. Soundy et al[27] emphasize multidimensional support: "four functional dimensions of social support (informational, tangible, esteem and emotional) and the one structural dimension (importance of group exercise)." Physical therapists and other team members can provide this support by giving useful information, facilitating meeting of material needs, building up patients, and validating their emotional experiences in the context of individual or group exercise.

One mind-body technique, basic body awareness therapy (BBAT), is an option for patients with schizophrenia by physical therapists in Europe; analogous techniques in the United States include occupational therapy, sports psychology, and therapeutic recreation. Probst et al[28] overviews BBAT and its parent, psychomotor physical therapy. In Europe, psychomotor physical therapy is a common adjunct to psychiatric treatment for many mental health conditions, with a growing knowledge base for each. While the rationale for psychomotor physical therapy is primarily psychological due to few (if any) acute physical functional impairments, it does address:

> [F]ine and gross motor abilities, eye-hand coordination, balance, time and space, perception, attention, interaction with materials, recognition of stimuli ... learning how to relax, acquiring a good physical condition, and learning the basic rules of communication.[28]

Strategies used by psychomotor physical therapists to address psychiatric, emotional, and movement-related symptoms include setting short- and long-term goals at a challenge level just right for mastery, focusing on modeling effective group interaction (as small a group as the patient and therapist), allowing maximal choice for the patient, validating the patient's symptoms, and asking the patient to summarize each session's feelings and experiences. Additional strategies specific to schizophrenia include stress reduction, habitual physical activity to decrease drug-induced metabolic abnormalities, and group problem solving and participation.

Hedlund and Gyllensten[29] explored 3 themes related to this technique:

1. Encountering: at evaluation, therapists seek to become aware of important aspects of a patient's identity.
2. Discovery: during treatment, therapists guide patients to become aware of their own bodies and experiences, which can decrease feelings of dissociation in patients.
3. "Inner space towards outer world": once patients are more somatically aware, therapists help them summarize positive changes over the course of therapy and then "turn their attention to the outside world."[29]

Randomized controlled trials evaluating the effectiveness of BBAT as an adjunct to medical treatment for schizophrenia and major depression found positive effects on depressive symptoms, balance, posture, somatic awareness and control, self-efficacy, sleep quality, attitude toward one's body, and utilization of social services in outpatient settings, with up to a year's maintenance of gains.[30-33]

Physical Activity Interventions

Physical activity has wide clinical support in patients with schizophrenia spectrum disorders, affording the clinician considerable choice for interventions. Most approaches involve a social or educational component. A meta-analysis of 39 trials evaluated interventions including "structured exercise programs; exercise counselling [sic]; lifestyle interventions in which physical activity was a major component; Tai Chi; or physical yoga."[34] Regardless of the dosage of these interventions, the meta-analysis found large effects on psychotic symptoms and moderate effects on aerobic capacity and quality of life. Thus, **almost any physical activity a patient enjoys is appropriate to prescribe, as long as it is intense enough to address metabolic risk factors**, including body mass index, blood glucose levels, and cholesterol levels. Supervision by a physical therapist increases adherence.[21]

Dance movement therapy has moderate quality evidence for patients with schizophrenia with the goals of "emotional, social, cognitive, and physical integration" of participants.[35] Yoga, while reducing depressive symptoms, can also manage psychotic symptoms adjunct to pharmacotherapy.[36] Aerobic exercise improves cognitive performance and fitness parameters in isolation or in combination with progressive resistance exercise.[37,38] Supporting the critical importance of social support in patients with schizophrenia spectrum disorders, the authors note that group exercise has better efficacy and adherence.[37,38]

Under current payment systems, insurance coverage for ongoing physical therapy is limited. To get around this obstacle, the physical therapist can offer options such as a wellness program or referral to low-cost fitness services, with continued state- and national-level advocacy for changes to the payment landscape. A friend of the author of this text highlights the benefits of a continued vs fragmented intervention (I. Johnson, written communication, January 22, 2017):

> A sixty-three-year-old woman who has been saddled with schizoaffective disorder (bipolar type) since her teens, who was married, had four children, been divorced, and now lives in a ramshackle apartment, penniless and dependent on the state combined with support from her church, has become my friend. For several years now I've been with her as she battles on in her difficult life, and have observed the impact of physical therapy and the lack of it.
>
> To describe her, she is mildly obese, uses a walker due to bone-on-bone arthritis in both knees, has many medical problems exacerbated by her sedentary lifestyle, is on multiple medications, and experiences continual difficulties with depression and the internal voices that plague her. She has received electric shock treatments every other week for several years now. These alleviate her depression yet also cause forgetfulness.
>
> Physical therapy is not part of her normal medical or psychiatric help—a psychiatrist once a week, a counselor once a week, and medical doctors as needed. Yet when she is hospitalized—on average two to three hospitalizations per year—she receives physical therapy. The hospitalizations happen typically when her depressive voices overpower her and she forgets good hygiene and diet, falls because of walking bent forward leaning on her walker, and incurs other problems such as dehydration or various infections. When things become too difficult she calls 911 and enters the hospital for a few days.
>
> During her hospital stays and sometimes rehab afterward, she receives physical therapy to strengthen her muscles, improve balance, move her joints, and walk more safely. When she gets home there is home therapy for a week or so. As a result, she is better both physically and mentally, since she thrives on the people contact. She loves her therapists!

The effectiveness of this therapy, however, is lost as time goes on, when her depressive thoughts take over, and also some of her "voices" convince her that it is all useless. Then the process needing hospitalization starts again, as she spirals downward mentally, forgets the healthy lifestyle including physical activity, becomes ill and/or mentally so distraught that she cannot function, and calls 911 to go to the hospital once more.

Seeing this process of repeated hospitalizations due in part to lack of physical therapy indicates to me that continual regular physical therapy would be a life-saver for this lady in many ways. She sees her psychiatrist and a counselor once a week. A physical therapist once a week would give her the lifestyle help and reminders she needs, be another person in her life to prevent the depression coming with loneliness, help avoid the falls she has when depressed and physically depleted, and help prevent the hospitalizations and rehab care which may be unnecessary, and also are of much greater cost than paying a therapist for once-a-week visits. If the medical system could see the benefit of such ongoing therapy and make it part of the prescribed treatment for patients with schizophrenia, much good would be done for the system, and especially for people like my friend!

Summary

Schizophrenia spectrum disorders, previously classified as distinct types of schizophrenia (eg, paranoid, residual, and catatonic), are now considered manifestations of a common set of factors including genetics, neurological abnormalities, and extreme life stressors. While underlying causes are not yet fully understood, the clinician should be aware of the common cognitive, social, and emotional deficits, as well as the higher risk of death from comorbid medical disorders including metabolic syndrome. Just as causes and effects of symptoms are diverse, so also treatment options are broad for the physical therapist, with evidence favoring interventions that are supervised and group-based to facilitate psychosocial support for this population.

Key Points

- Metabolic syndrome is an important area of knowledge for clinicians. Marked by at least 3 of the following risk factors: abdominal obesity, elevated triglycerides, decreased HDL cholesterol, hypertension, and fasting blood sugar over 100 mg/dL. Treatment can include slowly introducing education, encouragement of memory aids, and simplified presentation of messages in text and picture form.
- Almost any supervised aerobic-intensity physical activity is appropriate for treatment and prevention of metabolic syndrome in persons with schizophrenia spectrum disorders.

Review Questions

- Why is metabolic syndrome so prevalent in persons with schizophrenia spectrum disorders? Why is it often difficult to address?
- What are some barriers to physical activity in persons with schizophrenia?

- Recall several recent patients you or a coworker/fellow student have worked with who had diagnoses of schizophrenia spectrum disorders.
  - How did their presentations differ based on their individual psychiatric and social backgrounds?
  - How did you or your colleague address these different psychosocial aspects of care?
- What group exercise classes are available in your community? In a small group, evaluate their potential appropriateness for referral for a patient with schizophrenia, based on research presented in this chapter. If you work in a setting where group therapy is discouraged or disallowed by a patient's insurance, what steps might you take to address this?
- What strategies can you incorporate as an individual student or physical therapist with how you approach the following components of the therapy episode of care with future patients with schizophrenia?
  - Initial interview, for examination and evaluation
  - Plan of care, including aspects of communication and care coordination
  - Follow-up and exercise program prescription
  - Other procedural interventions, including aspects of physical setting and your mental state
- Given an example of a patient with medication-treated schizophrenia, obesity, sedentary lifestyle, depression, and hypertension, how would you tailor your plan of care to address medication side effects and potential interaction of conditions?

Case Studies: First Impressions

As you review the following case studies, you may want to consider these questions for thought or discussion:

- What standardized tests and measures (including psychiatric, for example, a depression screen) would you select for this patient? Why?
- Based on available data, what short- and long-term goals would you write for your plan of care? Consider using the acronyms SMART (specific, measurable, attainable, realistic, and timely) or ABCDE (actor, behavior, conditions, degree, and expected time frame) to guide your goal writing.
- What elements (procedures, psychosocial aspects, communication aspects, etc) would you make sure to include or omit in your plan of care for this patient? Why?
- What are your anticipated needs, if any, for consultation and referral for this patient?
- How will you transition this patient toward lasting health behavior change following discharge (eg, recommending a YMCA membership trial)?

Case 1

A 44-year-old male self-referred to outpatient physical therapy for whiplash-associated disorder 3 weeks after a motor vehicle accident. His goal is to eliminate neck pain and headaches, so he can return to recreational tennis.

- Social history: he lives in a 2-story house with his wife, who cares for their 3 children and completes cooking, cleaning, and laundry. He works on a factory floor but is currently on light duty.
- Medical/psychiatric history: type 2 diabetes, hypertension, and schizoaffective disorder. He is currently trying to manage his medical conditions with dietary and lifestyle changes.

- Impairments, activity limitations, and participation restrictions found on initial interview and examination
  - Neck pain rated 7/10, and headaches that occur with prolonged postures and abrupt movements
  - Active and passive neck range of motion 50% limited in all directions
  - Verbalizes a fear of making his condition worse
  - Unable to drive without a passenger to assist in scanning

Case 2

A 28-year-old female was hospitalized with a right tibial fracture and seen in inpatient physical therapy. Her goal is to return to her job as a technician in a biology lab.

- Social history: she lives in a 2-story house with her husband, who works 2 jobs and is thus unable to help significantly with home maintenance activities. She takes the bus to work and needs to stand for 20 to 30 minutes at a time for her job.
- Medical/psychiatric history: right shoulder instability with dislocation, panic disorder, and recently diagnosed schizophreniform disorder (has had symptoms for the past 2 months)
- Impairments, activity limitations, and participation restrictions found on initial interview and examination
  - Weightbearing-as-tolerated surgical restriction for 6 weeks
  - Pain rated 6/10 in weightbearing with axillary crutches
  - Standing tolerance 5 minutes due to pain and sensation of foot heaviness
  - Unable to manage stairs with crutches while carrying a purse or other bag

Case 3

A 70-year-old male living in a long-term care facility was referred to therapy by nursing staff due to increased shortness of breath and assistance required during ambulation and transfers. His goal is to move around the facility as independently as possible.

- Social history: he lives in a semi-private room near the nurses' station and has family members who visit several times per week. He is a retired college professor.
- Medical/psychiatric history: congestive heart failure, chronic obstructive pulmonary disease, schizophrenia with paranoia (diagnosed at age 30), urinary retention requiring a Foley catheter (placed 2 months ago during a brief hospitalization), and knee and hip osteoarthritis
- Impairments, activity limitations, and participation restrictions found on initial interview and examination
  - Dyspnea on mild exertion
  - Thirty-degrees hip and knee flexion contractures
  - Verbal outbursts with a low threshold for verbal aggression
  - Cardiovascular response to exercise consistent with deconditioning
  - Currently self-transfers from a wheelchair with poor safety awareness
  - Requires assistance of 2 people to stand and ambulate using a 2-wheeled walker
  - Refuses medication approximately 25% of the time
  - Sleeps in stretches of 2 to 3 hours during all shifts, thus missing most meal times

Quick Reference

- Possible diagnoses and their signs/symptoms:
  - Paranoia: unwarranted suspicion of others, sensitivity to criticism, difficulty working in a team, social isolation, irritability, defensiveness
  - Disorganized behavior: aimless behavior, anhedonia, poor motivation, delusions, hallucinations, grimacing, inappropriate laughter
  - Catatonic behavior: prolonged lack of motion, lack of response to stimuli, aimless movement, acute autonomic instability (malignant catatonia)
  - Schizophreniform disorder: less than 6 months' duration of hallucinations, delusions, poor hygiene and energy, odd behavior, social withdrawal, anhedonia
  - Schizoaffective disorder: cyclic symptom exacerbations and improvement, combining symptoms of schizophrenia and anxiety, depression, or bipolar
- Questions to ask the patient (or friend/family member):
  - Do you often feel any of the symptoms (listed previously)?
  - Have you ever been diagnosed with a schizophrenia spectrum disorder (listed previously)? What was going on in your life around the time of that diagnosis?
  - How do you deal with your schizophrenia? How well does that work for you?
  - What should I know about your schizophrenia?
- Referral options:
  - Psychiatrist for diagnosis, behavioral and pharmacological management
  - Social worker for care and resources to facilitate continued independence
  - Support group for persons with schizophrenia spectrum disorders

References

1. Stubbs B, Soundy A, Probst M, et al. The assessment, benefits and delivery of physical activity in people with schizophrenia: a survey of members of the International Organization of Physical Therapists in Mental Health. *Physiother Res Int.* 2014;19(4):248-256. DOI:10.1002/pri.1592
2. Vancampfort D, Probst M, Helvik Skjaerven L, et al. Systematic review of the benefits of physical therapy within a multidisciplinary care approach for people with schizophrenia. *Phys Ther.* 2012;92(1):11-23.
3. Vera-Garcia E, Mayoral-Cleries F, Vancampfort D, Stubbs B, Cuesta-Vargas AI. A systematic review of the benefits of physical therapy within a multidisciplinary care approach for people with schizophrenia: an update. *Psychiatry Res.* 2015;229(3):828-839.
4. Shusterman N. *Challenger Deep.* New York, NY: HarperCollins; 2015.
5. Sue D, Sue DW, Sue S. *Understanding Abnormal Behaviors.* 6th ed. Boston, MA: Houghton Mifflin; 2000.
6. American Psychiatric Association. *Diagnostic and Statistical Manual of Mental Disorders.* 5th ed. Washington, DC: American Psychiatric Association; 2013.
7. Tandon R, Gaebel W, Barch DM, et al. Definition and description of schizophrenia in the DSM-5. *Schiz Res.* 2013;150(1):3-10.
8. Drench ME, Noonan AC, Sharby N, Ventura SH. *Psychosocial Aspects of Health Care.* 3rd ed. Upper Saddle River, NJ: Pearson; 2012.
9. Lundy-Ekman L. *Neuroscience: Fundamentals for Rehabilitation.* 3rd ed. St. Louis, MO: Saunders; 2007.
10. Vancampfort D, Probst M, De Hert M, et al. Neurobiological effects of physical exercise in schizophrenia: a systematic review. *Disabil Rehabil.* 2014;36(21):1749-1754.
11. Vancampfort D, De Hert M, Knapen J, et al. State anxiety, psychological stress and positive well-being responses to yoga and aerobic exercise in people with schizophrenia: a pilot study. *Disabil Rehabil.* 2011;33(8):684-689.
12. Olesen J, Gustavsson A, Svensson M, Wittchen HU, Jönsson B; CDBE2010 study group; European Brain Council. The economic cost of brain disorders in Europe. *Eur J Neurology.* 2012;19(1):155-162.

13. Murru A, Pacchiarotti I, Amann BL, Nivoli AMA, Vieta E, Colom F. Treatment adherence in bipolar I and schizoaffective disorder, bipolar type. *J Affect Disord.* 2013;151(3):1003-1008.
14. Rastad C, Martin C, Åsenlöf P. Barriers, benefits, and strategies for physical activity in patients with schizophrenia. *Phys Ther.* 2014;94(10):1467-1479.
15. Lynn SA, Plant RD. Dyskinesia in chronic schizophrenia: an examination of the psychiatric nurse's perspective and its implications for physiotherapy. *Clin Rehabil.* 1995;9(2):97-101.
16. Fujino J, Tanaka H, Taniguchi N, Tabushi K. Effectiveness of aripiprazole in a patient with presumed idiopathic Parkinson's disease and chronic paranoid schizophrenia. *Psychiatry Clin Neurosci.* 2010;64(1):107-109.
17. Craddock B, Craddock N. Contractures in neuroleptic malignant syndrome. *Am J Psychiatry.* 1997;154(3):436.
18. Brown S, Inskip H, Barraclough B. Causes of the excess mortality of schizophrenia. *Br J Psychiatr.* 2000;177:212-217.
19. US Department of Health & Human Services. What is metabolic syndrome? *National Institute of Health: National Heart, Lung, and Blood Institute.* https://www.nhlbi.nih.gov/health/health-topics/topics/ms. Accessed February 21, 2018.
20. Littrell KH, Hilligoss NM, Kirshner CD, Petty RG, Johnson CG. The effects of an educational intervention on antipsychotic-induced weight gain. *J Nurs Scholarsh.* 2003;35(3):237-241.
21. Poulin MJ, Chaput JP, Simard V, et al. Management of antipsychotic-induced weight gain: prospective naturalistic study of the effectiveness of a supervised exercise programme. *Aust N Z J Psychiatry.* 2007;41(12):980-989.
22. Nyboe L, Vestergaard CH, Moeller MK, Lund H, Videbech P. Metabolic syndrome and aerobic fitness in patients with first-episode schizophrenia, including 1-year follow-up. *Schizophr Res.* 2015;168(1-2):381-387.
23. Cimo A, Stergiopoulos E, Cheng C, Bonato S, Dewa CS. Effective lifestyle interventions to improve type II diabetes self-management for those with schizophrenia or schizoaffective disorder: a systematic review. *BMC Psychiatry.* 2012;12:24.
24. Vancampfort D, De Hert M, Helvik Skjerven L, et al. International Organization of Physical Therapy in Mental Health consensus on physical activity within multidisciplinary rehabilitation programmes for minimising cardio-metabolic risk in patients with schizophrenia. *Disabil Rehabil.* 2012;34(1):1-12.
25. Ventegodt S, Andersen NJ, Kandel I, Merrick J. Effect, side effects and adverse events of non-pharmaceutical medicine. A review. *Int J Disabil Hum Dev.* 2009;8(3):227-235.
26. Cai C, Yu L, Rong L, Zhong H. Effectiveness of humor intervention for patients with schizophrenia: a randomized controlled trial. *J Psychiatr Res.* 2014;59:174-178.
27. Soundy A, Freeman P, Stubbs B, Probst M, Vancampfort D. The value of social support to encourage people with schizophrenia to engage in physical activity: an international insight from specialist mental health physiotherapists. *J Ment Health.* 2014;23(5):256-260.
28. Probst M, Knapen J, Poot G, Vancampfort D. Psychomotor therapy and psychiatry: what's in a name? *Open Complement Med J.* 2010;2:105-113.
29. Hedlund L, Gyllensten AL. The physiotherapists' experience of Basic Body Awareness Therapy in patients with schizophrenia and schizophrenia spectrum disorders. *J Bodyw Mov Ther.* 2013;17(2):169-176.
30. Danielsson L, Papoulias I, Petersson EL, Carlsson J, Waern M. Exercise or basic body awareness therapy as add-on treatment for major depression: a controlled study. *J Affect Disord.* 2014;168:98-106.
31. Gyllensten AL, Hansson L, Ekdahl C. Outcome of basic body awareness therapy. A randomized controlled study of patients in psychiatric outpatient care. *Adv Physiother.* 2003;5(4):179-190.
32. Gyllensten AL, Hansson L, Ekdahl C. Patient experiences of basic body awareness therapy and the relationship with the physiotherapist. *J Bodyw Mov Ther.* 2003;7(3):173-183.
33. Gyllensten AL, Ekdahl C, Hansson L. Long-term effectiveness of basic body awareness therapy in psychiatric outpatient care. A randomized controlled study. *Adv Physiother.* 2009;11(1):2-12.
34. Rosenbaum S, Tiedemann A, Sherrington C, Curtis J, Ward PB. Physical activity interventions for people with mental illness: a systematic review and meta-analysis. *J Sci Med Sport.* 2014;18(suppl 1):e150.
35. Ren J, Xia J. Dance therapy for schizophrenia. *Cochrane Database Syst Rev.* 2013;(10):CD006868.
36. Balasubramaniam M, Telles S, Doraiswamy PM. Yoga on our minds: a systematic review of yoga for neuropsychiatric disorders. *Front Psychiatry.* 2013;3(117):1-16.
37. Oertel-Knöchel V, Mehler P, Thiel C, et al. Effects of aerobic exercise on cognitive performance and individual psychopathology in depressive and schizophrenia patients. *Eur Arch Psychiatry Clin Neurosci.* 2014;264(7):589-604. DOI 10.1007/s00406-014-0485-9.
38. Marzolini S, Jensen B, Melville P. Feasibility and effects of a group-based resistance and aerobic exercise program for individuals with severe schizophrenia: a multidisciplinary approach. *Ment Health Phys Act.* 2009;2(1):29-36.

Personality Disorders

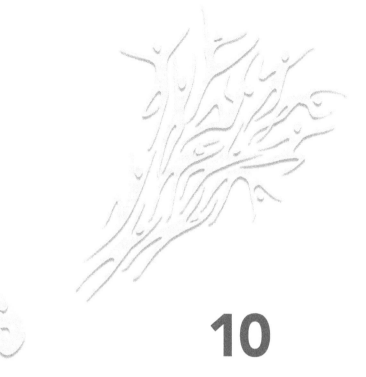

10

Outline

- Scope and Classification of Personality Disorders
- Neurophysiological Background, Etiology, and Risk Factors
- Comorbid Medical and Psychosocial Issues
- Specific Clinical Approaches to Improve Physical Therapy Outcomes
- Summary
- Key Points
- Review Questions
- Case Studies: First Impressions
- Quick Reference

Learning Objectives

- Demonstrate awareness of various personality disorder diagnoses per the *Diagnostic and Statistical Manual of Mental Disorders, 5th Edition (*DSM-5) classification
- Summarize research related to changes in the human movement system for personality disorders
- Incorporate risk factor assessment for personality disorders into the patient/client interview
- Delineate impact of common comorbidities on patient care per the patient management model
- Propose changes to the physical therapist's approach, based on a personality disorder diagnosis, into assessments, exercise prescription, home exercise programs, building/maintaining rapport, and clinical documentation to improve outcomes

Johnson H.
Psychosocial Elements of Physical Therapy: The Connection of Body to Mind (pp 161-170).

Personality disorders occur when certain normal aspects of a person's identity are exaggerated to a pathological extent, impairing the ability to interact well with others. While the classification section of this chapter will survey major personality disorders per the DSM-5, the majority of the chapter will focus on borderline personality disorder (BPD), which is perhaps the most researched and most difficult disorder to address, and which most impacts the physical therapy plan of care[1]:

> In my first year working I had a patient who had what was likely undiagnosed [BPD]. He came to the [skilled nursing facility] as 911 was called because he lived in a very cluttered house and was heating it with the oven. One night some of his items caught fire from the open oven and 911 was called. As his place was not suitable for living he was admitted to the ER and then transitioned to the rehab department I worked in. Upon coming to the [skilled nursing facility] he fell his first day trying to take the battery out of the clock as he feared that there was a camera inside of it.
>
> In therapy he would become quickly agitated when given certain tasks, sometimes ones he had performed many times. There was one point where he was asked to hold onto a walker and he became very upset. He grabbed the walker and threw it at the volunteers who were sitting by the wall and yelled "I don't need this! I'm abled, not disabled." For everyone else's safety I told him it would be best to go back to his room. He was very unsteady and nearly fell multiple times on the walk to the elevator. However, when attempting to prevent him from falling he would swing at me stating he did not need any help.
>
> Following this incident we had a social worker begin to assist him in his care. It turns out the place he was living in did not belong to him and he did not have any keys to retrieve his items. The person whose name was on the apartment had actually passed away a year prior. We never found out how he came to be living here as he had an incident with a night staff [certified nursing assistant] and had to be removed from the building for the safety of the staff. (Z. Meineke, PT, DPT, written communication, January 7, 2017)

Scope and Classification of Personality Disorders

To learn about personality disorders, one needs to first know the classification of personality types. As described in Chapter 1, one way of classifying personality types is the Big 5, or 5-Factor Model, developed first in the 1940s. These factors are "neuroticism, extraversion, openness to experience, agreeableness, and conscientiousness."[2] Neuroticism, the tendency toward negative emotions, is involved with anxiety and well-being and is a risk factor for depression. Extraversion includes sociability, activity, and relative lack of introspection. Openness to experience combines creativity and a commitment to lifelong learning. Agreeableness involves cooperation and a gentle good nature. Finally, conscientiousness manifests itself in goal-directed behavior, dependability, and orderliness. A personality disorder in any domain is diagnosed by a psychiatrist when it is consistently observed and causes significantly impaired function or distress to the individual.

Sue et al[3] hypothesized that personality disorders are undesirable variants on the Big 5 personality traits. Saulsman and Page[4] confirmed this hypothesis while leaving the potential for other means of classification, while Kotov et al[5] linked the factors to depressive disorders (high neuroticism, low extraversion, and conscientiousness), anxiety disorders (high neuroticism), and substance use disorders (high neuroticism and disinhibition with low agreeableness). Given these complex relationships between types of psychological conditions, classification can be difficult. To simplify this issue, the reader may refer to the 3-cluster system from the DSM-5 in Table 10-1, being aware that individuals might have more than one overlapping disorder.

Table 10-1

Cluster Classification of Personality Disorders

CLUSTER A	CLUSTER B	CLUSTER C
Odd or eccentric behaviors,[6] including social awkwardness, withdrawal, and distorted thought process	Dramatic, emotional, or erratic behaviors, involving deficits in "impulse control and emotional regulation"[7]	Anxious or fearful behaviors,[8] with underlying high anxiety levels
• **Paranoid:** individuals are suspicious and distrustful of others, preventing close relationships. • **Schizoid:** individuals are socially detached and do not express a full range of emotions, rarely seeking out or enjoying close relationships. • **Schizotypal:** individuals are uncomfortable in social settings and express odd beliefs, such as thought broadcasting (see Chapter 5 for definition), with low ability to keep close relationships.	• **Antisocial:** individuals ignore others' rights and demonstrate deceit, manipulation, hostility, and a lack of real remorse for illegal actions. • **Borderline:** individuals have "intense and unstable emotions and moods," causing impulsive behaviors (including substance abuse), tendency to see the world in black and white, and propensity for self-destructive behavior as a coping mechanism for high distress levels.[7] • **Histrionic:** individuals show excessive but shallow emotion, seeking attention, and being depressed when not the center of attention; close relationships are difficult. • **Narcissistic:** individuals have strong feelings of entitlement, fantasies of being exceptional in all things, tendency toward superficial relationships, and anger on realizing their limitations.	• **Avoidant:** individuals have "social inhibition, feelings of inadequacy, and a hypersensitivity to negative evaluation" causing avoidance of social situations.[8] • **Dependent:** individuals feel "a strong need to be taken care of by other people," which can unfortunately make them prone to abuse and manipulation by others.[8] • **Obsessive-compulsive personality disorder:** individuals are inflexibly adherent to rules and orderliness, and are unable to delegate tasks or complete projects due to excess attention to detail.

BPD, the focus of this chapter, is "characterized by difficulties in regulating emotion. This difficulty leads to severe, unstable mood swings, impulsivity and instability, poor self-image and stormy personal relationships," which can result in "destructive behavior, such as self-harm (cutting) or suicide attempts."[9] Indicators of this emotional instability include:

- Massive effort expended to avoid real or perceived abandonment
- Interpersonal relationships that are "split" between idealizing and devaluing the other person
- Inaccurate and fluctuating perception of self, affecting values, goals, and moods
- Impulsive and potentially dangerous patterns of behavior, such as substance abuse
- Hours- to days-long bouts of depression, irritability, and anxiety with "feelings of boredom or emptiness"[9]
- Feelings of dissociation and paranoia, with potential for short psychotic episodes if stress is high enough

Neurophysiological Background, Etiology, and Risk Factors

BPD, perhaps one of the most difficult personality disorders to work with, has multifaceted causes. Some literature relevant to the physical therapist's approach to BPD exists, but very limited to no research relative to other personality disorders. BPD may develop as early as one's teens; risk factors include prior attention-deficit hyperactivity disorder and oppositional defiant disorder.[10] According to the National Alliance on Mental Illness, other risk factors include "traumatic life events, such as physical or sexual abuse during childhood or neglect and separation from parents," as well as underlying neurological changes with possible genetic basis.[9] Burgess[11] hypothesized that the timing of traumatic childhood events may coincide with frontotemporal lobe development.

These changes affect neurological areas and circuits influencing emotional regulation and good judgment. Kraus et al[12] noted decreased orbitofrontal cortex and midcingulate activation, but increased dorsolateral prefrontal cortex activation in subjects who imagined self-injurious behavior (a common maladaptive coping mechanism for the emotional pain of BPD). Dell'Osso et al[13] note that both volume and activity level change in "the prefrontal and cingulate cortex, amygdala and hippocampus," which are areas involved in memory and fear reactions. Frontotemporal deficits manifest themselves in test results for "delayed memory, serial sevens [subtraction], rhythm reproduction, and perseveration."[11]

Chemical changes also underlie BPD. Persons with BPD "ascribe anger to ambiguous facial expressions and exhibit enhanced and prolonged reactions in response to threatening social cues, associated with enhanced and prolonged amygdala responses."[14] When oxytocin was administered in this study, if subjects were not on other medications for BPD symptoms, it normalized these abnormal emotional responses. Dell'Osso et al[13] add that circuits using the neurotransmitters glutamine, dopamine, and serotonin are abnormal in BPD.

Comorbid Medical and Psychosocial Issues

People with BPD are like people with third degree burns over 90% of their bodies. Lacking emotional skin, they feel agony at the slightest touch or movement.

—Marsha M. Linehan[15]

Personality disorders as a whole cause high costs to the medical system, as well as lost productivity when the disorder impairs the individual's function. Olesen et al[16] estimate at least

27.3 billion euros ($29.3 billion in 2017) were spent in 2010 to address personality disorders and related problems in Europe. This high cost is associated with numerous comorbid medical issues, psychosocial problems, and medication effects.

Psychiatric comorbidities for BPD include anxiety, posttraumatic stress disorder, bipolar disorder, depression, bulimia nervosa or other eating disorder, other personality disorders, and substance use disorders.[9] Specific substances include alcohol, non-prescribed drugs, and tobacco.[17] Other psychiatric comorbidities include obsessive-compulsive and impulse-control disorders, attention-deficit hyperactivity disorder, potentially undiagnosed seizure disorder, and increased risk of suicide.[3,13]

Multiple medical issues also exist. Having a personality disorder, or even a high level of neuroticism, predicts the lack of success of fusion surgery (vs conservative care, including physical therapy) for persistent low back pain and poor adherence to oral medication treatment for comorbid bipolar I or schizoaffective disorder (bipolar type).[18,19] Additionally, the patient is more likely to have "arteriosclerosis or hypertension, hepatic disease, cardiovascular disease, gastrointestinal disease, arthritis, [and] venereal disease" if BPD is present.[20] Dell'Osso et al[13] add chronic fatigue syndrome, fibromyalgia, temporomandibular joint dysfunction, hypertension, low back pain, urinary incontinence, and more emergency room and hospital visits. More comorbidities also predict greater suicide risk. BPD is not, however, significantly associated with metabolic diseases such as type 2 diabetes, obesity, and history of stroke.[13]

There is no pharmacological treatment for "the core symptoms of emptiness, abandonment and identity disturbance" in BPD.[9] However, mood stabilizers, antidepressants, and antipsychotics decrease other symptoms of the condition. An efficacy study of medications for BPD found that "the mood stabilisers [sic] topiramate, lamotrigine, and valproate semisodium, and the second-generation antipsychotics aripiprazole and olanzapine" work best.[21]

Medication side effects of special interest to the physical therapist include:

- Topiramate: drowsiness, dizziness, and impaired coordination
- Lamotrigine: dizziness, drowsiness, back pain, and double vision
- Valproate: sleepiness, dry mouth, and gastrointestinal distress
- Aripiprazole: dysphagia, dizziness, anxiety, and drowsiness
- Olanzapine: weight gain, sedation, impaired memory, back or extremity pain

Psychosocial issues, especially suicide risk, are common in personality disorders. Antisocial personality disorder predicts job termination in the 1-year period following interprofessional rehabilitation for job-related injuries.[22] High stress levels, poor social support, and legal or interpersonal problems are associated with personality disorders as a group.[17] Several authors, though, noted high remission rates (causes unspecified) for BPD: 85% over 10 years with 12% relapse; 56% recovery within 2 years of diagnosis with typical normalization by age 40, although social function may remain impaired in others.[23,13]

Specific Clinical Approaches to Improve Physical Therapy Outcomes

It is easy for the clinician to become frustrated and burned out by personality disorders, especially BPD. This problem has several possible solutions. One is to have another team member treat the patient for a short period of time, if possible, which the author has seen to be effective. Another option is to refer the patient to psychiatric evaluation services if the patient is willing.[24] This referral can help the patient cope with impaired adaptation skills and flawed interpersonal relationships. Additionally, the clinician should be familiar with concepts of cognitive behavioral therapy and its subtypes (see Chapter 4) as these can help treat individuals with BPD.[25]

For many mental health issues, as explored in Chapters 6 through 12, judicious use of groups and other psychosocial supports is supported by research literature. Two strong studies support intensive multicomponent individualized and group psychotherapy, which **includes a walking program and training to improve body awareness.**[26,27] If group members are educated in what to expect from themselves and others, groups give the patient a variety of other people with whom to interact and receive support from. Thus, for a person with BPD, the characteristic feelings of aloneness and emptiness may decrease in an exercise group.

Regardless of the specific physical activity component in a physical therapy plan of care, the therapist should practice "being empathetic, performing an ongoing assessment of cases, self-disclosing, making explicit treatment contracts, validating patients' experiences and promoting awareness of psychological experience" for effective personality disorder treatment.[28] The following are examples from the author's personal experience. This validation can compensate for the difficulty persons with BPD have "in actively suppressing irrelevant information when it is of an aversive nature."[13] Thus, the clinician should educate simply and clearly, especially when it includes content the patient may not want to hear but needs to hear anyway.

One patient with whom the author worked did not have a clinical diagnosis of BPD, but displayed signs of the condition. These included intense and rapid apparent mood swings, splitting of relationships with therapists on the team in the subacute rehabilitation setting, and reactions suggesting intense anger when the patient did not understand an instruction or other communication. Maintaining a mindset of intent to validate the patient's feelings and insecurities, the author typically approached this patient in a more public area of the rehabilitation unit, so that another staff member or therapist who happened to be nearby could be a neutral party.

As often as possible, the author also encouraged the patient to come to the therapy gym for healthy interpersonal interactions. Due to the patient's additional cognitive impairments, the author used consistency and written participation expectations in patient instruction, especially for follow-through of strengthening exercises and a gradually increased activity level to speed postoperative recovery. Ultimately, the patient was discharged due to a verbal incident between the patient, the author's supervisor, and the facility's medical director. While these factors prevented the discharge from being ideal in terms of lead time for planning purposes, the team members came together to maximize the patient's safety in her discharge setting by providing assistive and adaptive equipment.

Another patient, also not formally diagnosed with BPD, was seen for physical deconditioning, complicated by amputations of parts of both legs. When the author first walked into her room on a long-term care unit for the physical therapy evaluation, the patient emphatically stated "I don't want a psych evaluation!" and displayed indicators of mood swings, split relationships, and bouts of intense anger throughout the episode of care. One physical therapist assistant (PTA) typically worked with the patient, with limited patient participation influenced by the patient verbalizing a lack of acceptance of the functional implications of her amputations. During supervisory visits by the author, the patient was alternately friendly, tearful, and complaining about the PTA. A home visit was provided by the PTA and treating occupational therapist for safety and to improve carryover of discharge recommendations. The patient was finally discharged home with caregiver support, and a wheelchair was provided for mobility.

Summary

While personality disorders are not as common as other psychological conditions, nor as detrimental to function, their presence may complicate the physical therapy plan of care especially related to rapport, burnout prevention, and adherence to treatment. In particular, BPD is difficult for many professionals to work with and requires the support of the interdisciplinary team/

interprofessional team and the clinician's personal network. This chapter covered strategies to help the clinician and patient deal with the difficulties of a personality disorder and its many potential comorbid conditions.

Key Points

- Research supports a walking program and body awareness training as part of multicomponent psychotherapy and physical therapy for persons with BPD and other mental illnesses.
- Keep education simple, clear, and non-confrontational due to BPD's associated cognitive deficits.

Review Questions

- Recall a recent patient with eccentric, dramatic, or fearful behaviors (Cluster A, B, or C) that negatively impacted your plan of care.
  - Might these behaviors, based on the earlier criteria, qualify as consistent with a personality disorder? Where might you refer for a diagnosis if the patient was willing?
  - How did you address these behaviors? How might you change your approach next time?
- If applicable, review a case from you, a coworker, or friend concerning someone with a diagnosed personality disorder.
  - What risk factors were present in the person's social history?
  - What comorbidities were present in the person's medical history?
  - If this patient came to you for a physical therapy evaluation, how would you approach the case? Consider the patient management model (see Figure 5-1) and the *International Classification of Functioning, Disability and Health* domains.
  - Given the importance of therapist-patient rapport, how would you address the roadblocks presented by the personality disorder and common impairments in interpersonal relationships?

Case Studies: First Impressions

As you review the following case studies, you may want to consider these questions for thought or discussion:

- What standardized tests and measures (including psychiatric, for example, a depression screen) would you select for this patient? Why?
- Based on available data, what short- and long-term goals would you write for your plan of care? Consider using the acronyms SMART (specific, measurable, attainable, realistic, and timely) or ABCDE (actor, behavior, conditions, degree, and expected time frame) to guide your goal writing.
- What elements (procedures, psychosocial aspects, communication aspects, etc) would you make sure to include or omit in your plan of care for this patient? Why?
- What are your anticipated needs, if any, for consultation and referral for this patient?
- How will you transition this patient toward lasting health behavior change following discharge (eg, recommending a YMCA membership trial)?

Case 1

A 32-year-old female was referred to outpatient physical therapy for lateral epicondylalgia. Her goal is to return to recreational tennis, where she attributes the epicondylalgia to a tennis overuse injury.

- Social history: she has 2 children whom she cares for at home. When her husband can be home to watch the children, she works part time as a photographer, which requires carrying equipment and frequently changing position.
- Medical/psychiatric history: bilateral wrist fractures (10 years ago, in collegiate gymnastics), delivery of her first child via C-section (5 years ago), and narcissistic personality disorder
- Impairments, activity limitations, and participation restrictions found on initial interview and examination
  - Pain and paresthesia in right upper extremity; both symptoms are affected by sleep or prolonged resting position
  - Decreased proprioception in affected wrist and elbow
  - Standing tolerance 15 minutes due to subjective instability in low back

Case 2

A 44-year-old male was hospitalized and is in the intensive care unit with second- and third-degree burns to his upper body and face following a grill explosion at home. His goal is to return to work as an accountant.

- Social history: he lives in a 2-story house with a basement. Prior to injury, he completed approximately half of indoor and outdoor household tasks. His wife works as a school administrator; they have no children.
- Medical/psychiatric history: mild heart attack (2 years ago), hypertension, coronary artery disease, nicotine dependence (started 30 years ago), and paranoid personality disorder. He is compliant with medications for all cardiovascular conditions and currently smokes half a pack of cigarettes per day.
- Impairments, activity limitations, and participation restrictions found on initial interview and examination
  - Occasional pain reported in second-degree burn areas
  - Reluctance to move from the side of the hospital bed
  - Shortness of breath with 3 minutes of standing or short-distance ambulation
  - Requests that lights be left on in his room at all times
  - States to hospital staff that nurses are impersonating other personnel
  - Unsteady gait pattern even with a 2-wheeled walker (used no device prior to injury)

Case 3

A 66-year-old female was admitted to subacute rehabilitation following surgical repair of right hip fracture, with a non-weightbearing restriction imposed for 2 weeks following admission. Her goal is to move to a different state where she can be near family.

- Social history: limited information available from the patient and hospital records. Both her prior residence and intended discharge location have at least 4 steps to enter with a single railing.
- Medical/psychiatric history: obesity, congestive heart failure, major depressive disorder, and suspected BPD (refuses recommended psychiatric evaluation)

- Impairments, activity limitations, and participation restrictions found on initial interview and examination
  - Pain in right hip rated 10/10 without medication and 9/10 with medication
  - Pitting edema noted in surgically operated lower extremity
  - Shortness of breath at rest and increased with upright sitting or standing
  - Poor observed carryover of weightbearing restriction during transfers with a 2-wheeled walker
  - Standing tolerance 30 to 60 seconds with 50% assistance required
  - Prefers to stay in her wheelchair vs the elevating recliner in her room, despite medical recommendations to elevate both legs as much as possible due to edema
  - Unable to ambulate or hop with 2-wheeled walker at time of evaluation

Quick Reference

- Possible diagnoses and their signs/symptoms:
  - Paranoid personality disorder: mistrust of others, poor social life, suspiciousness
  - Schizoid personality disorder: avoidance of close relationships, limited emotional range, indifference to praise
  - Schizotypal personality disorder: social discomfort, odd beliefs or thoughts, social anxiety and isolation, rambling speech, inappropriate emotional response
  - Antisocial personality disorder: deceitfulness, irresponsibility, boredom, anger, impulsivity, irritability, substance dependence
  - BPD: compulsiveness, impulsivity, antisocial behavior, loneliness, guilt, mood swings, suicidal thoughts, narcissism
  - Histrionic personality disorder: focus on appearance and being the center of attention, emotional lability, depression, treatment of relationships as closer than in reality, susceptibility to influence by others
  - Narcissistic personality disorder: callousness, grandiosity, social isolation, excessive need for approval and recognition
  - Avoidant personality disorder: social isolation, inferiority complex, fear
  - Dependent personality disorder: passivity, conflict and decision avoidance, need to be with others, excessive grief when relationships end
  - Obsessive-compulsive personality disorder: excessive punctuality and perfectionism, rigid habits, working at the expense of relationships
- Questions to ask the patient (more typically a friend/family member, since persons with personality disorder may refuse psychiatric evaluation or diagnosis):
  - Do you often feel any of the symptoms (listed previously)?
  - Have you ever been diagnosed with a personality disorder (listed previously)? What was going on in your life around the time of that diagnosis?
  - How do you deal with your disorder? How well does that work for you?
  - What should I know about your personality disorder?
- Referral options:
  - Psychiatrist for diagnosis and behavioral treatment
  - Social worker for safe community discharge options if disorder impairs function
  - Support group for persons with personality disorders

References

1. American Psychiatric Association. *Diagnostic and Statistical Manual of Mental Disorders.* 5th ed. Washington, DC: American Psychiatric Association; 2013.
2. Judge TA, Higgins CA, Thoresen CJ, Barrick MR. The big five personality traits, general mental ability, and career success across the life span. *Pers Psychol.* 1999;52(3):621-652.
3. Sue D, Sue DW, Sue S. *Understanding Abnormal Behaviors.* 6th ed. Boston, MA: Houghton Mifflin; 2000.
4. Saulsman LM, Page AC. The five-factor model and personality disorder empirical literature: a meta-analytic review. *Clin Psychol Rev.* 2004;23(8):1055-1085.
5. Kotov R, Gamez W, Schmidt F, Watson D. Linking "big" personality traits to anxiety, depressive, and substance use disorders: a meta-analysis. *Psychol Bull.* 2010;136(5):768-821.
6. Hoermann S, Zupanick CE, Dombeck M. DSM-5: the ten personality disorders: cluster A. *Mentalhelp.* https://www.mentalhelp.net/articles/dsm-5-the-ten-personality-disorders-cluster-a/. Published December 6, 2013. Updated November 17, 2015. Accessed February 22, 2018.
7. Hoermann S, Zupanick CE, Dombeck M. DSM-5: the ten personality disorders: cluster B. *Mentalhelp.* https://www.mentalhelp.net/articles/dsm-5-the-ten-personality-disorders-cluster-b/. April 26, 2016. Accessed November 13, 2016.
8. Hoermann S, Zupanick CE, Dombeck M. DSM-5 the ten personality disorders: cluster C. *Mentalhelp.* https://www.mentalhelp.net/articles/dsm-5-the-ten-personality-disorders-cluster-c/. Published December 6, 2013. Updated April 26, 2016. Accessed February 22, 2018.
9. National Alliance on Mental Illness. Borderline personality disorder. *National Alliance on Mental Illness.* http://www.nami.org/Learn-More/Mental-Health-Conditions/Borderline-Personality-Disorder. Updated 2017. Accessed February 22, 2018.
10. Stepp SD, Burke JD, Hipwell AE, Loeber R. Trajectories of attention deficit hyperactivity disorder and oppositional defiant disorder symptoms as precursors of borderline personality disorder symptoms in adolescent girls. *J Abnorm Child Psychol.* 2012;40(1):7-20.
11. Burgess JW. Cognitive information processing in borderline personality disorder: a neuropsychiatric hypothesis. *Jefferson Journal of Psychiatry.* 1990;8(2):34-49.
12. Kraus A, Valerius G, Seifritz E, et al. Script-driven imagery of self-injurious behavior in patients with borderline personality disorder: a pilot FMRI study. *Acta Psychiatr Scand.* 2010;121(1):41-51.
13. Dell'Osso B, Berlin HA, Serati M, Altamura AC. Neuropsychobiological aspects, comorbidity patterns and dimensional models in borderline personality disorder. *Neuropsychobiology.* 2010;61(4):169-179.
14. Bertsch K, Gamer M, Schmidt B, et al. Oxytocin and reduction of social threat hypersensitivity in women with borderline personality disorder. *Am J Psychiatry.* 2013;170(10):1169-1177.
15. Greenstein L. Understanding borderline personality disorder. *National Alliance on Mental Illness.* https://www.nami.org/Blogs/NAMI-Blog/June-2017/Understanding-Borderline-Personality-Disorder. Published June 5, 2017. Accessed May 2, 2018.
16. Olesen J, Gustavsson A, Svensson M, Wittchen HU, Jönsson B; CDBE2010 study group; European Brain Council. The economic cost of brain disorders in Europe. *Eur J Neurology.* 2012;19(1):155-162.
17. Trull TJ, Jahng S, Tomko RL, Wood PK, Sher KJ. Revised NESARC personality disorder diagnoses: gender, prevalence, and comorbidity with substance dependence disorders. *J Pers Disord.* 2010;24(4):412-426.
18. Daubs MD, Norvell DC, McGuire R, et al. Fusion versus nonoperative care for chronic low back pain. *Spine.* 2011;36(suppl 21):S96-S109.
19. Murru A, Pacchiarotti I, Amann BL, Nivoli AMA, Vieta E, Colom F. Treatment adherence in bipolar I and schizoaffective disorder, bipolar type. *J Affect Disord.* 2013;151(3):1003-1008.
20. El-Gabalawy R, Katz LY, Sareen J. Comorbidity and associated severity of borderline personality disorder and physical health conditions in a nationally representative sample. *Psychosom Med.* 2010;72(7):641-647.
21. Lieb K, Völlm B, Rücker G, Timmer A, Stoffers JM. Pharmacotherapy for borderline personality disorder: Cochrane systematic review of randomised trials. *Br J Psychiatry.* 2010;196(1):4-12.
22. Brede E, Mayer TG, Gatchel RJ. Prediction of failure to retain work 1 year after interprofessional functional restoration in occupational injuries. *Arch Phys Med Rehabil.* 2012;93(2):268-274.
23. Gunderson JG, Stout RL, McGlashan TH, et al. Ten-year course of borderline personality disorder. *Arch Gen Psychiatry.* 2011;68(8):827-837.
24. Lundy-Ekman L. *Neuroscience: Fundamentals for Rehabilitation.* 3rd ed. St. Louis, MO: Saunders; 2007.
25. Stoffers JM, Völlm B, Rücker G, Timmer A, Huband N, Lieb K. Psychological therapies for people with borderline personality disorder (Review). *Cochrane Database Syst Rev.* 2012;(8):CD005652.
26. Solbakken OA, Abbass A. Intensive short-term dynamic residential treatment program for patients with treatment-resistant disorders. *J Affect Disord.* 2015;181:67-77.
27. Solbakken OA, Abbass A. Symptom- and personality disorder changes in intensive short-term dynamic residential treatment for treatment-resistant anxiety and depressive disorder. *Acta Neuropsychiatr.* 2016;28(5):257-271. DOI: 10.1017/neu.2016.5
28. DiMaggio G, Salvatore G, Fiore D, Carcione A, Nicolò G, Semerari A. General principles for treating personality disorder with a prominent inhibitedness trait: towards an operationalizing integrated technique. *J Pers Disord.* 2012;26(1):63-83.

Dementias
Neurocognitive Disorders

11

Outline

Johnson H.
Psychosocial Elements of Physical Therapy: The Connection of Body to Mind (pp 171-198).

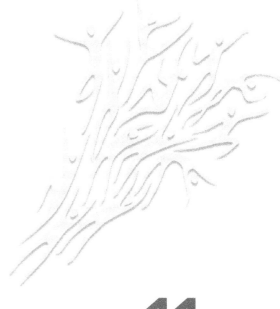

Learning Objectives

- Describe various neurocognitive disorders (*Diagnostic and Statistical Manual of Mental Disorders, 5th Edition* [DSM-5] term) in terms of affected neurological structures, signs and symptoms, prognosis for improvement with physical therapy, and treatment approaches
- Summarize research related to alterations in the human movement system for dementias
- Develop a patient interview format incorporating risk factor assessment for dementias
- Understand the effect of dementias' common co-occurring conditions into patient evaluation, treatment, and outcomes
- Propose changes to the physical therapist's approach, based on a diagnosis of dementia, to assessment, exercise prescription, home exercise programs, building and maintaining rapport, and documentation

Dementias, called *neurocognitive disorders* by the DSM-5, require a room full of books to explain their scope, etiology, comorbid movement-related disorders, psychosocial issues, and evidence-based physical therapy approaches.[1] Many useful books already exist on the subject; the goal of this text is to provide essential background and clinical reference with attention to the psychiatric aspects of various dementias. The reader may refer to such resources as Lewis and Bottomley's classic text for more treatment ideas.[2]

Physical therapy has demonstrated benefits for persons with dementia, in part because the insurance and medical landscape has vastly improved regarding other professionals' opinions of the benefits of physical therapy. However, significant education to stakeholders is still indicated because therapy services are far less likely to be used in long-term care and palliative care.[3,4] In the geriatric population as a whole, **"structured, individualized, higher intensity, longer duration, and multicomponent [exercise programs] show promise for preserving cognitive performance."**[5]

In persons with dementia, functional weightbearing exercise programs in particular are beneficial, especially when tailored to challenge the individual's physical capabilities and medical conditions (including hip fracture).[6] For persons with dementia, program duration may need to last at least several months.[7] As a whole, rehabilitation services, including physical and occupational therapy, show promise for delaying placement in a skilled nursing facility for non-progressive dementias; literature is inconclusive about effects on progressive dementias.[8]

Scope and Classification of Dementias and Other Neurocognitive Disorders

As noted in Chapter 5, dementia is a cluster of symptoms of cognitive and motor impairment with gradual onset, normal level of consciousness, minimal fluctuation, potential for delusions and hallucinations, and disorientation to time and place. According to the DSM-5,[1] dementias include:

- Alzheimer's disease (AD)
- Dementia with Lewy bodies, or Lewy body dementia (DLB)
- Vascular-associated dementia (VAD)
- Pick's disease and other types of frontotemporal dementia (FTD)
- Wernicke-Korsakoff syndrome, or alcoholic dementia (WKS)
- Dementia related to other medical conditions including normal pressure hydrocephalus (NPH), Huntington's disease (HD), Parkinson's disease (PD), HIV-AIDS, and multiple sclerosis

While the public may think only of AD when hearing the term dementia, it is important for the health care provider to educate other people about the various types, presentations, progression, and prognosis. However, there is a commonality among the various kinds of dementia, for which Lewis and Bottomley offer the acronym JAMCO for remembering dementia's general characteristics[2]:

- J: judgment is impaired.
- A: affect is altered. Friends and spouses may say that the person is not the person they once knew.
- M: memory is impaired to varying degrees.
- C: cognition and problem-solving abilities prevent safe independent living.
- O: orientation is diminished. Generally, the person with dementia knows his or her name and date of birth, but knowledge of other aspects such as social roles, place, and time disappear.

AD is diagnosed in 3% of people 65 to 74 years old, 19% between 75 and 84 years old, and 47% over 85 years old. Risk factors include depression, genetics, poor nutrition, physical inactivity, low education level, and head trauma. Symptoms and signs unique to this form of dementia include impaired memory, thinking, behavior, initiative, word-finding, environmental navigation, and a return to primitive motor reflexes over an average of 8 to 10 years, at which point, the cause of death is typically a secondary condition, such as aspiration pneumonia. Symptoms may begin up to 20 years before diagnosis.[9,10] Gras et al[11] determined norms for measures of balance and ambulation ability in adults with very mild AD, as measured by the Timed Up and Go (TUG), 10-Meter Walk, and Sharpened (tandem-stance) Romberg tests.

As shown in Table 11-1, balance and gait deteriorate early in AD. The minimally detectable change (MDC) is not attributable to measurement variance or error. These impairments are amenable to physical therapy, with high-intensity functional exercises that incorporate attention to the individual's specific impairments.[7,12,13]

DLB comprises about 20% of all cases of dementia. Lewy bodies are abnormal protein accumulations in the substantia nigra, correlating with Parkinsonian symptoms because PD also affects this area. The condition begins earlier than AD, typically around 60 to 70 years old, with variable cognition and alertness; repeated falls; fainting; visual hallucinations; and Parkinsonian signs, which actually worsen with the administration of anti-Parkinsonian medications, due to frequent misdiagnosis of this condition as PD. Cognitive impairments are milder than those in AD but may still be significant. Despite milder cognitive impairments, DLB progresses rapidly over 5 to 7 years until death from similar causes.[9,14]

VAD, a late effect of stroke, covers 10% to 20% of dementias in the United States and Europe, including 1% of all people over 65 years old. Often mixed with one or more other types of dementia, its unique features are stepwise and variable cognitive decline; focal neurological signs, including facial droop and difficulty in swallowing; gait abnormalities and urinary incontinence at an early stage; and changes in personality and emotional regulation. Risk factors include prior stroke, hypertension, type 2 diabetes, history of myocardial infarction, smoking, and cardiac arrhythmias. Treatment and prognosis are similar to that of a stroke alone.[9]

Pick's disease, now classified as an FTD, is a relatively rare, inherited form of dementia, comprising less than 5% of all cases and with a much earlier onset of 50 to 65 years old. Abrupt aphasia occurs early on, with reemergence of grasping and sucking reflexes, as well as a tendency for the patient to put objects in his or her mouth; this requires environmental adaptation and monitoring by caregivers. At this stage, the patient may spend up to 14 hours per day walking continuously. Later in the disease, the patient's ability to transfer, walk, and complete activities of daily living (ADL) rapidly declines, although memory remains until relatively late.[9] Progressively worse attention deficits also occur.[15] Other types of FTD affect personality, emotional lability, or motor coordination more strongly than language; all impair frontal lobe functions.

Table 11-1

Functional Tests Indicating Gait Impairments in Early Alzheimer's Disease

FUNCTIONAL TEST (MDC)	NORMAL VALUES FOR OLDER ADULTS	VALUES INDICATING FALL RISK IN HEALTHY ADULTS	TYPICAL VALUES IN MILD ALZHEIMER'S DISEASE
Sharpened Romberg (15.52 s with EO)	Females 60 to 69 years old: 56.15 s EO Females 70 to 79 years old: 44.13 s EO Males 60 to 90 years old: 46.53 to 54.7 s EO Females 60 to 69 years old: 28.08 s EC Females 70 to 79 years old: 19.16 s EC Males 60 to 90 years old: 15.46 to 24.62 s EC	Females: 34.28 to 38.5 s EO 8.24 to 10.51 s EC	24.5 s EO 6.5 s EC
TUG (2.77 s)	60 to 69 years old: 8.1 s 70 to 79 years old: 9.2 s	16 s or greater	8.1 s or greater
10-Meter Walk (0.125 m/s comfortable speed, 0.21 m/s fast speed)	60 to 69 years old: 1.24 m/s comfortable speed, 1.84 m/s fast speed 70 to 79 years old: 1.09 to 1.25 m/s comfortable speed, 1.86 m/s fast speed	N/A	1.21 m/s comfortable speed 1.82 m/s fast speed

s: seconds; EO: eyes open; EC: eyes closed

WKS, also known as *alcoholic dementia*, is caused by vitamin B1 (thiamine) deficiency after years of prolonged heavy drinking; secondary causes can include HIV-AIDS, chronic malnutrition, and infection. This syndrome can occur in younger individuals, depending on medical and substance use history. Unique symptoms include confabulation, or making up stories to compensate for severe and persistent loss of both past and currently forming memories[15]; a manipulative personality; confusion and memory impairment that persist until at least 1 year of abstinence from alcohol; and an ataxic slow gait pattern. Little research exists on long-term outcomes and prognosis for WKS.[9]

NPH, in which enlarged ventricles impinge on the brain, is a dementia with origins internal to the cerebral cortex. Although pressure of cerebrospinal fluid (CSF) remains within normal limits, the ventricles enlarge due to multiple possible causes, including "meningitis, head injury, subarachnoid hemorrhage, or encephalitis," while the majority of cases are idiopathic.[16] Symptoms common to all subcortical dementias include "a decline in immediate and delayed recall with preserved memory storage, impaired complex information processing, and psychomotor slowing."[16] About 5% of dementias are caused by NPH, with long-term care settings having a relatively higher proportion of 14%. Many cases are misdiagnosed, and thus poorly managed; early shunt placement helps 50% of patients, but the shunt can easily become obstructed. The classic symptom triad is wet, wild, and wobbly, with urinary incontinence as a first symptom (as compared to tremor as initial symptom in PD and cognitive impairment initially in AD). Specific gait deviations, not responsive to auditory cues and oral levodopa, include "bradykinesia, apraxia, shuffling, shorter stride length, broad base of support, difficulty turning, decreased foot clearance, and external rotation of the legs with poor balance," which looks like a magnetic attraction between the patient and the floor.[16]

PD is another type of subcortical dementia, with damage mostly in dopamine-producing areas of the brain. In 20% to 50% of cases, the disease leads to dementia, with depression as a common comorbidity. This dementia has milder memory impairments compared to other types, but the individual is still unable to learn new information or names.[9] Specific cognitive impairments include decreased planning, decision making, and goal-oriented behaviors.[14]

In rare cases, dementia can occur in other medical conditions, including HIV-AIDs (where dementia may be the initial sign),[17] HD, Creutzfelt-Jakob disease, and multiple sclerosis. More resources listed prior to this chapter's references are a starting point for the reader to deepen knowledge about any type of dementia. Regardless of the type of dementia, the clinician should maintain awareness of the key features of the dementias discussed in this chapter to tailor the plan of care, as well as educate patients, family, members of the public, and other stakeholders.

Neurophysiological Background, Etiology, and Risk Factors

Not all activities are equal in this regard. Those that involve genuine concentration—studying a musical instrument, playing board games, reading, and dancing—are associated with a lower risk for dementia. Dancing, which requires learning new moves, is both physically and mentally challenging and requires much concentration. Less intense activities, such as bowling, babysitting, and golfing, are not associated with a reduced risk of Alzheimer's.

—Norman Doidge[18]

Dementias have varied causes, just as they have varied presentation depending on the underlying disorder. AD remains a "black box" etiologically, with several hypotheses under investigation (namely, a viral infection or heavy metal toxicity); the causes of other types of dementia are better understood. This section discusses the known and suspected risk factors and neurological changes in major neurocognitive disorders.

AD is well-researched due to its progressive nature and relatively high prevalence, causing severe functional deficits with high burden on caregivers and finances. Microscopically, the disease is associated with buildup of abnormal tau and beta-amyloid proteins, with a third copy of chromosome 21 in some cells.[14] Trisomy 21 is not surprising, as persons with Down syndrome develop AD by age 40. These cell-level changes are associated with a patient's decreased ability to navigate the environment, track motion, and regulate emotions.

At an organ level, AD "starts in myelinated (white matter) structures in the brain (eg, hippocampus, corpus callosum, and olfactory bulb), and slowly (over years) progresses into the unmyelinated (grey matter) lobes of the cerebral cortex (eg, frontal, temporal, parietal, occipital)."[19] This progression, though not always linear, correlates to a staging system to help the clinician educate patients, family members, and other caregivers. This system combines the Global Deterioration Scale and the Functional Assessment Staging Tool (FAST; Table 11-2).[19]

Table 11-2

Functional Staging System for Alzheimer's Disease

STAGE	STRUCTURES AFFECTED	CLINICAL PRESENTATION	PHYSICAL THERAPIST ROLE
1	None	Cognition normal; medical risk factors present (diabetes, depression)	• Treat as cognitively normal • Address impact of medical risk factors
2	Mild damage to memory structures	Mild forgetfulness but no functional impairment	• Screen health risks, sensory deficits, and signs of cognitive impairment • Monitor vitals • Promote health literacy
3	Severe damage to corpus callosum, hippocampus, and olfactory bulb	Mildly impaired daily routine, long-term memory, sense of smell, ability to navigate familiar environment, factual recall, and balance	• Address caregiver needs • Track weight/cognition • Use multisensory cues • Adapt pain assessment • Continue stage 1 to 2 treatment
4	Centers for smell, taste, and touch damaged	Poor recall of personal history; impaired complex ADL (eg, writing a check or using a microwave)	• Track complex ADL, as well as continue stage 3 treatment • Monitor for signs of neglect and abuse • Use and teach procedural memory cues (to caregiver as well)
5	More severe damage to all structures above	Disorientation to time; impaired procedural memory (for familiar tasks)	• Modify stage 4 services • Track orientation/dressing ability • Use orienting cues
6	Severe damage to sensory processing areas	Delusions, hallucinations, and possibly perseveration; unable to live alone; basic ADL impairment	• Modify stage 5 services • Teach caregiver body mechanics for assisting patient with ADL
7	Autonomic centers	Impaired breathing, swallowing, speaking, walking, sitting balance, and facial expression	• Modify stage 6 services • Train caregivers for equipment (eg, a Hoyer lift for transfers) • Refer to hospice if needed

AD can also be inherited with an autosomal dominant pattern, with onset before 55 to 60 years old. In this case, the primary risk factor is an abnormal variant in 1 of 3 genes. The clinical course is the same, although death often occurs much earlier. The inheritance pattern requires only one parent to have the condition to give the child a 50% risk of developing it.[15]

VAD is closely related to AD in etiology and risk factors, particularly metabolic syndromes. Hypertension is a significant risk factor,[20] as are insulin resistance, dyslipidemia, type 2 diabetes, and obesity.[21] However, Ligthart et al[22] have found some evidence that treating cardiovascular risk factors prevents cognitive decline. Regarding relationships between metabolic and cognitive abnormalities, one review found that "treatments for one class of [metabolic] disorders affect the expression of other disorders; for example, some antihypertensives reduce the risk of diabetes and some antidiabetic agents improve blood pressure."[21] Other, modifiable, risk factors for VAD and AD include physical activity and cognitive stimulation.[23] This phenomenon, termed *cognitive reserve*, is built by higher levels of education or intelligence, extensive social networking, and complex leisure-time activities. However, if dementia does occur in persons with greater cognitive reserve, more extensive brain damage occurs prior to the onset of symptoms.[24]

Pick's disease is a type of FTD, affecting the frontal and temporal lobes. This dementia encompasses between "12-15% of all dementias and 30-50% [of] early onset ones."[25] Clinical presentation varies, though non-fluent aphasia frequently occurs. Initially, "the most common early manifestation is reduced speech output, followed by stuttering and a hesitant quality in utterance, paraphrasis, and apraxis [sic] of speech."[26] These speech impairments can progress quickly to total aphasia.

Research is conflicting about risk factors and specific accumulations and abnormalities of brain proteins in Pick's disease vs Alzheimer's and other dementias; these proteins may be abnormal without symptoms, depending on cognitive reserve and other factors.[27] Macroscopically, the brain atrophies markedly, sometimes asymmetrically between left and right sides. Ventricles dilate, and the corpus callosum narrows and thins.[26]

WKS, a combination of Wernicke encephalopathy and Korsakoff's syndrome, can occur at younger ages than other dementias. Its primary cause is acute-to-chronic thiamine (vitamin B1) depletion in the central nervous system[28]; this depletion can be due to alcoholism, anorexia, bariatric surgery, and possible genetic disposition.[29,30] Wernicke encephalopathy first presents as edema in "the mammillary bodies, periaqueductal and periventricular gray matter, collicular bodies and thalamus" with neuronal loss, scarring of glial cells, and small brain hemorrhages.[28,30] However, the patient may not have typical signs of thiamine deficiency, which can lead to underdiagnosis and undertreatment. If the health care provider notes anorexia, weakness, shortness of breath, impaired coordination, neuropathy, and pain or swelling in the extremities, prompt assessment of thiamine levels is vital.[31]

If untreated by administration of thiamine, Wernicke encephalopathy can advance to Korsakoff's syndrome, with the most common symptom being global amnesia (ie, the person cannot form new memories or recall old ones). As with other dementias, this global amnesia can be compensated for by implicit motor learning (automatic by repeated movement), alerting the patient to new information, total abstinence from alcohol for at least 1 year, and "a calm and well-structured environment."[30] Two cautionary case reports of WKS presenting with comorbid psychiatric disorders include one young adult with bipolar and somatization disorders, and another with schizophrenia with paranoia who "developed delusions that food and water were harmful." In both cases, the thalamus was severely damaged before caregivers recognized the underlying thiamine deficiency, leaving both patients "with persistent cognitive and physical disabilities."[29]

NPH, another relatively rare dementia, can present with a triad of symptoms: wet, wild, and wobbly. Urinary incontinence is present first, with altered mental status and unsteady gait; psychiatric symptoms of apathy, anxiety, and aggression are less prominent than in AD.[32] However, differential diagnosis is still difficult, resulting in 80% of patients improperly diagnosed and treated. Comorbidities in 75% of patients include another dementia, usually AD or VAD. Gait deviations include slow shuffling steps (10-meter walk lasting greater than 10 seconds and with more than 13 steps), narrow base of support, frequently incorrect foot placement, and impaired turns (at least 4 to 6 steps to complete a 360-degree rotation).[33]

Nervous system changes in NPH include impaired flow of CSF, causing poor blood circulation and damage to axons (but only mild damage to the more superficial cerebral cortex) in the frontal lobes.[33] Thus, surgical insertion and monitoring of a shunt is the preferred and often successful treatment. Metabolic changes underlie alterations in CSF circulation, as shown by pre-to-postshunting changes in levels of neurofilament light protein, amyloid precursor protein, tau proteins, and albumin.[34]

PD and DLB are similar clinically but require different treatment; as noted previously, anti-Parkinsonian medications increase symptoms in a person with DLB. Microscopically, DLB involves accumulation of tau and alpha-synuclein proteins in neurons, causing cognitive impairment, Parkinsonian symptoms, and visual hallucinations.[14]

In PD, alpha-synuclein proteins are also abnormal and, along with other proteins, cause neuronal degeneration and formation of Lewy bodies; predisposition to this dementia involves changes in chromosomes 4 and 12 and oxidative stress.[15] Also, dopamine-producing cell death increases the activity of neural pathways that inhibit movement and decreases activity of pathways facilitating movement, resulting in overall loss of movement quantity and size. Movement system impairments in PD include:

- Slow, low-amplitude tremor in extremities and sometimes the trunk
- Rigidity, feeling like a lead pipe or a cogwheel when the therapist attempts to move a limb
- Bradykinesia, slow movement that fatigues the patient rapidly
- Freezing of gait when the patient encounters surface or lighting changes (eg, doorways)
- Stooped posture and poor righting reactions, causing shuffling gait (festination) and backward falls
- Syncope, fainting due to orthostatic hypotension

In animal studies, vigorous habitual physical activity protects dopamine-producing cells from toxins via a temporary increase in brain-derived neurotrophic factor and neuroplasticity. Also, starting or continuing exercise at midlife reduces the risk for PD, dementia, and mild cognitive impairment, though research is unclear as to the amount of neuroprotection. In patients with PD, it is important to time administration of movement-facilitating medications, such as levodopa, to maximize the patient's ability to participate in exercise intense enough to gain neuroprotective benefits.[35]

Differential diagnosis by risk factors and clinical signs is important for the clinician working with patients over 65 years old. **Delirium, depression, and dementia are related conditions but are often misdiagnosed**, causing inadequate prevention and incorrect treatment. While depression is an independent risk factor for any type of dementia, it is a distinct condition.[36] While delirium may present with either increased or decreased activity levels, in geriatric populations a lethargic presentation is more common. Only 54% of geriatric patients with delirium in the hospital recover fully while 29% have symptoms for months.[37] See Table 11-3 for a clinical comparison of delirium, dementia, and depression.

Comorbid Medical and Psychosocial Issues

Regardless of etiology, dementia puts individuals at higher risk for medication- and symptom-related side effects that the therapist should address proactively through the treatment plan. Ways the therapist can address these side effects include: exercise interventions, communication, care coordination, education of the patient and stakeholders, and advocacy. Common in acute care, subacute rehabilitation, and long-term care is the potential for comorbid delirium or depression, which can be confused with dementia.[38]

Table 11-3

Clinical Comparison of Delirium, Dementia, and Depression

FEATURE	DELIRIUM	DEMENTIA	DEPRESSION
Development	Abrupt and obvious start	Insidious and unclear start	Clear start
Cause	Medical instability (eg, infection)	Any subtype of dementia	Drug overdose or recent emotional stress
Early Symptoms	Periods of decreased alertness, poor attention	Loss of long- and short-term memory	Anhedonia (inability to experience joy)
Effect at Night	Worsened symptoms	May worsen symptoms (sundowning)	More sleep during day, less at night
Level of Consciousness	Varies	Normal until late and end stages	Usually normal
Effect on Communication	Speech and thought lack organization and go off on tangents	Difficulty in naming things and people, resulting in slow and less frequent speech	Decreased speech but preserved language skills
Memory	Varies	Short- more than long-term memory loss	Recall may be decreased
Progression	Fluctuates	Slowly progressive	May be stable or worsen
Need for Treatment	Urgent	Needed, not urgent	Needed, urgent if person has suicidal thoughts
Effect of Treatment	Usually resolves symptoms, but many cases can persist up to 6 months	Slows worsening but cannot undo damage	Can resolve with treatment

Adapted from Fischer MG, Harb J, Josef KL. Delirium prevention, assessment and treatment by the physical therapist. *GeriNotes*. 2016;23(6):28-32.

Falls interest many therapists, especially in settings serving geriatric clients. In persons with dementia, some medications increase fall risk (although memantine, used to slow cognitive decline, is a rare exception in that it reduces risk of fractures). Cholinesterase inhibitors, commonly used to treat cognitive symptoms, increase the patient's risk of fainting (syncope).[39] The disease process itself can also cause gait abnormalities, especially in early AD.[38] Although this can increase fall risk during such activities as cardiopulmonary exercise testing, cardiovascular risk itself was not significantly different solely due to presence or absence of cognitive impairment; thus, with careful guarding, the physical therapist can safely test aerobic capacity in persons with dementia.[40]

Because many persons with dementia have age-related osteoporosis or osteopenia, hip fractures either causing or following a fall are common. Since cognitive impairments decrease carryover and rate of progress during rehabilitation, functional outcomes, such as safe discharge to home, are poorer.[41-43] More comorbidities may include "depression, cardiovascular and pulmonary diseases, infections, arthritis, other neurological disorders, sleep disturbances ... incontinence, and drug-related adverse effects" that worsen cognitive status even more.[44] Unless members of the interdisciplinary team/interprofessional team (IDT/IPT)—particularly rehabilitation professionals (physical, occupational, and speech therapists)—apply skilled and individualized interventions for those with cognitive impairments, economic costs may be higher for rehabilitation and long-term care for persons with dementia.[45]

This higher cost relates to decreased use of community-based resources in favor of more expensive medical-based resources.[46] Persons with cognitive impairments have a significantly higher prevalence of diabetes and 6 other common chronic diseases than do persons without cognitive limitations.[47] These conditions can flare up without proper management, although the first line of flare-up prevention should be community supports. The resource-utilization discrepancy can be lessened by case management, which facilitates communication between stakeholders and resources in the community to allow patients to discharge home if possible.[48] These resources include "home health, day care, meal preparation, transportation, counseling, support groups, respite care, [and] physical therapy."[46]

Physical dependence and combativeness are 2 other common issues in dementia care. Dependence may take the form of inability to follow cues for transfers and bed mobility, leading to greater amounts of required physical assistance that can injure caregivers. This is an opportunity for education by the physical therapist on body mechanics.[49] Besides physical injury and joint pain, caregivers often develop stress-related illnesses, including fractures, ulcers, and myocardial infarction. Caregiver education, therefore, is an important issue and is addressed in the section on clinical approaches. Also, cognitive dependence due to decreased self-awareness frequently leads to patient wandering, requiring constant supervision.[50,51]

Combativeness, a behavioral and psychological symptom of dementia (BPSD), is common in the early to middle stages of dementia as the person's awareness of his or her deficits starts to decrease.[52,53] Common medications for BPSD are short-term antipsychotics, memantine, and cholinesterase inhibitors.[44] While combativeness and other BPSD can burn out caregivers and increase risk of elder abuse, BPSD can be prevented in many cases with strategies described in the following section.

Lastly, dementia can indirectly cause death. In 2004, the top 10 causes of death in the United States were, in order, heart disease, cancer, cerebrovascular accident (stroke), chronic obstructive pulmonary disease, accidents, type 2 diabetes, AD, influenza, pneumonia, chronic kidney disease, and septicemia (blood infection). If a person has AD or another dementia, he or she cannot manage well other acute chronic conditions without assistance. Additionally, listed conditions that affect the heart, lungs, and blood vessels (all except cancer and accidents) slowly starve the brain of its needed oxygen and glucose, which can cause or worsen dementia.

Specific Clinical Approaches to Improve Physical Therapy Outcomes

Even though people experiencing dementia become unable to recount what has just happened, they still go through the experience—even without recall ... The moods and actions of people with dementia are expressions of what they have experienced, whether they can still use language and recall, or not.

—Judy Cornish[54]

Based on the prior descriptions of clinical presentations and underlying neurological deficits in persons with dementia, the reader may already be thinking of ways to adjust clinical approaches. This section is based on literature and the author's experience, and is organized by the physical therapy patient management model. More thorough information can be found in dementia-specific texts, but this section presents essential information.

Examination, Evaluation, and Diagnosis

Although dementia's clinical presentation varies by etiology and the person's baseline personality, the clinician should focus on 4 key areas in the initial examination; these areas are the patient's decision-making capacity, social communication style, pain, and fall risk factors. Decision-making capacity can be affected by superimposed delirium, or by its risk factors: pain, lower baseline level of function, disturbed sleep-wake cycles, dehydration, polypharmacy (more than 4 medications), lack of cognitive stimulation, and sensory deprivation (eg, misplaced glasses or hearing aids). Addressing these risk factors can prevent 30% to 40% of cases of delirium, which can otherwise persist up to 6 months beyond acute hospitalization.[55]

Regardless of delirium's presence or absence, the clinician should respect the patient's decision-making capacity as much as possible. Many caregivers and health care providers assume that dementia automatically eliminates the person's decision-making capacity. However, patients remain decisional in a late stage of dementia; this ability needs to be continually respected. Indeed, "informed consent is a legal requirement in all 50 states and is a process for communication between the patient and provider to discuss diagnosis, treatment, risk/benefits, and alternatives."[56]

Communication strategies to facilitate informed consent include:

- Recognize: discover the person's preferences, greet him or her by name, and make open-ended conversation to acknowledge the person's personal history
- Negotiate: use yes/no questions to find needs/preferences; propose alternatives if needed
- Facilitate: soften therapeutic requests, converse during ADL, offer verbal or physical assistance for tasks. "Open-ended questions facilitate initiation of a task or conversation; closed-ended questions facilitate task completion."[56] Examples of open-ended questions or prompts include "What would you like to do today?" and "Tell me about your pain," while closed-ended questions include "Can you move from your bed to your chair?" and "What number is your pain?"
- Validate: respond to the person's feelings more than his or her altered reality; use ample non-verbal communication, including gentle touch on the hand or shoulder and face the patient directly

Non-verbal communication is more important as dementia progresses and verbal abilities decline. Strategies to facilitate patient participation in an evaluation, including impairment and functional testing, are adding visual or tactile cues (eg, pat the surface where the patient is to sit), coming to the patient's eye level (eg, sitting if the patient is in a wheelchair), maintaining a gentle smile and hand contact (site of hand contact may vary depending on the patient's cultural background), and demonstrating the task repeatedly (eg, sit to stand without upper extremity support when assessing components of the Berg Balance Scale). Other changes to the patient exam include[57]:

- Use the caregiver's presence to encourage the patient to function at his or her or true baseline, since isolating the patient in an unfamiliar clinic location can cause the patient psychological discomfort and mask true abilities
- Screen strength and range of motion during voluntary movement in functional tasks vs manual muscle testing and goniometry, as the patient may not be able to follow cues for these tests
- Document outcome measures used for referral as needed to other medical professionals, including neuropsychologists, if signs appear consistent with undiagnosed medical or psychiatric conditions

Maintaining an inner calm is important, too, as patients may pick up subtle signs of anxiety or anger in the practitioner and become agitated themselves. In the patient:

> [A]ctions signifying anxiety include furrowed brow, motor restlessness, repeated motions, sighing, hand wringing, crying, hyperventilation, and clinging. Signals of depression include crying, sad facial expression, slowness to respond, turning away, slow motor activity, and downcast eyes.[38]

Risk factors for these behaviors in dementia include environmental, medical, or pharmacological stressors; each patient's routine is important to maintain and respect. More strategies for behavioral management and fall risk assessment during examination and throughout the episode of care include[38]:

- Use the Geriatric Depression Scale for persons with mild to moderate dementia. Depression can decrease activity levels, which can cause deconditioning and falls.
- Be aware that antidepressant selective serotonin reuptake inhibitors increase fall risk
- Lengthen the episode of care, if possible, to facilitate rapport and progress, since patients with dementia and related conditions tend to progress more slowly
- Assess contractures, balance, weight shifting, and gait characteristics in early-stage AD. In middle-stage AD, assess contractures, gait speed, stride length, and step variability. Reliable standardized tests include the 6-Minute Walk Test (for endurance and gait characteristics) and TUG, while timing separately the components of coming to a standing position and walking 25 feet with a single turn.
- Train specific functional tasks, repeatedly and with positive feedback, in a familiar environment, to translate into safe performance of these activities in the patient's discharge environment
- Maximize patient autonomy by respecting each patient's personalized living space, offering choices for "activities, clothing, or time of treatment,"[38] and recruiting higher-functioning patients to help monitor patients with greater deficits (particularly in long-term care settings)

Pain assessment in persons with dementia requires experience and keen observation skills. Health care providers tend to misinterpret delirium symptoms as pain, leading to potential overuse of opioid or other pain medications that may prolong the delirium.[58] Patients may misunderstand traditional pain assessment tools such as the horizontal visual analogue scale or Wong-Baker FACES pain scale, thus invalidating them for clinical use. **Instead, after obtaining a Mini-Mental State Exam (MMSE) score, if possible, use the patient's self-report in a consistent environment over time, corroborating with observational scales**, such as the Pain Assessment in Advanced Dementia (PAINAD, online) or Doloplus-2 (with few statistics on reliability and validity at time of this text's writing). During functional task assessment, note the timing and potential movement-related cause of pain behaviors. If caregivers are available, ask about environmental and social factors.[59]

Finally, fall risk factors in persons with and without dementia include muscle power; balance, including single-limb stance and multidirectional functional reach; environmental factors, including lighting, surface changes, or carpet texture; and use of assistive device for ambulation or transfers. While functional outcome measures are discussed in the Outcomes Assessment section, it is worth noting that the 7-item version of the Physical Performance Test, commonly used to assess ADL in geriatric patients, does not predict future falls despite identifying a history of falls in persons with mild AD.[60] History of falls or near-falls in the preceding 6 months, though, does predict future falls.[61] Time of day is important in fall risk assessment, since the phenomenon of sundowning (the worsening of confusion or agitation later in the day) increases fall risk as the day progresses.[2]

Prognosis

For persons with dementia, the episode of care may need to be lengthened for better outcomes. Several authors have investigated the impact of dementia-related cognitive deficits on length of stay in inpatient acute and subacute rehabilitation settings. An MMSE score of 17 or less (indicating moderate to severe cognitive impairment) predicts a shorter acute care stay and less rehabilitation for an older patient with a surgically repaired hip fracture.[62] In a sample of patients with surgery for hip fracture in the subacute rehabilitation setting, surgeons' weightbearing restrictions impacted length of rehabilitation as well as return to independent ambulation in patients with and without dementia[63]:

- Non-weightbearing or 50% weightbearing status.
  - Entire study sample: 53 days in rehabilitation; 41% of patients regaining independent ambulation.
  - Persons with dementia: 73.5 days in rehabilitation; 8% of patients regaining independent ambulation, while 44% of all patients with dementia did not ever return home.
- No surgical restriction and patient self-selects how much weight to place on the limb.
  - Entire study sample: 38 days in rehabilitation; 84% of patients regaining independent ambulation.
  - Persons with dementia: 45.5 days in rehabilitation; 83% of patients regaining independent ambulation. Prior to hip fracture, 81% of persons with dementia lived at home.

The person's chances for recovering physical function, regardless of rehabilitation or living setting, can be increased by a high activity level; few physical or chemical restraints, including seat belts in wheelchairs or tranquilizing medications to reduce BPSD; a familiar and structured environment with calming music and high visual contrasts; and minimal new assistive devices, since the patient often cannot recall sequencing and hand placement for safe use of a walker or other device. **Something as simple as a daily supervised walking or wheelchair-propulsion program can prevent secondary musculoskeletal and cardiopulmonary impairments; Lewis and Bottomley[2] suggest that it can also improve or minimize decline in judgment.** The physical therapist and other members of the IDT/IPT can also focus on good nutrition, less medication use, and more sensory stimulation, especially in the early stages of the disease.

Interventions

Patient-Related Interventions

Almost any intervention that keeps the patient active in a supervised environment can achieve good outcomes in a physical therapy episode of care. **Vigorous-intensity activity seems to exert a protective effect on residual cognitive capacity in PD and potentially other dementias[35]**; other studies investigated effects of exercise programs for various types of dementia. Evidence supporting a cognition-protecting role is not clear,[64] though one study noted that a 6-month program of aerobic training at 3 times per week appeared to protect cognition as well as increase cardiopulmonary endurance in persons with mild vascular-related cognitive impairment.[65]

Although therapy might not protect cognitive capacity in persons with dementia, other studies show that physical function[66]; gait performance, including fast gait speed necessary for continued physical independence; balance; and a positive attitude toward exercise by both patients and caregivers, do improve with multimodal exercises in an interprofessional setting.[67-69] Depending on the impairments and functional deficits found on initial examination and evaluation, the plan of care may include strength training, cardiopulmonary activities, functional balance tasks, and retraining of safe mobility patterns. Individualization and skilled supervision by the clinician show superior outcomes over an unsupervised, non-specific exercise program.

Research on motor learning principles for persons with dementia supports implicit (procedural) learning for single tasks to capitalize on the patient's remaining cognitive strengths, and avoidance of a secondary task with the mobility activity. Implicit learning uses repeated task practice vs front-loading the patient with detailed instructions. The clinician can give visual feedback to increase the rate of learning via modeling, gestural cues, or technology, and may have the patient practice the task dozens of times in a row (with ample rest for fatigue) to maximize the level of consistent performance. If the patient has more severe cognitive deficits, the clinician should not add a secondary task (eg, reciting one's shopping list while walking) so that the patient can focus cognitive reserves on the motor task at hand for reduced fall risk.[70]

Errorless learning, spaced retrieval, and guided repetition of practice are 3 research-supported ways to improve implicit motor learning and memory.[71] Errorless learning occurs where the clinician structures the task to minimize errors; this can include modeling task performance, using small steps, correcting with encouragement, and gradually decreasing the frequency of verbal or visual cues. Spaced retrieval has all providers interacting with the patient, asking for active recall of a given strategy with a consistent cue; the time between successive prompts for this active recall should gradually increase to maximize the patient's use of short- and long-term memory capabilities. A sample prompt, given by the care provider just prior to the patient sitting down, is "What do you do before you sit down?" The patient should answer, "I reach back for my chair," while actually reaching back, and then sitting down. Finally, guided practice is best in a structured environment that also gives patients interesting activity choices and compassionate supervision.[72]

As discussed earlier, one's interpersonal approach can make or break patient-clinician rapport for participation and success in the physical therapy plan of care. If possible, therapy should take place in a realistic, personalized, and quiet environment: limit background noise to a conversational level; decrease the number of residents a staff member must supervise; and incorporate familiar items, such as pictures of a patient's loved ones in a memory book.[72] The therapist should also allow more time for command processing, use mostly positive feedback, shorten sentences, and communicate using information from the patient's social history to encourage reminiscence.[73] Some patients prefer a familiar functional activity over formal therapeutic exercises; several authors have had success by incorporating music into exercise routines or even salsa dancing, with attention to components such as weight shifting, trunk rotation, and foot placement.[74,75]

More treatment strategies for less common dementias include[9,76]:

- DLB: use written cues for exercise instruction
- VAD: rehabilitate as with an acute or chronic stroke, including fall risk factors
- Pick's disease: provide a safe environment with appropriate foods and a space to walk
- WKS: establish an alliance with the patient, bribe the patient with non-addictive substances (eg, chocolate), and allow at least 1 year of abstinence from alcohol for memory recovery
- PD: monitor for medication reactions and depression to minimize functional decline[77]; encourage positioning for an effective cough, since patients have a 50% risk of dysphagia and subsequent aspiration pneumonia

Caregiver-Related Interventions

Since physical abilities decline in most dementias, the clinician must include caregiver-related education in the plan of care. This can occur at home, where the caregiver may be an adult child or spouse of the patient, or in an institution, such as a skilled nursing facility (SNF) or a group home, where the caregiver may be a different nurse's aide during every shift. Since BPSD, such as agitation, combativeness, or resistance to care, can cause rapid caregiver burnout, injury, or elder abuse, clinicians in the IDT/IPT should educate caregivers on the causes and courses of dementia, so that the caregiver knows what to expect and can practice strategies to adapt to or prevent the behaviors.[78]

Physical activity is a key to managing BPSD and reducing fall risk in persons with dementia.[79] However, not all caregivers may share this view, but instead may accept an inactive lifestyle for their patients. In a home care situation with family caregivers, as well as paid outside caregivers, this is often complicated by poor communication between caregivers and severely limited resources for specialized physical activities (eg, quality resistance bands for strengthening exercises). Such barriers to physical activity are often based on a different view of physical activity, as well as a lack of knowledge about it.[80]

Thus, physical therapists can use personal experience and, if the caregiver is receptive, research evidence to promote increased physical activity (especially informal and integrated into daily habits) for persons with dementia. A combined daily home exercise program and a caregiver-supervised walking program for persons with AD still living in the community improved ADL independence, fall risk, and cognition.[81] One trial trained nurses' assistants to encourage their residents to participate more in daily activities vs completing the activities for them to get to the next resident faster. After this intervention in 4 SNFs, falls decreased from 50% to 28% of residents, and staff attitude remained positive toward this method of function-focused care due to high levels of initial training.[82]

Since many caregivers have internet access for information to help them and their patients with dementia, the physical therapist may direct them to evidence-based resources. Four such websites are as follows[83]:

- Alzheimer's Association: for facts on AD and other types of dementia (www.alz.org/index.asp)
- American Parkinson Disease Association: for PD resources, as this disease has frequent associated dementia (www.apdaparkinson.org)
- National Alliance on Mental Illness: addresses many mental health issues broadly and in a layperson-friendly way (www.nami.org)
- National Mental Health Association: for resources similar to National Alliance on Mental Illness (www.mentalhealthamerica.net)

Wandering

Wandering, the undesired mobility of a person with dementia, is a problem in many settings. If a patient who is ambulatory or independent in wheelchair mobility and living at home begins to wander, he or she is likely to get lost and may require hospitalization or die due to exposure to the elements. In an institution (assisted living or SNF), the patient might enter other residents' rooms or other areas, causing complaints and potential altercation, depending on the mental status of both residents. If the patient has mobility limitations such as low vision or balance problems, risk of injury increases.

Environmental adaptations and behavioral analysis are 2 ways to prevent wandering. The Alzheimer's Association website has many suggestions on ways to adjust lighting, flooring, doorways, and other features of the living environment to promote safe mobility, including universal design.[9,84] Behavioral analysis examines routines and reasons behind wandering, and honoring them (eg, checking if the person needs to use the toilet, is hungry, or bored). If neither strategy works, the therapist can give the patient another task (as simple as folding washcloths or going through a box of interesting objects) or use the wandering in a therapeutic way to tire the patient out and encourage a rest period.

Combativeness

Combativeness and resistance to care, 2 common BPSD, increase when caregivers and other residents or neighbors do not have dementia-specific training and knowledge in how to interact with the person with dementia. One example is a patient who shouts and strikes out when placed in a bath chair by nursing home staff for transportation to a shower room. Verbal and non-verbal communication are 2 opportunities to prevent, reduce, or redirect combative behaviors.[85]

There are 2 basic strategies that the physical therapist can model and verbalize to reduce combativeness:

1. Use of short instructions, positive feedback, a 5-second response delay, and avoidance of questions that challenge the patient's cognitive deficits ("Do you remember?")[86]
2. Treat the patient as an adult: face him or her; call by name; use a normal tone of voice; and offer choice questions, where any choice offered is appropriate to the task at hand ("Do you want to wear the blue top or the red top?")[87,88]

Outcomes Assessment

Many tests and measures used by physical therapists in cognitively intact patient populations are also appropriate for use for persons with dementia. However, these may require modified instructions as well as awareness of slightly different normative values. Table 11-4 summarizes some recommended functional tests.[57,89-95] **Including subjective data (eg, separate patient and caregiver interviews, in a non-distracting setting and with attention to the person's emotions) can lend more depth to the test results.**[89] Documentation of such test results can show the benefits of physical therapy for persons with dementia, as well as increase the odds of reimbursement for longer plans of care for Medicare and other payors.

Table 11-4

Outcome Measures Useful for Persons With Dementia

DOMAIN	TEST	CONSIDERATIONS	NORMS FOR DEMENTIA
Cognition	Mini-Cog	Screen; 3 minutes	
	Montreal Cognitive Assessment	Mild cognitive impairment or AD; 10 minutes	26 or above: normal cognition Add 1 point to score if person has under 13 years education
	MMSE	Use for more advanced dementia; under 10 minutes	24 or above: no impairment 18 to 23: mild impairment 17 or less: severe impairment
	Confusion Assessment Method	Assesses delirium; versions for intensive care unit, emergency department, or SNF	
	1-Minute Verbal Fluency for Animals	Assesses memory in dementia with verbal ability remaining	Name at least 14 animals in 60 seconds
	FAST	Assesses cognitive ability in persons with all stages of dementia	Refer to Neurophysiological Background, Etiology, and Risk Factors section of this chapter

(continued)

Table 11-4 (continued)

Outcome Measures Useful for Persons With Dementia

DOMAIN	TEST	CONSIDERATIONS	NORMS FOR DEMENTIA
Depression	Geriatric Depression Scale	Appropriate for persons with dementia; 1 to 5 minutes	8 or above: depression (mild cognitive impairment) 6 or above if dementia present 0 to 10: low risk of depression
	Beck Depression Inventory	Appropriate for persons with mild cognitive impairment (eg, status post cerebrovascular accident); 1 to 5 minutes	0 to 9: minimal depression 10 to 18: mild/moderate 19 to 29: moderate/severe 30 to 63: severe depression
	Cornell Scale for Depression in Dementia	30-minute caregiver and patient interview	
	Delirium Rating Scale	Can differentiate between delirium, dementia, depression, and schizophrenia	
Pain	PAINAD	Observational scale of pain behaviors that can correlate to numerical pain ratings (available for free online)	
Balance	TUG	Screen for fall risk; reliable in dementia but modify directions	MDC: 4.09 seconds
	Mini-Balance Evaluation Systems Test (BESTest)	Short version (10 to 15 minutes) of BESTest; appropriate for mild cognitive impairment	
	Berg Balance Scale (can modify)	Reliable, with single-step directions; takes 10 to 15 minutes	MDC: 16.66 points

(continued)

Table 11-4 (continued)

Outcome Measures Useful for Persons With Dementia

DOMAIN	TEST	CONSIDERATIONS	NORMS FOR DEMENTIA
Lower-Body Muscle Power	Chair Rise Test or 5 Times Sit to Stand	Requires ability to stand up and sit down without use of hands; patient completes as fast as safely possible	4.2 seconds or less for 5 Times Sit to Stand
Gait	Gait speed	Use straight 3- to 6-meter path	MDC: 9.4 cm/second improvement
	6-Minute Walk Test	Use consistent pathway of documented dimensions; allow assistive device and standing rests but no physical assistance	MDC: 33.5 meter increase
	Groningen Meander Walking Test	Assesses speed, stepping accuracy, and direction changes along a serpentine path 6 meters long and 0.15 meters wide, with 4 curves for 4.96-meter total length; divide oversteps and total time by 2	MDC: 2.96 seconds if no assistive device; 10.35 seconds if 4-wheeled walker used; 4.38 oversteps

Adapted from Blankevoort CG, van Heuvelen MJG, Scherder EJA. Reliability of six physical performance tests in older people with dementia. *Phys Ther.* 2013;93(1):69-78; Bossers WJR, van der Woude LHV, Boersma F, Scherder EJA, van Heuvelen MJG. The Groningen Meander Walking Test: a dynamic walking test for older adults with dementia. *Phys Ther.* 2014;94(2):262-272; Francis NJ. Assessment tools for geriatric patients with delirium, mild cognitive impairment, dementia, and depression. *Top Geriatr Rehabil.* 2012;28(3):137-147; McGough EL, Logsdon RG, Kelly VE, Teri L. Functional mobility limitations and falls in assisted living residents with dementia: physical performance assessment and quantitative gait analysis. *J Geriatr Phys Ther.* 2012;36(2):78-86; Muir-Hunter SW, Graham L, Odasso MM. Reliability of the Berg Balance Scale as a clinical measure of balance in community-dwelling older adults with mild to moderate Alzheimer disease: a pilot study. *Physiother Can.* 2015;67(3):255-262; Nash J, Ross C. Application and interpretation of functional outcome measures for testing individuals with cognitive impairment. *GeriNotes.* 2016;23(6):34-37; Ries JD, Echternach JL, Nof L, Gagnon Blodgett M. Test-retest reliability and minimal detectable change scores for the Timed "Up & Go" Test, the Six-Minute Walk Test, and gait speed in people with Alzheimer disease. *Phys Ther.* 2009;89(6):569-579; Warden V, Hurley AC, Volicer L. Development and psychometric evaluation of the Pain Assessment in Advanced Dementia (PAINAD) scale. *J Am Med Dir Assoc.* 2003;4(1):9-15.

Summary

Dementias, or neurocognitive disorders, are a collection of symptoms caused by degeneration of portions of the brain and central nervous system. Persons with dementias regress cognitively and physically, even with intervention, but skilled physical therapy and interprofessional intervention can slow functional decline; thus, saving costs, caregiver stress, and potentially delaying transfer to an institutional setting such as long-term care. Communication strategies and multifaceted approaches are critical to improving outcomes with this population.

Key Points

- Exercise programs for persons with dementia are best if they have many structured parts, are high intensity with long duration, and are tailored for the individual's cognitive performance.
- The geriatric practitioner should be able to tell between delirium, depression, and dementia.
- Facilitate informed consent of persons with dementia by recognizing the person as a unique individual, negotiating within his or her communicative capacity, facilitating conversation with open-ended requests, and validating the person's feelings and altered reality.
- Maintain an inner calm to minimize agitation in persons with dementia picking up non-verbal cues.
- Assess pain by observational scales and self-reports with baseline knowledge of the patient's cognition.
- Promote supervised aerobic mobility programs (walking or wheelchair propulsion) to prevent secondary impairments in musculoskeletal, cardiopulmonary, and potentially neurocognitive systems. More vigorous activity has a suspected neuroprotective effect in many dementias.
- Improve implicit motor learning by errorless learning, spaced retrieval, and guided practice repetition.
- In outcomes assessment, combine subjective and objective data to deepen the test results.

Review Questions

- Recall at least one patient with dementia that you, a coworker, or a classmate has recently worked with.
  - What underlying medical condition(s) did this patient have?
  - How did the symptoms and signs relate to the underlying neurological degeneration?
  - Use the JAMCO acronym to help you describe this patient's symptoms of dementia.[2]
  - Given your new knowledge from this chapter, what aspects of patient management (examination, evaluation, diagnosis, prognosis, intervention, and outcomes) would you change?
- Where might you see persons with dementia living, depending on the FAST stage they are in?
- If you are unable to redirect the wandering of a patient with dementia, how might you use the wandering to facilitate clinical benefit to the patient?

- Develop a list of strategies for patient- and caregiver-related communication and education that you can use with subsequent persons with dementia to improve outcomes in your clinical practice setting.
- In a person without diagnosed dementia, what would you include in the initial interview and objective examination to incorporate assessment of common risk factors for dementia?

Case Studies: First Impressions

As you review the following case studies, you may want to consider these questions for thought or discussion:

- What standardized tests and measures (including psychiatric, for example, a depression screen) would you select for this patient? Why?
- Based on available data, what short- and long-term goals would you write for your plan of care? Consider using the acronyms SMART (specific, measurable, attainable, realistic, and timely) or ABCDE (actor, behavior, conditions, degree, and expected time frame) to guide your goal writing.
- What elements (procedures, psychosocial aspects, communication aspects, etc) would you make sure to include or omit in your plan of care for this patient? Why?
- What are your anticipated needs, if any, for consultation and referral for this patient?
- How will you transition this patient toward lasting health behavior change following discharge (eg, recommending a YMCA membership trial)?

Case 1

A 50-year-old male was admitted to acute care with pneumonia. His goal is to return home with family.

- Social history: he lives in a single-story house with one porch step to enter; his wife is his primary caregiver, and his daughter is attending graduate school locally.
- Medical/psychiatric history: early-onset AD (diagnosed 5 years ago), coronary artery disease, and prehypertension. He is on medications for cognitive symptoms and cardiovascular conditions, and was started on antibiotics for pneumonia on admission to the hospital.
- Impairments, activity limitations, and participation restrictions found on initial interview and examination
  - Shortness of breath and mild hypoxemia in supine and sitting
  - Currently requires oxygen via nasal cannula
  - Agitation that starts at the staffing change from first to second shift
  - Sporadic sleeping pattern noted
  - Refuses to try to transfer or ambulate with anyone except his wife or daughter

Case 2

A 60-year-old male was referred to outpatient physical therapy, 6 weeks after 2 thoracic compression fractures and an increasing frequency of falls. His goal is to resume daily neighborhood walks with his wife.

- Social history: he lives in a 2-story house with his wife, who reports bilateral upper extremity and low back pain from a recently increased level of assistance the patient requires for stair negotiation.

- Medical/psychiatric history: DLB (symptomatic for 5 months), lumbar spinal stenosis, generalized anxiety disorder, osteopenia, and stage 3 chronic kidney disease
- Impairments, activity limitations, and participation restrictions found on initial interview and examination
  - Stooped posture in sitting and standing
  - Pain in middle and lower back rated 3/10 with standing greater than 5 minutes
  - Slow shuffling gait with a 4-wheeled walker
  - Requires assistance of one person to negotiate steps
  - Ambulates 200 feet prior to needing to sit due to fatigue
  - Wife reports that patient has had visual hallucinations that have contributed to several falls at home

Case 3

A 70-year-old female was referred to home health physical therapy, after discharge from subacute rehabilitation, for a stroke with mild left hemiparesis and residual expressive aphasia. Her goal is to manage her apartment independently with occasional support from her children, as prior.

- Social history: she lives in a low-income apartment with elevator access and sleeps in a recliner. She is able to use a weekly reminder box for medication management once her daughter fills the daily boxes.
- Medical/psychiatric history: postpartum depression (beginning 50 years ago and worse with the birth of each of her 5 children), type 2 diabetes with distal sensory polyneuropathy (feet are affected more than hands), hypertension, and mid-stage AD
- Impairments, activity limitations, and participation restrictions found on initial interview and examination
  - Requires 25% assistance for safe ambulation with a 2-wheeled walker, indoors and outdoors
  - Mild confusion that worsens after lunch
  - Requires home health nursing for blood sugar checks and insulin administration due to safety concerns (noted by speech therapist during subacute rehabilitation stay medication teaching)
  - Requires contact guard assistance for transfers
  - Spends time daily searching for her house keys
  - Mild apraxia noted during meal preparation using a microwave

Case 4

A 73-year-old female was referred to outpatient physical therapy, 4 weeks after a surgical repair of a right rotator cuff tear sustained in a fall down steps at home. Her goal is to keep living at home with her daughter.

- Social history: daughter provides transportation. The patient lives in a ranch house with her daughter, who also completes shopping, meal preparation, laundry, and heavy cleaning.
- Medical/psychiatric history: VAD, major depressive disorder, hypertension, type 1 diabetes, generalized anxiety disorder, peripheral artery disease, coronary artery disease, hyperlipidemia, and congestive heart failure. Her daughter facilitates compliance with all medications.
- Impairments, activity limitations, and participation restrictions found on initial interview and examination
  - Shortness of breath with transfers and ambulation greater than 50 feet
  - Requires 25% assistance for safe use of her 4-wheeled walker (has had for 3 years)
  - Dynamic balance deficits during ambulation and standing with head turns
  - Uneven step length and width on walk into clinic
  - Easily distracted during the initial interview
  - Often defers questions to her daughter

Case 5

An 80-year-old male was readmitted to a memory care unit after a hospitalization for an exacerbation of chronic kidney disease. His goal is to "walk normal," and nursing staff request evaluation for potential reduction of current restraints, per federal law.

- Social history: he has lived in memory care for 8 years, and prior to hospitalization ambulated with a single-point cane or no device. He prefers to sleep during the day and be more active at night, due to a long work history of third-shift manufacturing jobs. Despite nursing staff and family members voicing opposition, another resident provides him with alcohol occasionally.
- Medical/psychiatric history: congestive heart failure, knee and lumbar spine osteoarthritis, cocaine use (stopped 30 years ago), alcohol dependence, WKS, AD, peripheral artery disease, and history of slowly-healing lower extremity vascular wounds
- Impairments, activity limitations, and participation restrictions found on initial interview and examination
  - Bed and chair alarms in place due to a 25% incidence of falls during self-transfers and ambulation between his bed and the room's toilet
  - Wide-based antalgic gait requiring 25% assistance for safety
  - Use of single-point cane noted as unsafe, so nursing provided a manual wheelchair for mobility
  - Impaired Romberg scores and unable to perform sharpened Romberg

Quick Reference

- Possible diagnoses and their signs/symptoms:
  - AD: short- and long-term memory loss, word-finding issues, poor sequencing of tasks or inappropriate object use, and cautious gait pattern
  - DLB: visual hallucinations, Parkinsonian gait pattern, and paranoia
  - VAD: symptoms of a new or worse stroke, abrupt change in personality and continence
  - FTD: impaired reasoning, personality change, and aphasia
  - WKS: habitual lying, ataxic slow gait, resistance to assistive device prescription, and ongoing alcohol abuse
  - NPH: abrupt onset of urinary incontinence, behavioral lability, and wide-based unsteady gait
  - HD: impaired cognitive processing, athetoid movement, and falls
  - PD: bradykinesia, shuffling gait, stooped posture, "mask" face, soft voice, increased incidence of falls, and pneumonia
  - HIV-AIDS dementia: previous HIV infection (risk factors including unprotected sex, intravenous drug use, and other exposure to body fluids)
  - Multiple sclerosis dementia: long duration of multiple sclerosis, short-term memory loss, word-finding difficulty, and poor concentration
- Questions to ask the patient (or friend/family member if the patient cannot remember):
  - Do you often feel any of the symptoms (listed previously)?
  - Have you ever been diagnosed with dementia (listed previously)? What kind? What was going on in your life around the time of that diagnosis?
  - How do you deal with your dementia? How well does that work for you?
  - What should I know about your dementia?
- Referral options:
  - Neurologist for diagnosis, behavioral and pharmacological treatment
  - Support group for patients and their caregivers
  - Adult day care or continuing care communities
  - Occupational therapist for cognitive and home safety evaluation
  - Exercise group for persons with dementia

Additional Resources

- Fritsch MJ, Meier U, Kehler U. *Normal Pressure Hydrocephalus: Pathophysiology - Diagnosis - Treatment*. Stuttgart, Germany: Thieme; 2014.
- Gogia PP, Rastogi N. *Clinical Alzheimer's Rehabilitation*. New York, NY: Springer; 2009.
- Leatherdale L. *Korsakoff's or Wernicke Korsakoff Syndrome Explained. Is it Alcohol Induced Dementia?* IMB Publishing; 2013.
- Ravdin LD, Katzen HL. *Handbook on the Neuropsychology of Aging and Dementia*. New York, NY: Springer; 2013.
- Umphred DA, Lazaro RT, Roller M, Burton G. *Umphred's Neurological Rehabilitation*. 6th ed. St. Louis, MO: Elsevier; 2013.

- *Special Olympics Wisconsin.* www.specialolympicswisconsin.org. Accessed February 22, 2018.
  - This Special Olympics organization is one of several state chapters that offers regular informational sessions on how to encourage participation of persons with AD and other dementias.
- National Council on Aging. Evidence-based falls prevention programs. *National Council on Aging.* www.ncoa.org/healthy-aging/falls-prevention/falls-prevention-programs-for-older-adults. Accessed February 22, 2018.
  - Refer especially to A Matter of Balance, the Otago Exercise Program, Stepping On, and Tai Ji Quan as dementia-friendly programs.

References

1. American Psychiatric Association. *Diagnostic and Statistical Manual of Mental Disorders.* 5th ed. Arlington, VA: American Psychiatric Publishing; 2013.
2. Lewis CB, Bottomley JM. *Geriatric Rehabilitation: A Clinical Approach.* 3rd ed. Upper Saddle River, NJ: Pearson; 2008.
3. McArthur C, Hirdes J, Berg K, Giangregorio L. Who receives rehabilitation in Canadian long-term care facilities? A cross-sectional study. *Physiother Can.* 2015;67(2):113-121.
4. Montagnini M, Lodhi M, Born W. The utilization of physical therapy in a palliative care unit. *J Palliat Med.* 2003;6(1):11-17.
5. Kirk-Sanchez NJ, McGough EL. Physical exercise and cognitive performance in the elderly: current perspectives. *Clin Interv Aging.* 2014;9:51-62.
6. Muir SW, Yohannes AM. The impact of cognitive impairment on rehabilitation outcomes in elderly patients admitted with a femoral neck fracture: a systematic review. *J Geriat Phys Ther.* 2009;32(1):24-32.
7. Littbrand H, Stenvall M, Rosendahl E. Applicability and effects of physical exercise on physical and cognitive functions and activities of daily living among people with dementia: a systematic review. *Am J Phys Med Rehabil.* 2011;90(6):495-518.
8. McLaren AN, LaMantia MA, Callahan CM. Systematic review of non-pharmacologic interventions to delay functional decline in community-dwelling patients with dementia. *Aging Ment Health.* 2013;17(6):655-666.
9. Alzheimer's Association. What is dementia? *Alzheimer's Association.* http://www.alz.org/what-is-dementia.asp. Updated 2018. Accessed February 22, 2018.
10. Crowther J. Factsheet: the later stages of dementia. *Alzheimer's Society.* https://www.alzheimers.org.uk/download/downloads/id/1762/factsheet_the_later_stages_of_dementia.pdf. Reviewed May 2017. Accessed May 2, 2018.
11. Gras LZ, Kanaan SF, McDowd JM, Colgrove YM, Burns J, Pohl PS. Balance and gait of adults with very mild Alzheimer's disease. *J Geriatr Phys Ther.* 2015;38(1):1-7.
12. Littbrand H, Rosendahl E, Lindelöf N, Lundin-Olsson L, Gustafson Y, Nyberg L. A high-intensity functional weight-bearing exercise program for older people dependent in activities of daily living and living in residential care facilities: evaluation of the applicability with focus on cognitive function. *Phys Ther.* 2006;86(4):489-498.
13. Manckoundia P, Taroux M, Kubicki A, Mourey F. Impact of ambulatory physiotherapy on motor abilities of elderly subjects with Alzheimer's disease. *Geriatr Gerontol Int.* 2014;14(1):167-175.
14. Lundy-Ekman L. *Neuroscience: Fundamentals for Rehabilitation.* 3rd ed. St. Louis, MO: Saunders; 2007.
15. McCance KL, Huether SE. (Eds.) *Pathophysiology: The Biologic Basis for Disease in Adults and Children.* Maryland Heights, MO: Mosby Elsevier; 2010.
16. Billek-Sawhney B, Jackson NA. Normal pressure hydrocephalus. *J Acute Care Phys Ther.* 2012;3(2):182-188.
17. Sue D, Sue DW, Sue S. *Understanding Abnormal Behaviors.* 6th ed. Boston, MA: Houghton Mifflin; 2000.
18. Doidge N. *The Brain that Changes Itself: Stories of Personal Triumph from the Frontiers of Pain Science.* New York, NY: Penguin Group; 2007.
19. McCarthy L. Cognitive-based functional assessment in Alzheimer's disease: a focus on the GDS/FAST staging system. *GeriNotes.* 2016;23(6):6-10.
20. Sharp SI, Aarsland D, Day S, Sønnesyn H; Alzheimer's Society Vascular Dementia Systematic Review Group, Ballard C. Hypertension is a potential risk factor for vascular dementia: systematic review. *Int J Geriatr Psychiatry.* 2011;26(7):661-669.
21. Craft S. The role of metabolic disorders in Alzheimer's disease and vascular dementia. *Arch Neurol.* 2009;66(3):300-305.
22. Ligthart SA, Moll van Charante EP, Van Gool WA, Richard E. Treatment of cardiovascular risk factors to prevent cognitive decline and dementia: a systematic review. *Vasc Health Risk Manag.* 2010;6:775-785.

23. Aarsland D, Sardahaee FS, Anderssen SA, Ballard C; Alzheimer's Society Systematic Review group. Is physical activity a potential preventive factor for vascular dementia? A systematic review. *Aging Ment Health.* 2010;14(4):386-395.
24. Meng X, D'Arcy C. Education and dementia in the context of the cognitive reserve hypothesis: a systematic review with meta-analyses and qualitative analyses. *PLoS ONE.* 2012;7(6):e38268.
25. Kertesz A. Frontotemporal dementia, Pick's disease. *Ideggyogy Sz.* 2010;63(1-2):4-12.
26. Munoz DG, Morris HR, Rossor M. Pick's disease. In: Dickson D, Weller RO, eds. Neurodegeneration: *The Molecular Pathology of Dementia and Movement Disorders.* 2nd ed. Oxford, United Kingdom: Wiley-Blackwell; 2011.
27. Van Eersel J, Bi M, Ke YD, et al. Phosphorylation of soluble tau differs in Pick's disease and Alzheimer's disease brains. *J Neural Transm.* 2009;116(10):1243-1251.
28. Sullivan EV, Pfefferbaum A. Neuroimaging of the Wernicke-Korsakoff syndrome. *Alcohol Alcohol.* 2009;44(2):155-165.
29. McCormick LM, Buchanan JR, Onwuameze OE, Pierson RK, Paradiso S. Beyond alcoholism: Wernicke-Korsakoff syndrome in patients with psychiatric disorders. *Cogn Behav Neurol.* 2011;24(4):209-216.
30. Kopelman MD, Thomson AD, Guerrini I, Marshall EJ. The Korsakoff syndrome: clinical aspects, psychology and treatment. *Alcohol Alcohol.* 2009;44(2):148-154.
31. Isenberg-Grzeda E, Kutner HE, Nicolson SE. Wernicke-Korsakoff syndrome: under-recognized and under-treated. *Psychosomatics.* 2012;53(6):507-516.
32. Kito Y, Kazui H, Kubo Y, et al. Neuropsychiatric symptoms in patients with idiopathic normal pressure hydrocephalus. *Behav Neurol.* 2009;21(3):165-174.
33. Kiefer M, Unterberg A. The differential diagnosis and treatment of normal-pressure hydrocephalus. *Dtsch Arztebl Int.* 2012;109(1-2):15-26.
34. Jeppsson A, Zetterberg H, Blennow K, Wikkelsø C. Idiopathic normal-pressure hydrocephalus: pathophysiology and diagnosis by CSF biomarkers. *Neurology.* 2013;80(15):1385-1392.
35. Ahlskog JE. Does vigorous exercise have a neuroprotective effect in Parkinson disease? *Neurology.* 2011;77(3):288-294.
36. Da Silva J, Gonçalves-Pereira M, Xavier M, Mukaetova-Ladinska EB. Affective disorders and the risk of developing dementia: systematic review. *Br J Psychiatry.* 2013;202(3):177-186.
37. Cole MG, Bailey R, Bonnycastle M, et al. Frequency of full, partial and no recovery from subsyndromal delirium in older hospital inpatients. *Int J Geriatr Psychiatry.* 2016;31(5):544-550.
38. Williams AK. Psychosocial issues in long-term care. *Top Geriatr Rehabil.* 1999;15(2):14-21.
39. Kim DH, Brown RT, Ding EL, Kiel DP, Berry SD. Dementia medications and risk of falls, syncope, and related adverse events: meta-analysis of randomized controlled trials. *J Am Geriatr Soc.* 2011;59(6):1019-1031.
40. Billinger SA, Vidoni ED, Greer CS, et al. Cardiopulmonary exercise testing is well-tolerated in people with Alzheimer's-related cognitive impairment. *Arch Phys Med Rehabil.* 2014;95(9):1714-1718.
41. Buddingh S, Liang J, Allen J, Koziak A, Buckingham J, Beaupre LA. Rehabilitation for long-term care residents following hip fracture: a survey of reported rehabilitation practices and perceived barriers to delivery of care. *J Geriatr Phys Ther.* 2013;36(1):39-46.
42. Landi F, Bernabei R, Russo A, et al. Predictors of rehabilitation outcomes in frail patients treated in a geriatric hospital. *J Am Geriatr Soc.* 2002;50(4):679-684.
43. Beaupre LA, Cinats JG, Jones CA, et al. Does functional recovery in elderly hip fracture patients differ between patients admitted from long-term care and the community? *J Gerontol A Biol Sci Med Sci.* 2007;62(10):1127-1133.
44. Hort J, et al.; EFNS Scientist Panel on Dementia. EFNS guidelines for the diagnosis and management of Alzheimer's disease. *Eur J Neurol.* 2010;17(10):1236-1248.
45. Olesen J, Gustavsson A, Svensson M, Wittchen HU, Jönsson B; CDBE2010 study group; European Brain Council. The economic cost of brain disorders in Europe. *Eur J Neurology.* 2012;19(1):155-162.
46. Weber SR, Pirraglia PA, Kunik ME. Use of services by community-dwelling patients with dementia: a systematic review. *Am J Alzheimers Dis Other Demen.* 2011;26(3):195-204.
47. Reichard A, Stolzle H, Fox MH. Health disparities among adults with physical disabilities or cognitive limitations compared to individuals with no disabilities in the United States. *Dis Health J.* 2011;4(2):59-67.
48. Reilly S, Miranda-Castillo C, Malouf R, et al. Case management approaches to home support for people with dementia. *Cochrane Database Syst Rev.* 2015;(1):CD008345.
49. Cornman-Levy D, Gitlin LN, Corcoran MA, Schinfeld S. Caregiver aches and pains: the role of physical therapy in helping families provide daily care. *Alzheimers Care Q.* 2001;2(1):47-55.
50. Yokoi T, Aoyama K, Ishida K, Okamura H. Conditions associated with wandering in people with dementia from the viewpoint of self-awareness: five case reports. *Am J Alzheimers Dis Oth Demen.* 2012;27(3):162-170.
51. Yokoi I, Okamura H. Why do dementia patients become unable to lead a daily life with decreasing cognitive function? *Dementia.* 2012;12(5):551-568.
52. Guideline Adaptation Committee. Clinical practice guidelines and principles of care for people with dementia. Sydney. Guideline Adaptation Committee;2016

53. National Institute for Health and Care Excellence. Dementia: supporting people with dementia and their carers in health and social care. *National Institute for Health and Care Excellence.* https://www.nice.org.uk/guidance/cg42. Published November 2006. Updated September 2016. Accessed February 22, 2018.
54. Cornish J. *The Dementia Handbook: How to Provide Dementia Care at Home.* North Charleston, SC: CreateSpace Independent Publishing Platform; 2017.
55. Fischer MG, Harb J, Josef KL. Delirium prevention, assessment and treatment by the physical therapist. *GeriNotes.* 2016;23(6):28-32.
56. Criss M, Heitzman J, Wharton MA. Legal and ethical reasoning to enhance compassionate care in patients experiencing cognitive decline. *GeriNotes.* 2016;23(6):18-22.
57. Francis NJ. Assessment tools for geriatric patients with delirium, mild cognitive impairment, dementia, and depression. *Top Geriatr Rehabil.* 2012;28(3):137-147.
58. Mah K, Rodin RA, Chan VWS, Stevens BJ, Zimmermann C, Gagliese L. Health-care workers' judgments about pain in older palliative care patients with and without delirium. *Am J Hosp Pall Care.* 2017;34(10):958-965.
59. Hadjistavropoulos T, Fitzgerald TD, Marchildon GP. Practice guidelines for assessing pain in older persons with dementia residing in long-term care facilities. *Physiother Can.* 2010;62(2):104-113.
60. Ryan JJ, McCloy C, Rundquist P, Srinivasan V, Laird R. Fall risk assessment among older adults with mild Alzheimer disease. *J Geriatr Phys Ther.* 2011;34(1):19-27.
61. Farrell MK, Rutt RA, Lusardi MM, Williams AK. Are scores on the Physical Performance Test useful in determination of risk of future falls in individuals with dementia? *J Geriatr Phys Ther.* 2011;34(2):57-63.
62. Bellelli G, Frisoni GB, Pagani M, Magnifico F, Trabucchi M. Does cognitive performance affect physical therapy regimen after hip fracture surgery? *Aging Clin Exp Res.* 2007;19(2):119-124.
63. Raivio M, Korkala O, Pitkälä K, Tilvis R. Rehabilitation outcome in hip-fracture: impact of weight-bearing restriction—a preliminary investigation. *Phys Occup Ther Geriatr.* 2005;22(4):1-9.
64. Forbes D, Forbes SC, Blake CM, Thiessen EJ, Forbes S. Exercise programs for people with dementia. *Cochrane Database Syst Rev.* 2015;(4):CD006489.
65. Liu-Ambrose T, Best JR, Davis JC, et al. Aerobic exercise and vascular cognitive impairment: a randomized controlled trial. *Neurology.* 2016;87(20):2082-2090.
66. Rao AK, Chou A, Bursley B, Smulofsky J, Jezequel J. Systematic review of the effects of exercise on activities of daily living in people with Alzheimer's disease. *Am J Occup Ther.* 2014;68(1):50-56.
67. Hageman PA, Thomas VS. Gait performance in dementia: the effects of a 6-week resistance training program in an adult day-care setting. *Int J Geriatr Psychiatry.* 2002;17(4):329-334.
68. Telenius EW, Engedal K, Bergland A. Long-term effects of a 12 weeks high-intensity functional exercise program on physical function and mental health in nursing home residents with dementia: a single blinded randomized controlled trial. *BMC Geriatrics.* 2015;15:158.
69. Frederiksen KS, Sobol N, Beyer N, Hasselbach S, Waldemar G. Moderate-to-high intensity aerobic exercise in patients with mild to moderate Alzheimer's disease: a pilot study. *Int J Geriatr Psychiatry.* 2014;29(12):1242-1248.
70. Van Tilbourg IADA. *Procedural learning in cognitively impaired patients and its application to clinical practice* [dissertation]. Nijmegen, Netherlands: Radboud University; 2011.
71. White L, Ford MP, Brown CJ, Peel C, Triebel KL. Facilitating the use of implicit memory and learning in the physical therapy management of individuals with Alzheimer disease: a case series. *J Geriatr Phys Ther.* 2014;37(1):35-44.
72. Hardy J, Morgan NA. Dementia: improving function and quality of life with a biopsychosocial approach. *GeriNotes.* 2016;23(6):24-27.
73. Mirolsky-Scala G, Kraemer T. Fall management in Alzheimer-related dementia: a case study. *J Geriatr Phys Ther.* 2009;32(4):181-189.
74. Johnson L, Deatrick EJ, Oriel K. The use of music to improve exercise participation in people with dementia: a pilot study. *Phys Occup Ther Geriatr.* 2012;30(2):102-108.
75. Abreu M, Hartley G. The effects of salsa dance on balance, gait, and fall risk in a sedentary patient with Alzheimer's dementia, multiple comorbidities, and recurrent falls. *J Geriatr Phys Ther.* 2013;36(2):100-108.
76. Lewis CB. Rehabilitation strategies for dementia: therapy that works. Presentation at: GREAT Seminars and Books; May 2015; Green Bay, WI.
77. Pontone GM, Bakker CC, Chen S, et al. The longitudinal impact of depression on disability in Parkinson disease. *Int J Geriatr Psychiatry.* 2016;31(5):458-465.
78. Olazarán J, Reisberg B, Clare L, et al. Nonpharmacological therapies in Alzheimer's disease: a systematic review of efficacy. *Dement Geriatr Cogn Disord.* 2010;30(2):161-178.
79. D'Amico F, Rehill A, Knapp M, et al. Cost-effectiveness of exercise as a therapy for behavioural and psychological symptoms of dementia within the EVIDEM-E randomised controlled trial. *Int J Geriatr Psychiatry.* 2016;31(6):656-665.
80. Cartwright L, Reid M, Hammersley R, Walley RM. Barriers to increasing the physical activity of people with intellectual disabilities. *Br J Learning Disabil.* 2016;45(1):47-55.
81. Vreugdenhil A, Cannell J, Davies A, Razay G. A community-based exercise programme to improve functional ability in people with Alzheimer's disease: a randomized controlled trial. *Scand J Caring Sci.* 2012;26(1):12-19.

82. Galik E, Resnick B, Hammersla M, Brightwater J. Optimizing function and physical activity among nursing home residents with dementia: testing the impact of function-focused care. *Gerontologist.* 2013;54(6):930-943.
83. Haber D. *Health Promotion and Aging: Practical Applications for Health Professionals.* 4th ed. New York, NY: Springer; 2007.
84. Hometime Video Publishing, Inc. Universal design. *PBS.* http://www.pbs.org/hometime/house/udesign.htm. Accessed April 25, 2018.
85. McCallion P. An evaluation of a family visit education program. *J Am Geriatr Soc.* 1999;47(2):203.
86. Dijkstra K. Effects of a communication intervention on the discourse of nursing home residents with dementia and their nursing assistants. *J Med Speech-Lang Pathol.* 2002;10(2):143.
87. Ripich DN. Alzheimer's disease caregivers: the focused program. A communication skills training program helps nursing assistants to give better care to patients with disease. *Geriatr Nurs.* 1995;16(1):15.
88. Williams C. Elderspeak communication: impact on dementia care. *Am J Alzheimer's Dis Other Dem.* 2009;24(1):11-20.
89. Nash J, Ross C. Application and interpretation of functional outcome measures for testing individuals with cognitive impairment. *GeriNotes.* 2016;23(6):34-37.
90. Warden V, Hurley AC, Volicer L. Development and psychometric evaluation of the Pain Assessment in Advanced Dementia (PAINAD) scale. *J Am Med Dir Assoc.* 2003;4(1):9-15.
91. Blankevoort CG, van Heuvelen MJG, Scherder EJA. Reliability of six physical performance tests in older people with dementia. *Phys Ther.* 2013;93(1):69-78.
92. Ries JD, Echternach JL, Nof L, Gagnon Blodgett M. Test-retest reliability and minimal detectable change scores for the Timed "Up & Go" Test, the Six-Minute Walk Test, and gait speed in people with Alzheimer disease. *Phys Ther.* 2009;89(6):569-579.
93. McGough EL, Logsdon RG, Kelly VE, Teri L. Functional mobility limitations and falls in assisted living residents with dementia: physical performance assessment and quantitative gait analysis. *J Geriatr Phys Ther.* 2012;36(2):78-86.
94. Muir-Hunter SW, Graham L, Odasso MM. Reliability of the Berg Balance Scale as a clinical measure of balance in community-dwelling older adults with mild to moderate Alzheimer disease: a pilot study. *Physiother Can.* 2015;67(3):255-262.
95. Bossers WJR, van der Woude LHV, Boersma F, Scherder EJA, van Heuvelen MJG. The Groningen Meander Walking Test: a dynamic walking test for older adults with dementia. *Phys Ther.* 2014;94(2):262-272.

Substance Use Disorders

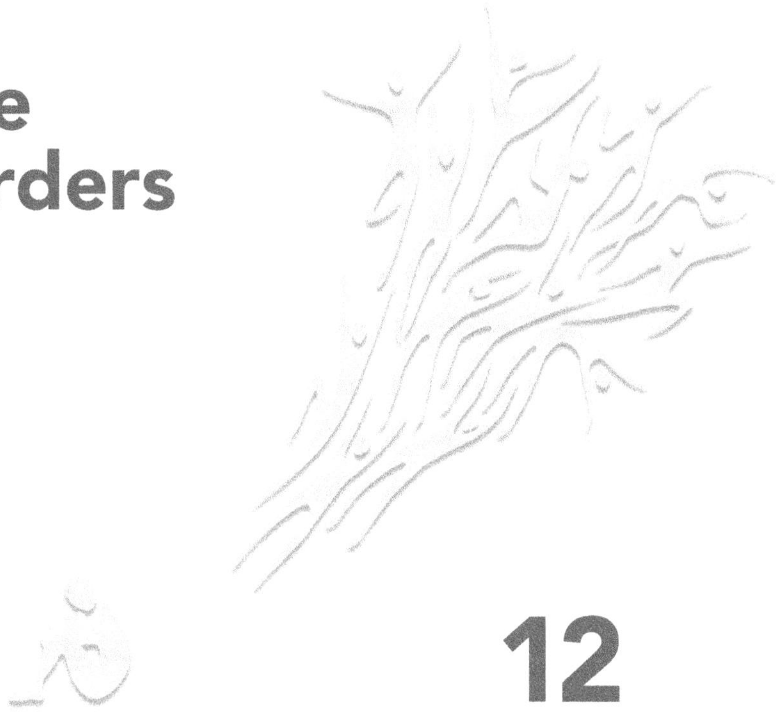

12

Outline

- Scope and Classification of Substance Use Disorders
- Neurophysiological Background, Etiology, and Risk Factors
- Comorbid Medical and Psychosocial Issues
- Focus Issue: Opioid Epidemic
- Specific Clinical Approaches to Improve Physical Therapy Outcomes
    - Psychosocial Approaches
    - Physical Activity-Based Approaches
- Summary
- Key Points
- Review Questions
- Case Studies: First Impressions
- Quick Reference

Learning Objectives

- Articulate major causative factors for substance use disorders
- Identify and note effects of common medical and psychosocial issues that occur in persons with substance dependence
- Develop clinical strategies to assess and treat impairments, functional limitations, and participation restrictions, related to substance dependence, in various age groups

Johnson H.
Psychosocial Elements of Physical Therapy: The Connection of Body to Mind (pp 199-209).

You are not an alcoholic or an addict. You are not incurably diseased. You have merely become dependent on substances or addictive behavior to cope with underlying conditions that you are now going to heal, at which time your dependency will cease completely and forever.

—Chris Prentiss[1]

Substance use disorders (SUDs) are the misuse of prescription medications, tobacco, alcohol, street drugs, and other psychoactive chemicals. Their prevalence varies depending on the local and national culture, but regardless of practice setting, the clinician is likely to see patients with SUDs. For example, tobacco use causes decreased aerobic capacity and bone and tissue healing, impeding a patient's progress in physical therapy. Survey results of academic coordinators of clinical education indicate that only about 60% of doctor of physical therapy programs in 2012 included 1 to 2 hours of tobacco cessation counseling training, and about half of these programs included training for applying relevant clinical practice guidelines.[2]

As part of a physical therapist's scope of practice, educating these patients through support groups or other interventions to break their patterns of substance use is not only reasonable but vital to health promotion. Health promotion should address persons without disability, with risk factors for disability, and with disabling conditions; therapists should steer patients toward community-based fitness resources whenever possible.[3] This chapter presents scope, risks, comorbidities, and clinical approaches for persons with SUDs, since SUDs combined with conditions such as chronic pain are a barrier to physical therapy success.[4]

Scope and Classification of Substance Use Disorders

SUDs are often classified with psychological conditions. Globally, mental illness and SUDs account for 7.4% of disability-adjusted life years (ie, the number of years lost to a person's illness or disability that can cause early death). Most mental illnesses and SUDs start between 10 and 29 years old, including illicit drug use (10.9% of this global burden), alcohol use (9.6%), tobacco use, and prescription drug misuse. These conditions also shorten absolute as well as disability-free life expectancy, and the combined mental health and SUD burden has increased by 37.6% between 1990 and 2010, mainly due to aging and population growth.[5]

The geriatric population in particular has a high risk for medication-related SUDs, due to polypharmacy (ie, more than 4 medications taken at the same time). Adding more medications dramatically increases the risk of side effects, including other illnesses caused by medications themselves. Women are at higher risk for polypharmacy; worldwide, persons over 60 years old are projected to increase from 605 million in 2000 to 2 billion by 2050. In the United States, by 2020 SUDs in the elderly are projected to triple to 5 million needing treatment. However, even brief interventions such as cognitive behavioral therapy, individual psychologist sessions, and interdisciplinary team/interprofessional team care coordination can reduce prevalence and disability related to geriatric SUDs.[6]

Other populations at risk include military veterans and persons with persistent pain (see Chapter 13).[7] Opioid analgesics are inherently addictive, leading to a push in the United States and elsewhere to reduce unnecessary prescriptions, thus preventing premature death due to opioid addiction. From 2011 to 2013, illicit use of opioids did decrease slightly, but much progress remains to be made.[8] Interventions in any case may benefit from team-based care coordination, since SUDs make patients more psychosocially complex and difficult for only one health care provider to help.[9]

Neurophysiological Background, Etiology, and Risk Factors

These aren't just physical allergies, they're obsessions of the mind and maladies of the spirit. It's a threefold disease. And if it's partly a spiritual malady, then there's a spiritual cure.

—Anthony Kiedis[10]

SUDs typically occur along with other medical or psychiatric conditions because many persons use chemical substances illicitly to manage pain, stress, mood changes, and other similar daily occurrences. One study found that 20% of military veterans who were prescribed opioids for pain management had additional SUDs, but only one-third of them were treated for the substance dependence, even though the SUD itself increased the risk of mental health comorbidities.[11]

Certain populations, including children with motor or mental health disorders and adolescents with certain personality traits, are also at a higher risk for SUDs. Children with attention-deficit hyperactivity disorder are 6 times more likely to have a comorbid SUD than typically developing children.[12] Developmental coordination disorder, motor incoordination in children that does not typically have neurological or intellectual impairment, is associated with SUDs, social anxiety, and criminal offenses.[13] Once a child reaches adolescence, personality traits and underlying brain chemistry influence his or her use of alcohol, psychoactive medications, and marijuana (cannabis)[14]:

- Impulsivity increases the odds of using cocaine and other stimulants.
- Sensation seeking increases the odds of using alcohol and cannabis.
- Anxiety sensitivity and hopelessness increase the odds of using alcohol, sedatives, opioids, and other central nervous system depressants.

In crowded cities and places with uncertain economies in the United States, substance abuse often causes hospital admissions. In a study of a large hospital system, predominant characteristics of hospital outpatients with SUDs were African American ethnicity; male sex; homeless status; and use of heroin, cocaine, and alcohol. Complications of SUDs listed in this study included "infectious endocarditis, abscess or nonhealing ulcer, and osteomyelitis with intravenous antibiotic."[15] Typically, these patients stayed for 12 days, had 63% to 70% rates of completion of treatment for complications, and appropriate referral to an SUD management program. Their chances of success increased with proximity of available medical care and amount of social support. Outside the United States, however, SUD risk was low in an analysis of 90 African refugee camps completed with data gathered between 2009 and 2013.[16]

Comorbid Medical and Psychosocial Issues

SUDs may occur with other mental health issues and are related to medical conditions including lifestyle-related diseases (ie, diseases related to behaviors that the person can change). Diseases and conditions co-occurring with SUDs include HIV-AIDS, chronic pain, spinal cord injury, and pressure injuries depending on the patient's past medical history.[17,18]

Mental health conditions that may cause or be caused by SUDs include:

- Depression: SUDs increase the risk of depression relapse.[19]
- Schizophrenia: SUDs combined with poor diet and physical inactivity increase cardiovascular illness and death in this population.[20]
- Borderline personality disorder: SUDs are among psychiatric comorbidities, occurring more in men than in women.[21]

Outside of the United States, Poudel et al[22] present a broader view of psychosocial issues faced by persons with SUDs. Studying Nepalese subjects, the authors noted that the younger the age at which a person starts to use addictive substances, the more likely he or she is to have severe educational and psychological problems, with variation based on gender and substance. Congruent with other literature, these subjects typically developed their SUDs early, before age 20, and typically abused alcohol and cannabis, with other street drugs and prescription medications coming in close second.

The following is a list of common domains of psychosocial issues[22]:

- Substance use: most people used alcohol or other substances more than 3 times per day.
- School performance: SUDs typically impaired grades or caused premature dropout.
- Behavior pattern: the need to have another "hit" made the person seek that substance above all else.
- Peer relationship: undesirable behavior changes cost the person previous friendships, while attracting the user to people with a bad influence.
- Social competence: especially while under the influence, the users were less likely to conform to social norms of communication and follow-through.
- Psychiatric disorder: the SUD itself typically influenced the development of mental health conditions.
- Family system: the user prioritized the substance above family, causing fractured relationships. Also, many persons with SUDs had enabling family members who nurtured the substance-seeking behavior by giving money or easy access to the substance. These family members sometimes even developed the same SUD.
- Work adjustment: behavior changes influenced unemployment or underemployment.

Focus Issue: Opioid Epidemic

By most measurements, rates of opioid misuse and addiction in the United States are at epidemic proportions. Vowles et al[23] found that misuse occurs in 21% to 29% and addiction in 8% to 12% of persons receiving opioids for chronic pain. More generally, in a 2010 national survey, "an estimated 22.6 million, or 8.9% of Americans, aged 12 and older, were current or past month illicit drug users."[24] Sources of these drugs, including opioids, were friends and relatives (66.4%), one or more doctors (17.3%), dealers (4.4%), and the internet (0.4%). Due to this public health epidemic, opioid overdose death exceeds the prevalence of suicide and motor vehicle death. Besides overdose, opioid misuse can cause low birth weight and has a high rate of comorbidity with anxiety, depression, and other serious mental illnesses.[25,26]

Another source of addiction, besides intentional diversion of drugs, is iatrogenic (ie, persons who use the medications as prescribed but still become addicted). While the clinical picture is slowly improving, most health care providers do not have a clear understanding of this aspect of pain education. In the 1980s, medical education led doctors to believe that the risk of iatrogenic addiction was low to nil; to date, there are no reliable data about its prevalence. Due to conflicting and ambiguous evidence, the Joint Commission on Accreditation of Healthcare Organizations recommends non–narcotic first-line treatments for pain such as psychosocial interventions, mindfulness, exercise, and alternative medications.[27]

In response to the education and perception gap, Volkow and McLellan[28] compiled a set of corrected misconceptions and mitigation strategies for opioid abuse in persons with chronic pain.

Acute or chronic pain affects over one-third of persons in the United States and over 40% of older adults; however, prescribed opioids are commonly diverted, causing almost 40% of overdose-related deaths in 2013. Misconceptions common among providers include[28]:

- Equating addiction with physical tolerance or dependence (this leads to under-prescription of opioids where they would be appropriate treatments)
- Attributing addiction to a series of poor choices (this leads to discrimination)
- Assuming that pain would protect from addiction (this ignores iatrogenic addiction)
- Targeting chronic pain alone as an addiction risk (actually, most diverted opioids are those prescribed for acute pain)
- Discounting the usefulness of medication-assisted therapies (actually, slow opioid agonists do minimize abuse-related risks while allowing recovery)

Most mitigation strategies involve prescribing alternative forms or combinations of medications, as well as drafting medication use contracts and more systematic screening for SUDs.

Specific Clinical Approaches to Improve Physical Therapy Outcomes

As with other mental health issues, physical therapy for a patient with an SUD involves a blend of psychosocial techniques, exercise prescription, and a team approach. One example is a patient with chronic pain (typically defined as pain of any intensity lasting more than 3 months) who has become addicted to prescription opioids. Since "chronic pain … is associated with increased psychological distress, decreased mobility, obesity, decreased physical function, social isolation, financial loss, and development of chronic disability,"[29] the clinician must be able to refer the patient to other specialists. This can facilitate social and financial support as well as rehabilitate the movement system-related issues within the therapist's scope of practice.

In this example, the patient's addiction to opioid pain medications complicates the therapist's management of the case by adding "lowered pain thresholds, increased social stress … depression, anxiety … and decreased coping skills,"[29] which may require additional referral and specialized pain knowledge to address the central sensitization caused by the opioids (see Chapter 13). Management of this combined pain and SUD includes engaging the patient psychosocially (eg, by cognitive behavioral therapy or mindfulness-based stress reduction; see Chapter 4), emphasizing physical function and higher mobility levels (eg, including yoga or other enjoyable activity in the plan of care), weight management (eg, dietary and exercise counseling; discussed in Chapter 4), managing substance use itself, and careful medication prescription for symptom management. Pharmacological knowledge is essential because even non-steroidal anti-inflammatory drugs and selective serotonin reuptake inhibitors, both commonly prescribed for chronic pain, have side effects and potential interactions.

The following subsections discuss discrete psychosocial and physical activity interventions based on current literature. As a side note, since several states in the United States have liberalized marijuana use, clinicians should be aware of a patient's use of marijuana and other cannabinoids. Several clinically relevant cannabinoids include THC (delta-9-tetrahydrocannabinol) and CBD (cannabidiol), which are not psychoactive. Various other forms, however, have less predictable effects, depending on the route of administration (tea, spray, tablet, or other). Cannabinoids have some benefits for "chronic pain, inflammation, spasticity, and other conditions" for which research is ongoing. However, potential side effects can affect "cognition, coordination, balance, and cardiovascular and pulmonary function."[30] Cannabinoid and other substance use should be part of the patient's medical history, as reviewed by the clinician, to minimize adverse effects and facilitate referral to other professionals as needed.

Psychosocial Approaches

A systematic review of 45 randomized controlled trials and cohort studies found that several types of treatments are effective for persons with comorbid severe mental illness and SUDs. For the SUD itself, Drake et al[31] recommend "group counseling, contingency management [ie, planning for potential unforeseen events], and residential dual diagnosis treatment [a short-term placement at a facility outside the person's home to address both conditions]." To allow the patient to remain safely in the community, a case management approach is helpful, and the legal system can improve the patient's participation in treatments.

The clinician's approach to each patient needs to be sensitive to causes of the SUD, which can include childhood abuse. Schachter et al[32] note that childhood sexual abuse happens in 10% to 30% of persons under 18 years old and can result in diverse physical and mental health issues, including chronic pain, dissociation, and SUDs to cope with pain and boundary violation. Therapists may not know which patients were abused as children, but **all sessions should include**[32]:

- A culture of safety and respect, including private and public treatment spaces depending on a patient's needs that may change during a session
- Rapport, emphasizing gentleness, communication, and interpersonal connection
- Therapeutic alliance, including offering a therapist of the same sex as the patient if possible, asking verbal consent for each intervention, sharing control with the patient, and respecting boundaries
- Patient education on psychosocial and physical factors influencing effects of their past abuse
- Holistic practice, treating the whole person and referring to community services as needed, while respecting the patient's level of self-disclosure

Education to patients and their social support systems should include accurate information on SUDs. Acceptance and commitment therapy, with a trained therapist or via a smartphone app, is a relatively new approach to SUDs that asks the patient to notice, accept, and process cravings instead of performing the addictive behavior.[33-36] For alcoholism and other SUDs, the following websites may be useful[37]:

- Alcoholics Anonymous: www.aa.org
- Hazelden Betty Ford Foundation for outpatient and residential treatment programs: www.hazelden.org
- Smart Recovery: www.smartrecovery.org
- National Institute on Alcohol Abuse and Alcoholism: https://niaaa.nih.gov
- National Council on Alcoholism and Drug Dependence: www.ncadd.org

Besides these approaches, the clinician or other interdisciplinary team/interprofessional team member can directly deter substance abuse. One example of this comes from the author's experience. In a skilled nursing facility, the occupational therapist and a charge nurse saw a patient with a known history of alcoholism rummaging through an outdoor garbage bag. Inferring that the patient was being given alcohol by another resident through the hiding area of the bag, the charge nurse simply removed the extra bag.

Physical Activity-Based Approaches

Limited literature discusses physical therapy for persons with SUDs in isolation, but other approaches from mental health literature are appropriate. Persons with SUDs have increased risk of lifestyle-related diseases or noncommunicable diseases, including coronary artery disease. High-intensity interval training decreased risk and severity of noncommunicable diseases in persons with and without SUDs. The dosage in this study included four 4-minute intervals of aerobic activity on a treadmill "at 90-95% of maximal heart rate, 3 days a week for 8 weeks" to improve depression severity and aerobic capacity.[38]

Psychomotor physical therapy is another technique originally developed in mental health care that applies to SUDs, especially if the patient has more psychological than physical impairments. Key concepts are "body awareness and physical activities" individualized to the diagnosis and treatment setting, incorporating "medical, psychological, agogic [ie, dance- or music-related], kinesiological, and rehabilitative" interventions.[39] These coordinated approaches address "fine and gross motor abilities, eye-hand coordination, balance, time and space, perception, attention, interaction with materials, recognition of stimuli ... learning how to relax, acquiring a good physical condition, and learning the basic rules of communication."[37]

Within this approach, the team and the patient develop challenging short- and long-term goals to promote mastery. Patients have the maximal safe amount of choice. In the context of any physical activity chosen by the patient-therapist team, "the corrective emotional experience in a safe, containing, healing, and non-coercive social context through attachment to a predictable role model [ie, the therapist] is an important therapeutic leverage."[37] Thus, persons with SUDs should have one constant treating therapist, who can remain supportive and emotionally stable, while the patient is improving in physical condition and social function and lessening the craving for the substance(s) in question.

Summary

SUDs are on the rise in almost any population the physical therapist may interact with. Abused substances include alcohol, tobacco, opioid pain medications, street drugs, and prescription medications. Because the person with SUDs typically has multiple psychosocial and mental health issues, a solid team approach can be the most effective treatment.

Key Points

- A team approach is critical for physical therapy provided to persons with SUDs.
- For a patient with SUDs and a known or suspected history of abuse, clinicians should ensure a culture of safety, rapport, therapeutic alliance, psychosocial education, and holistic practice.

Review Questions

- What are risk factors noted in the text that can cause or worsen an SUD?
  - Does this match what you have seen in the clinic or in your social circles?
  - How can you improve your screening process for these risk factors?
- Have you seen any of the mentioned clinical effects of marijuana or other cannabinoid use in your clinical rotations or practice? What impact do they have on the plan of care for the patient?
- Recall a patient case where the patient had a diagnosed SUD.
  - What effects did the disorder have on the patient's physical function?
  - What medical conditions were present that could be impacted by the SUD?

  - How did the patient's social situation interact with the SUD?
  - How did the SUD affect your approach to the initial interview? The plan of care (including frequency and duration of sessions)? The short- and long-term results of the episode of care?
- Based on the text, and insights from classmates or colleagues, list clinical strategies to assess and treat impairments, functional limitations, and participation restrictions related to substance dependence in the age groups you have worked with or currently work with.

Case Studies: First Impressions

As you review the following case studies, you may want to consider these questions for thought or discussion:

- What standardized tests and measures (including psychiatric, for example, a depression screen) would you select for this patient? Why?
- Based on available data, what short- and long-term goals would you write for your plan of care? Consider using the acronyms SMART (specific, measurable, attainable, realistic, and timely) or ABCDE (actor, behavior, conditions, degree, and expected time frame) to guide your goal writing.
- What elements (procedures, psychosocial aspects, communication aspects, etc) would you make sure to include or omit in your plan of care for this patient? Why?
- What are your anticipated needs, if any, for consultation and referral for this patient?
- How will you transition this patient toward lasting health behavior change following discharge (eg, recommending a YMCA membership trial)?

Case 1

A 22-year-old male was referred to outpatient physical therapy 1 week after a left ankle sprain. His goal is to return to recreational contact sports.

- Social history: he goes to college full time and lives in a dormitory with elevator access. He must walk approximately one-quarter mile to get to his nearest class.
- Medical/psychiatric history: asthma and weekly episodes of severe alcoholic intoxication
- Impairments, activity limitations, and participation restrictions found on initial interview and examination
  - Pain in left ankle rated 3/10 at rest and 6/10 with partial weightbearing
  - Moderate inflammation and bruising noted on lateral aspect of ankle
  - Requires a single axillary crutch and unweighting boot to walk more than 10 feet
  - Increased postural sway noted with eyes closed on a firm surface
  - Shortness of breath and verbalization of frustration when talking about pain and other stressors

Case 2

A 34-year-old female was hospitalized after a motor vehicle accident where speed was a factor. Her goal is to return home and be able to take care of her children.

- Social history: she lives with her husband and 2 children in a 2-story condominium. Both she and her husband work first shift positions, while the children are in school.
- Medical/psychiatric history: acute diagnoses include whiplash-associated neck pain, mild traumatic brain injury with loss of consciousness at the accident site, and bilateral grade 2 posterior cruciate ligament sprain from knees being thrust into the dashboard during the accident. Past diagnoses include oxycodone dependence for chronic neck and low back pain, delivery of both children via C-section, obesity, and generalized anxiety disorder.
- Impairments, activity limitations, and participation restrictions found on initial interview and examination
  - Neck pain and dizziness with head turns in any position (does not rate numerically)
  - Impaired balance reactions during multidirectional seated and standing reach
  - Bilateral knee pain during weightbearing tasks and transfers
  - Requires 50% assistance for safe transfers and short-distance ambulation in the hospital room with a 2-wheeled walker
  - Requests pain medications more frequently than prescribed dosages allow

Case 3

A 48-year-old male was admitted to subacute rehabilitation following extended hospitalization for complications of diabetes, resulting in a left above-knee amputation. His goal is to return home and work with family support as needed.

- Social history: he works as a collegiate athletic director and lives alone in a third-floor apartment with a single railing on the stairs. His parents live nearby, and he has no significant other or children.
- Medical/psychiatric history: tobacco dependence, type 2 diabetes with distal sensory polyneuropathy (diagnosed at age 30), obstructive sleep apnea on BiPAP with 50% compliance, obesity, alcohol use disorder, hypertension, and history of low back and knee pain from collegiate sports
- Impairments, activity limitations, and participation restrictions found on initial interview and examination
  - Mild hypoxemia with exertion
  - Requires 25% to 50% assistance and a 2-wheeled walker to transition from sitting to standing and hop 5 feet from bed to chair
  - One near-fall in the hospital due to an attempted self-transfer
  - Mild deficits in upper and lower-extremity coordination tests
  - Unable to negotiate stairs
  - Standing tolerance 3 minutes with a 2-wheeled walker

Quick Reference

- Possible diagnoses and their signs/symptoms:
  - Alcohol: slurred speech, craving, dizziness, sweating, labile mood, aggression, compulsive behavior, delirium
  - Cannabis: impaired coordination and perception, poor problem solving and memory, productive cough, hunger, tachycardia, anxiety, dry mouth
  - Opioids: craving, euphoria, sweating, discontent, constipation, small pupils, pain sensitivity, slurred speech, shallow breathing
  - Tobacco: irritability, anger, mood symptoms, craving, poor concentration
  - Stimulants: overconfidence, alertness, rapid speech, dilated pupils, confusion, irritability, hallucinations, paranoia
  - Other substances: cocaine, methamphetamine, over-the-counter cough medicine, anabolic steroids, heroin, bath salts, ketamine, inhalants, hallucinogens
- Questions to ask the patient (or friend/family member):
  - Do you often feel any of the symptoms (listed previously)?
  - Have you ever been diagnosed with an SUD (listed previously)? What was going on in your life around the time of that diagnosis?
  - How do you deal with your SUD? How well does that work for you?
  - What should I know about your SUD?
- Referral options:
  - Primary care provider first, for diagnosis, behavioral and medication prescription
  - Outpatient or inpatient treatment programs
  - Support group for recovering users
  - Exercise group to capitalize on craving-reduction effects, especially of aerobics

References

1. Prentiss C. *The Alcoholism and Addiction Cure: A Holistic Approach to Total Recovery.* Malibu, CA: Power Press; 2007.
2. Pignataro RM, Gurka MJ, Jones DL, et al. Tobacco cessation counseling training in US entry-level physical therapist education curricula: prevalence, content, and associated factors. *Phys Ther.* 2014;94(9):1294-1305.
3. Rimmer JH. Health promotion for people with disabilities: the emerging paradigm shift from disability prevention to prevention of secondary conditions. *Phys Ther.* 1999;79(5):495-502.
4. Fritz JM, Kim J, Thackeray A, Dorius J. Use of physical therapy for low back pain by Medicaid enrollees. *Phys Ther.* 2015;95(12):1668-1679.
5. Whiteford HA, Degenhardt L, Rehm J, et al. Global burden of disease attributable to mental and substance use disorders: findings from the Global Burden of Disease Study 2010. *Lancet.* 2013;382(9904):1575-1586.
6. Bhatia U, Nadkarni A, Murthy P, Rao R, Crome I. Recent advances in treatment for older people with substance use problems: an updated systematic and narrative review. *Eur Geriatr Med.* 2015;6(6):580-586.
7. Van Til L, Fikretoglu D, Pranger T, et al. Work reintegration for veterans with mental disorders: a systematic literature review to inform research. *Phys Ther.* 2013;93(9):1163-1174.
8. Dart RC, Surratt HL, Cicero TJ, et al. Trends in opioid analgesic abuse and mortality in the United States. *N Engl J Med.* 2015;372(3):241-248.
9. Grant RW, Ashburner JM, Hong CS, et al. Defining patient complexity from the primary care physician's perspective. *Ann Intern Med.* 2011;155(12):797-804.
10. Kiedis A. *Scar Tissue.* New York, NY: Hyperion; 2004.
11. Morasco BJ, Duckart JP, Dobscha SK. Adherence to clinical guidelines for opioid therapy for chronic pain in patients with substance use disorder. *J Gen Intern Med.* 2011;26(9):965-961.

12. Zaso MJ, Park A, Antshel KM. Treatments for adolescents with comorbid attention-deficit/hyperactivity disorder and substance use disorder: a systematic review. *J Attention Disord.* 2015. doi: 10.1177/1087054715569280.
13. Barnhart RC, Davenport MJ, Epps SB, Nordquist VM. Developmental coordination disorder. *Phys Ther.* 2003;83(8):722-731.
14. Conrod PJ. Personality-targeted interventions for substance use and misuse. *Curr Addict Rep.* 2016;3(4):426-436.
15. O'Toole TP, Conde-Martel A, Young JH, et al. Managing acutely ill substance-abusing patients in an integrated day hospital outpatient program. *J Gen Intern Med.* 2006;21(6):570-576.
16. Kane JC, Ventevogel P, Spiegel P, et al. Mental, neurological, and substance use problems among refugees in primary health care: analysis of the Health Information System in 90 refugee camps. *BMC Medicine.* 2014;12:228.
17. Merlin JS. Chronic pain in patients with HIV infection: what clinicians need to know. *Top Antivir Med.* 2015;23(3):120-124.
18. Shields RK, Dudley-Javorski S. Musculoskeletal deterioration and hemicorporectomy after spinal cord injury. *Phys Ther.* 2003;83(3):263-275.
19. Malhi GS, Bassett D, Boyce P, et al. Royal Australian and New Zealand College of Psychiatrists clinical practice guidelines for mood disorders. *Aust N Z J Psychiatry.* 2015;49(12):1087-1206.
20. Vancampfort D, De Hert M, Helvik Skjerven L, et al. International Organization of Physical Therapy in Mental Health consensus on physical activity within multidisciplinary rehabilitation programmes for minimising cardio-metabolic risk in patients with schizophrenia. *Disabil Rehabil.* 2012;34(1):1-12.
21. Dell'Osso B, Berlin HA, Serati M, Altamura AC. Neuropsychobiological aspects, comorbidity patterns and dimensional models in borderline personality disorder. *Neuropsychobiology.* 2010;61(4):169-179.
22. Poudel A, Sharma C, Gautam S, Poudel A. Psychosocial problems among individuals with substance use disorders in drug rehabilitation centers, Nepal. *Subst Abuse Treat Prev Policy.* 2016;11(1):28.
23. Vowles KE, McEntee ML, Julnes PS, et al. Rates of opioid misuse, abuse, and addiction in chronic pain: a systematic review and data synthesis. *Pain.* 2015;156(4):569-576.
24. Manchikanti L, Helm II S, Fellows B, et al. Opioid epidemic in the United States. *Pain Physician.* 2012;15(suppl 3):ES9-ES38.
25. Patrick SW, Dudley J, Martin PR, et al. Prescription opioid epidemic and infant outcomes. *Pediatrics.* 2015;135(5):842-850.
26. Goldner EM, Lusted A, Roerecke M, Rehm J, Fischer B. Prevalence of Axis-1 psychiatric (with focus on depression and anxiety) disorder and symptomatology among non-medical prescription opioid users in substance use treatment: systematic review and meta-analyses. *Addict Behav.* 2014;39(3):520-531.
27. Beauchamp GA, Winstanley EL, Ryan SA, Lyons MS. Moving beyond misuse and diversion: the urgent need to consider the role of iatrogenic addiction in the current opioid epidemic. *Am J Public Health.* 2014;104(11):2023-2029.
28. Volkow BD, McLellan T. Opioid abuse in chronic pain—misconceptions and mitigation strategies. *N Engl J Med.* 2016;374(13):1253-1263.
29. Liebschutz J, Beers D, Lange A. Managing chronic pain in patients with opioid dependence. *Curr Treat Options Psychiatry.* 2014;1(2):204-223.
30. Ciccone CD. Medical marijuana: just the beginning of a long, strange trip? *Phys Ther.* 2017;97(2):239-248.
31. Drake RE, O'Neal EL, Wallach MA. A systematic review of psychosocial research on psychosocial interventions for people with co-occurring severe mental and substance use disorder. *J Subst Abuse Treat.* 2008;34(1):123-138.
32. Schachter CL, Stalker CA, Teram E. Toward sensitive practice: issues for physical therapists working with survivors of childhood sexual abuse. *Phys Ther.* 1999;79(3):248-261.
33. Boyko EJ, Trone DW, Peterson AV, et al. Longitudinal investigation of smoking initiation and relapse among younger and older US military personnel. *Am J Public Health.* 2015;105(6):1220-1229.
34. Heffner JL, McClure JB, Mull KE, Anthenelli RM, Bricker JB. Acceptance and commitment therapy and nicotine patch for smokers with bipolar disorder: preliminary evaluation of in-person and telephone-delivered treatment. *Bipolar Disord.* 2015;17(5):560-566.
35. Heffner JL, Vilardaga R, Mercer LD, Kientz JA, Bricker JB. Feature-level analysis of a novel smartphone application for smoking cessation. *Am J Drug Alcohol Abuse.* 2015;41(1):68-73.
36. Schuck K, Otten R, Kleinjan M, Bricker JB, Engels RC. Self-efficacy and acceptance of cravings to smoke underlie the effectiveness of quitline counseling for smoking cessation. *Drug Alcohol Depend.* 2014;142:269-276.
37. Haber D. *Health Promotion and Aging: Practical Applications for Health Professionals.* 4th ed. New York, NY: Springer; 2007.
38. Flemmen G, Unhjem R, Wang E. High-intensity interval training in patients with substance use disorder. *BioMed Research International.* 2014;616935. doi: 10.1155/2014/616935.
39. Probst M, Knapen J, Poot G, Vancampfort D. Psychomotor therapy and psychiatry: what's in a name? *Open Complement Med J.* 2010;2:105-113.

Chronic Pain and Illness

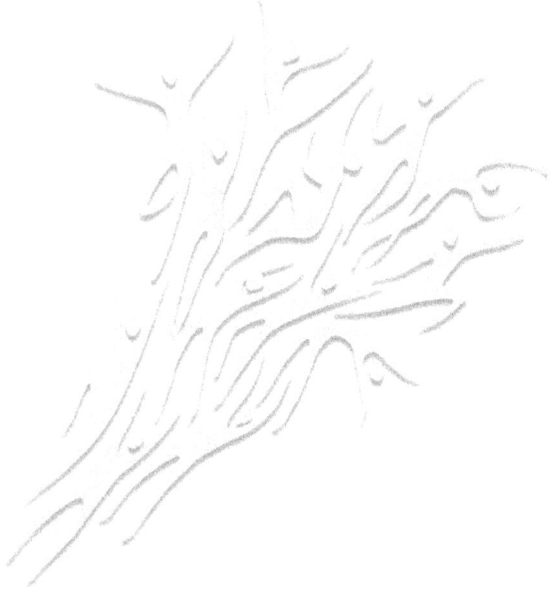

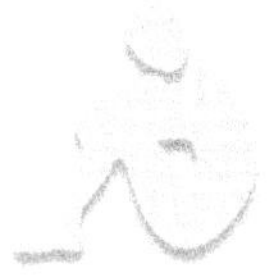

13

Outline

- Scope and Classification of Chronic Pain and Illness
- Persistent Pain: Neurophysiological Background, Etiology, and Risk Factors
  - Direct and Indirect Etiologies
  - Contributory and Risk Factors
  - Secondary and Tertiary Prevention
- Comorbid Medical and Psychosocial Issues
  - Disparities in Pain Management
  - Illness Interactions
  - Focus Issue: HIV-AIDS
- Specific Clinical Approaches to Improve Physical Therapy Outcomes
  - Interdisciplinary/Multidisciplinary Pain Clinics
  - Pain Neuroscience Education
  - Screening Tools and Outcome Measures
  - Other Opportunities for Physical Therapist Practice to Promote Health and Wellness
    - Exercise Adherence
    - Types of Activity
    - Modalities
    - Cognitive Behavioral Therapy
    - Other Psychosocial Considerations
    - Complementary and Alternative Medicine
- Summary
- Key Points
- Review Questions
- Case Studies: First Impressions

Johnson H.
Psychosocial Elements of Physical Therapy: The Connection of Body to Mind (pp 211-235).

Learning Objectives

- Identify known mechanisms of and risk factors for chronic (persistent) pain
- Propose impacts of chronic pain and illness on the physical therapist's plan of care
- Given the diversity and high prevalence of chronic pain and illness, outline strategies for management of these complex patients

For some reason the word "chronic" often has to be explained. It does not mean severe ... No, "chronic" means persistent over time, enduring, constant.

—Stephen Fry[1]

Chronic pain, chronic illness, and their overlap are perhaps the most common issues a physical therapist sees, especially in an aging population. This chapter will survey the range of chronic illnesses and pain with discussion of general strategies for secondary prevention, common comorbid medical and psychosocial issues, and several types of clinical approaches. These approaches include interprofessional pain clinics, pain neuroscience education (PNE), and selected screening tools and outcome measures to classify patients and track their progress in therapy.

Chronic conditions, also called *noncommunicable diseases* (NCDs), are a current research focus because they affect so many people; increase costs for all stakeholders; and are, for the most part, amenable to lifestyle changes. Common NCDs include arthritis, "heart disease, cancer, chronic lung disease, hypertension, stroke, type 2 diabetes mellitus, and obesity."[2] Physical therapists play an important part in NCD prevention and management. Doctor of physical therapy (DPT) curricula can reflect this by including examination techniques for health status and lifestyle; revising the minimum health competency requirements (related to smoking, nutrition, sitting, sleep, and mood symptoms, as well as physical activity); and encouraging lobbying for better reimbursement for patient wellness, regardless of the patient's ability to pay for services. **For reimbursement strategies, it is helpful for the therapist to cite studies demonstrating the cost-effectiveness of even 10 to 14 sessions of physical therapy for improving health and addressing both acute and chronic conditions.**[3,4]

With a focus on function, skilled physical therapy, as a component of an interdisciplinary team/interprofessional team (IDT/IPT) approach, is effective for many chronic musculoskeletal and neurologic conditions.[3,5,6] However, the attitudes of other medical professionals are inconsistent with these findings. In a study with an admittedly limited evidence base, Cottrell et al[7] concluded that general practitioners in Great Britain do not have consistent attitudes, beliefs, and professional behaviors about prescribing exercise for chronic knee pain related to osteoarthritis. Another study on chronic illness management found the educational system still in silos, while the medical world moves toward IDTs/IPTs. A school in New Zealand, however, used focus groups to suggest core competencies in "teams and teamwork, professional roles and responsibilities, interprofessional communication, cultural competence, better engagement with patients, families, and carers, and common systems, information sharing and confidentiality."[8]

Professional training programs in physical therapy, medicine, nutrition, and others can benefit from more interprofessional orientation. Areas to improve regarding chronic conditions include prioritization of chronic pain vs geriatrics and cognitive impairment for DPT students, and inclusion of persistent pain concepts including central sensitization and fear-avoidance in medical school curricula.[9,10] Additionally, the physical therapy profession can improve the public's knowledge of the usefulness of medically prescribed physical therapy and lifestyle modifications for persons with comorbid persistent low back pain and depression, and improve pain neurophysiology knowledge for medical and nutrition students.[11,12] Pain neurophysiology is a newer research area, discussed in greater depth later in this chapter.

Scope and Classification of Chronic Pain and Illness

Chronic conditions permeate all geographic settings and treatment specialties. One 2007 face-to-face study of persons over 18 years old in the United States indicated that over half of these adults had at least one mental or chronic physical illness. These illnesses caused a full month of vocation-related disability per year; the largest contributors to this additional disability were major depressive disorder and musculoskeletal conditions.[13] According to a set of surveys of 18 developed countries, if multiple mental and physical illnesses occur in the same person (comorbidity), the risk for severe disability increases; mental illness increased the risk for severe disability more than physical illness alone.[14]

This section focuses more on chronic or persistent pain, which is narrower in scope. Pain accompanies many chronic illnesses, particularly in geriatric clients.[15] On the other end of the lifespan, pediatric clients (girls more than boys) frequently have chronic pain that is best managed by an IDT/IPT; clinical practice guidelines are in development.[16]

Persistent pain can be classified by duration, part of body, intensity, functional impact, and mechanism (see Pain Neuroscience Education section). A multinational survey of adults in Israel and 15 European countries examined prevalence, impact on daily life, and adequacy of treatment. Of those participating, 19% reported pain for over 6 months at least a 5/10 intensity on the Numeric Pain Rating Scale. Of those persons with chronic pain, 66% had moderate and 34% had severe; 46% constant, 54% intermittent, and 59% lasting for 2 to 15 years; 21% with subsequent diagnosed depression; 61% with subsequent decreased work ability, 19% job loss, 13% job change; and 60% with 2 to 9 physician visits in last 6 months due to pain.

Regarding treatment, "only 2% were currently treated by a pain management specialist" with one-third undergoing no treatment.[17] Two-thirds of those treated used non-pharmacological treatments (physical therapy or massage) and half used non-prescription medications (non-steroidal anti-inflammatory drugs [NSAIDs] or weak opioids), two-thirds prescription meds (NSAIDs, weak or strong opioids, or COX-2 inhibitors). "Forty percent had inadequate management of their pain" depending on cultural factors.[17] Inadequate pain management is also a problem in cancer treatment, due to "health care providers' lack of training, fear of side effects and addiction, and reimbursement issues."[17]

Chronic low back pain (cLBP) is a worldwide problem for many people. In the United States alone, it costs over $600 million while affecting 100 million adults, about 31% of the population. Worldwide, cLBP affects approximately 39% of people, or 2.9 billion people. In a report by a National Institutes of Health Task Force to guide research standards to better understand, diagnose, and treat cLBP, one basic issue is the lack of a standardized definition of what is "chronic."[18] Since research authors use different time durations to define chronic, it is hard to determine by study parameters which interventions work best. Besides this lack of clarity, cLBP has many direct and indirect causes, including psychosocial aspects of the patients and their cultures. For researchers, the report recommended the following:

- Use a standardized screen to define cLBP
    - "How long has back pain been an ongoing problem for you?" with expected answer being more than 3 months
    - "How often has low-back pain been an ongoing problem for you over the past 6 months?" with expected answer being more than half the days in that 6-month time frame
- Classify cLBP by its functional impact, whether physically, in pain intensity, or the degree to which pain interferes with daily activities
- Gather study participant data about demographics, medical history, self-reported function, and symptoms
- Measure outcomes in all possible patients, but report available outcomes in all patients

Thus, there is more than one way to classify persistent pain. Since many, if not all, DPT programs now specifically teach principles of research and evidence evaluation as part of evidence-based practice, current and recent students should be familiar with using high-quality articles to guide patient care. All clinicians, however, need consistent practice to keep up with research and evaluate it accurately to prevent inadequate or negative outcomes for the patients served. The American Physical Therapy Association has several relevant practice resources, including the *PT Now* database (accessible at www.ptnow.org/Default.aspx).

Persistent Pain: Neurophysiological Background, Etiology, and Risk Factors

Direct and Indirect Etiologies

Persistent pain, as noted earlier, has multiple causes. Microscopically, the neurotransmitter glutamate has been implicated in persistent pain and several chronic diseases including "depression, Parkinson's disease, [and] schizophrenia."[19] At the organ and system level, persistent pain occurs in such conditions as cerebral palsy, hemophilia, and cancer. These conditions are all amenable to physical therapy and IDT/IPT management for pain and associated symptoms. Physiological mechanisms of pain include inactivity, medication side effects, and trauma related to the disease process (eg, joint bleeds in hemophilia or organ injury in cancer).[20-22]

While persistent pain was once thought to be caused by biological factors only, now researchers recognize the powerful influences of the mind and a patient's psychosocial factors. Especially in persons with more medical conditions, persistent pain has at least 3 possible mechanisms; it is helpful for the clinician to classify a patient into one of these categories for better treatment[23]:

1. Nociceptive pain
    - Caused by more peripheral nociceptive nerve fiber activation (nociception is an unpleasant sensory stimulus that is typically interpreted by the person as pain)
    - Diagnosed by its limited, local nature, related to specific movements or positions that increase or decrease it. This pain is typically not sharp, burning, or shooting
    - Treated by postural stretching and retraining, lower-quadrant joint mobilizations, strengthening, and motor control exercises
2. Peripheral neuropathic pain
    - Caused by "a lesion or dysfunction in the dorsal horn or cervico-trigeminal nucleus or peripheral nerve"[23]
    - Diagnosed by its presentation in a dermatomal distribution (ie, a horizontal band of skin that corresponds to the sensory innervation by a single nerve root; symptoms are increased by postures or movements that increase the loading on the neural tissue)
    - Treated by trigger point therapy, neural and lumbar intervertebral joint mobilizations
3. Central sensitization
    - Caused by "amplification of neural signaling in the central nervous system that elicits pain hypersensitivity"[23]
    - Diagnosed by its widespread nature disproportionate to the original injury (the patient will have poor adaptation strategies and treat the pain as a very threatening thing that limits many normal daily activities)
    - Treated by cognitive behavioral therapy (CBT), aerobic conditioning, progressive strength training, and manual therapy techniques

Contributory and Risk Factors

Psychosocial factors impacting the success or failure of pain treatments include social support, country and culture of origin, illness uncertainty, and cognitive processing speed. Increasing stable social support in one's care is helpful with conditions such as complex regional pain syndrome, where a minor injury causes severe sensory, vascular, cardiopulmonary, and motor changes. Especially in cases in children, good management of complex regional pain syndrome involves social support systems such as parents.[24] Regarding one's cultural origin, one study found that "subjects from Iran and Iraq reported significantly higher levels of sensory and affective pain as well as pain intensity than the Swedish subjects did," while "the Swedish group had larger confidence than the Iran group and especially the Iraq group in physiotherapy as a treatment and as a method of improvement."[25] Kvarén and Johansson[25] found that Iraqi patients preferred rest-based treatments, contrary to a more activity-based approach promoted in the United States as noted in Hensley and Courtney[23] and other studies.

Illness uncertainty and cognitive processing speed are not necessarily causes of chronic illness or pain, but they are associated with outcomes of treatment. The theory of illness uncertainty "proposes that patients with chronic illness may have difficulty adjusting to the illness if there is significant diagnostic or prognostic uncertainty."[26] These patients are unhappy if their doctor does not believe their accounts of symptoms or provides unsatisfactory treatment. Regarding cognitive processing speed, a study of persons with persistent pain in the Netherlands found that a decreased speed was correlated to a higher pain intensity and lower level of physical function.[27]

Additional insight can be gained into the neurophysiological and psychosocial facets of persistent pain by ongoing research. In a study of patients in outpatient physical therapy, Hankin et al[28] found that psychosocial characteristics are often affected by a person's persistent pain. The Multidimensional Pain Inventory is useful to identify pain behavior profiles such as the Adaptive Coper, Interpersonally Distressed, and Dysfunctional profile so that the clinician can refer the patient to a multidisciplinary treatment program.[28]

Another study found that persons with acute and persistent pain, whether being treated by physical therapists alone or by interprofessional programs, were more attentive toward sensory-related words describing pain (eg, "flickering," "throbbing," or "pinching") but not to "affective, disability, or threat words" (eg, "vicious," "cruel," "terrifying," "harmful," "suffering," and "sick").[29] These words are used in standardized psychosocial pain assessment tools such as the McGill Pain Questionnaire. How a patient describes the pain yields insight into the causes behind it, for more sensitive and individualized treatment.

Secondary and Tertiary Prevention

At least 3 types of prevention in health promotion and health care exist: **primary** (keeping risk factors from developing for a disease or condition), **secondary** (preventing a disease or condition from developing in a population at risk), and **tertiary** (minimizing the secondary effects of a disease or condition). While many health care professionals are lobbying for more allocation of funds to primary prevention, since this is arguably the most efficient use of resources, the move of the system to match this is slow.

Parra et al[30] argue that the promotion of physical activity, whether as a primary, secondary, or tertiary prevention activity, should be a priority for all physical therapists. **Physical inactivity is a key factor in the development of NCDs; one-third of people worldwide do not engage in enough activity.** This lack of activity kills as many people as tobacco use does, and decreases life expectancy by approximately 1 year. According to the article, priorities for therapists include[30]:

- Staying informed about current NCDs related to physical inactivity
- Showing "commitment to prevention and health promotion" as well as rehabilitation
- Developing interprofessional education (IPE) and practice for change in population health

Multiple opportunities for secondary and tertiary prevention exist for physical therapists. Sedentary people living in assisted living facilities (ALFs) benefit from an individualized wellness program offered "as little as twice weekly for 9 [out] of 12 months" in terms of lower fall risk and preserved functional independence.[31] Examination of a person's social and physical environment, along with individualized physical activity prescription, can prevent most type 2 diabetes, a major public health concern that also needs local and national policy revision.[32] In aging persons with cerebral palsy, secondary impairments amenable to therapy include fatigue and persistent pain, which are associated with decreased long-term function.[33] Finally, in a skilled nursing facility, giving maximal opportunities for choice to residents increases their lifespan and quality of life.[34] These are just a few examples of how physical therapists can prevent outright disease symptoms or secondary effects of a chronic illness.

Several studies examined ways to prevent acute conditions from progressing to persistent pain and disability. One model combined elements of structure (health care system, health service organizations, physical therapists, patients, facilitators, and barriers), process (interactions between the preceding components and perceived patient needs), and outcomes (costs and quality influencing value).[35] Another study found that targeting psychosocial risk factors via a Progressive Goal Attainment Program helped to increase return to work from 50% to 75% of patients with whiplash in physical therapy.[36]

McCallum[37] took a broader view of medically underserved adults in Ohio. These adults generally cannot access physical therapy, and when they can, the services are not as comprehensive to refer to other professionals for chronic conditions.[37] Therapists and other professionals can work together around financial, systemic, and human limitations for more emphasis on prevention with underserved populations. Researchers involved need to allow for differences between the lab environment and the real world; the latter cannot offer as rigid a structure and as high an intensity of interventions, such as wellness programs. To improve function in actual populations, therapists and researchers should focus on improving each patient's self-efficacy.[38]

Comorbid Medical and Psychosocial Issues

This section differentiates pain and illness, and shows that their comorbidities overlap significantly. Type 2 diabetes mellitus is one example with many comorbidities, including obesity, hypertension, cognitive impairments, depression, secondary neuropathy, and amputation. Self-management of this or other chronic diseases involves "depression, pain, fatigue, lack of support from family, and poor communication with physicians," of which the physical therapist needs to be aware to counsel the patient.[34] One such resource is the Chronic Disease Self-Management Program at www.selfmanagementresource.com.

One common psychosocial issue in chronic conditions is underinsurance or uninsurance. This is particularly evident in different senior living settings, as assisted living facilities (ALFs) tend to accept residents with higher incomes because Medicare and Medigap insurances rarely cover expenses associated with better care in an ALF.[34] Thus, physical therapists should capitalize on health promotion for this population, especially earlier in the disease when money, as well as health can be saved.[39] Clinicians can also educate patients on alternative living situations, such as the Eden Alternative (with autonomy, a stimulating environment, and staff investment) and the Program of All-Inclusive Care for the Elderly.[34]

Persistent pain has many co-occurring psychosocial issues with medical issues that relate to their frequent activity restrictions. For various reasons, including medication seeking, persons with persistent pain may fake facial expressions of pain, which providers can be trained by immediate corrective feedback to discriminate from real pain behaviors.[40] Another issue is avoidance of beneficial activity due to fear of reinjury, inflexibility to change, or the abnormal thought pattern of catastrophizing (projecting the worst-case scenario all the time). Studies, such as Pincus et al,[41] examined behavioral interventions for such fear-related avoidance.

In older adults, persistent pain is often treated by NSAIDs because the aging body cannot handle opioids without serious adverse effects. However, NSAIDs also have risks "including renal failure, stroke, hypertension, heart failure exacerbations, and gastrointestinal complications."[41] The American Geriatrics Society therefore recommended changes to pain management in older adults, including a **broader range of pain management options**, especially for osteoarthritis and rheumatoid arthritis. These treatments "include **physical therapy**, topical nonsteroidals, capsaicin, topical lidocaine, intra-articular therapies, and judicious use of narcotics" in addition to safer COX-2 selective NSAIDs.[42]

Disparities in Pain Management

Few things a doctor does are more important than relieving pain ... pain is soul destroying. No patient should have to endure intense pain unnecessarily. The quality of mercy is essential to the practice of medicine; here, of all places, it should not be strained.

—Marcia Angell[43]

Despite efforts to provide quality pain management, certain populations are at risk for poorer management due to race and sex. In a study of persons with cLBP, medical students recommended antidepressants more often for White patients than for African American patients, but only half were aware of this race-related bias. About 30% of students also showed bias on the basis of sex when recommending physical therapy or opioid medications.[44] Another study of veterans using the Veterans Affairs hospital system in 2008 found that female veterans had greater odds of multiple pain diagnoses (including fibromyalgia, irritable bowel disease, and osteoarthritis), of an emergency-room visit related to pain, and of referral to a physical therapist, but they had lower odds of receiving long-term opioid therapy.[45] Finally, a study based in Sweden found that males were much more likely than females to be referred to physical therapy and medical imaging for pain management, regardless of age, ethnicity, work status, and mood symptoms.[46]

One shift in persistent pain management is physical activity as prescription, based on each patient's psychosocial factors, symptoms, and current level of physical activity. Persons with persistent pain have more activity-related obstacles; they also "found it difficult to distinguish between physical activity on prescription and physiotherapy and perceived that also the physicians could not tell the difference."[47] After a motivational interviewing session, a physician will write a prescription for physical activity to include at least one type of recommended physical activity with dosage and frequency, which is different from an order for a physical therapist evaluation and treatment. Therapists have an opportunity to educate physicians and patients on the differences between this and skilled therapy.

Another changing area in pain management is the opioid addiction epidemic. Recent efforts in the United States are aimed at reversing the trend of narcotic overprescription for pain, due to serious secondary effects including overdose-related deaths. Besides the comorbidities of persistent pain that include "increased psychological distress, decreased mobility, obesity, decreased physical function, social isolation, financial loss, and development of chronic disability," opioid dependence adds "lowered pain thresholds, increased social stress ... depression, anxiety ... and decreased coping skills."[48] Thus, management of persistent pain must also include management of opioid dependence. This can occur by **patient engagement** (by CBT or mindfulness-based stress reduction), **emphasis on physical function** and higher mobility levels (by physical therapy and yoga, among others), **weight management** (by diet and exercise), **management of substance use, and careful medication prescription** for symptom management. In addition to NSAIDs, selective serotonin reuptake inhibitors (both commonly prescribed for persistent pain) also have side effects and interactions. In particular, substance use disorders (SUDs) occur in 20% of veterans who are prescribed opioids and increase the odds of requiring mental health services; only one-third of these veterans with an SUD were treated for the disorder.[49]

Multidisciplinary intervention, discussed later, has moderate evidence support for addressing opioid dependence in persons with persistent pain. One study successfully decreased high-dose opioid therapy in veterans from 27.7% to 24.7% over 4 years, while increasing referrals to conservative interventions, such as physical therapy and chiropractic care.[50] Dorflinger et al[50] accomplished this by the Stepped Care Model of Pain Management, described by Rosenberger and Kerns.[51]

Illness Interactions

Both the patient's physiology and psychology are influenced by the interaction between chronic disease and persistent pain. Physiologically, pain is a barrier to physical activity in diseases such as osteoporosis, while the osteoporosis itself can be either a facilitator or a barrier, by inspiring efforts to increase bone density or by making the patient fearful of movement due to fracture risk.[52] Psychologically, persistent pain often coexists with mental health issues, or symptoms of disorders in persons without diagnosed mental illness. In a study of a 12-week pain management program centered around physical therapy, about 70% of subjects were diagnosed with a psychological, personality, or mental retardation disorder, which, thankfully, did not hinder recovery from pain.[53]

Depression, anxiety, and posttraumatic stress disorder (PTSD) are 3 interactions of persistent pain and psychological conditions. Depressive symptoms often weaken positive outcomes of physical therapy for musculoskeletal pain; women are more likely than men to have severe depression.[54] Also, pain severity after spinal cord injury is correlated to depressive symptoms and poor sleep.[55]

Regarding anxiety, a sample of 45 patients with cLBP, participating in an interprofessional pain management program, experienced near-panic levels of anxiety during the physical examination. "Catastrophic cognitions, behavioral displays of pain and somatic sensations measured during examination uniquely predicted anxiety experienced."[56] While this study did not indicate that anxiety negatively affected outcomes, the clinician should be aware of symptoms that the patient may be having to decrease anxiety levels proactively.

While little is known about the prevalence of comorbid pain and PTSD, the 2 are also associated with heart disease, metabolic syndrome, and various mental illnesses.[57] One study of veterans with comorbid PTSD and persistent pain examined a team-based approach that included medication monitoring, diagnostic imaging, physical therapy, and behavioral activation to "increase activation and engagement so patients will have more rewarding experiences in their lives."[58] Specific successful strategies included "motivational interviewing, relaxation strategies, time-based pacing, anger management, assertiveness training, activity scheduling, behavioral experiments, grounding, adaptive coping statements, and education."[58]

Focus Issue: HIV-AIDS

HIV and its chronic manifestation, AIDS, have been noted in the United States since the 1960s. Physical therapy literature is expanding related to secondary impairments of the syndrome, including persistent pain and chronic mental health disorders. As persons with HIV-AIDS frequently seek out medical treatment, physical therapy, and complementary and alternative medicine (CAM) for pain and other functional limitations, the clinician is responsible for their evidence-based treatment, as well as support of ongoing research.

Persons with HIV have a prevalence as high as 67% of distal sensory polyneuropathy (DSP), which affects sensation and movement quality of hands and feet, especially in cases of chronic

HIV infection. DSP impairs physical health and lower limb function, and thus overall mental and physical health.[59] Aerobic exercise, or yoga if the person so desires, is recommended to combat the associated impairments and disability.[60] Aerobic exercise is safe and effective for DSP alone or in conjunction with strength training.[61] With a high adherence rate of approximately 84%, such a combination also targets cardiopulmonary impairments and health-related quality of life in persons with HIV-AIDS.[62,63]

Persistent pain is another complication of HIV-AIDS. Physical therapy, with or without CBT, is a low-cost option for such pain management.[64] Clinicians should screen and refer for comorbid SUDs and psychiatric conditions in persons with HIV infection, since opioids are a risky treatment option:

> In the current HIV treatment area, an estimated 39% to 85% of individuals with HIV infection also suffer from chronic pain compared with only 20% to 30% of the general population. Chronic pain in HIV-infected individuals is often musculoskeletal, although pain associated with peripheral neuropathy is observed in approximately 20% to 30% of individuals.[65]

Disability risk increases with combined pain and risk factors such as anxiety, depression, catastrophizing, fear avoidance, poor health, high initial pain severity, and increased patient age.

Orthopedic complications of HIV include connective tissue changes, skeletal myopathies, and lipodystrophy syndrome, which lessen the ability to move skeletal muscle. Lipodystrophy, due to the HIV treatment of highly active antiretroviral therapy, increases cardiovascular risk and redistributes fat from the face and extremities to the trunk.[66] Such fat redistribution, combined with obesity, affects limits of stability, strategy and amplitude of sway, fast gait speed, 360-degree turn speed, single-limb support time, and time required to initiate gait. Clinicians can use the chair rise test and 360-degree turn test to assess balance and gait in patients with HIV infection, with or without obesity.[67] Finally, connective tissue changes occurring in older adults with HIV include shoulder adhesive capsulitis, carpal tunnel syndrome, osteoporosis, and osteonecrosis.[68]

At both ends of the lifespan, HIV causes unique complications. Unpredictable, episodic disability is common,[69] and HIV itself is in the top 5 causes of early death in Africa, the Caribbean, and North America; this is exacerbated by a lack of geriatric health care providers in countries that need them the most.[70,71] Although infants with HIV live longer now, they are approximately 7.6 months behind typically developing counterparts in cognition and 9.6 months behind in motor milestones.[72] As persons with HIV age into their 50s and beyond, they may seem better at coping with disability, but they still have health needs related to adequate viral testing; depression; SUDs; and periodic neurological manifestations of opportunistic infections, such as Chagas disease (caused by a parasite).[73,74]

Researchers and educators are realigning priorities to stay abreast of the changing demographics and sequelae of HIV-AIDS. Six key research priorities identified include:

> (1) [D]isability and episodic disability, (2) concurrent health conditions living with HIV ... (3) HIV and the brain ... (4) labour [sic] force and income support issues, (5) access to and effect of rehabilitation, and (6) development and evaluation of outcome measurement tools.[75]

Likewise, health care providers in all geographic areas need to have a comprehensive knowledge base. Recommended curricular areas include types of and risk factors for HIV, impacts of infection on psychosocial and socioeconomic systems, dosage and side effects of antiretroviral therapy, primary and secondary effects on body systems, physical therapists' roles in disability management, and therapeutic attitudes and behaviors.[76]

Specific Clinical Approaches to Improve Physical Therapy Outcomes

If your body is screaming in pain, whether the pain is muscular contractions, anxiety, depression, asthma or arthritis, a first step in releasing the pain may be making the connection between your body pain and the cause. Beliefs are physical. A thought held long enough and repeated enough becomes a belief. The belief then becomes biology.

—Marilyn Van Derbur[77]

In DPT programs, students are taught to treat what they find in terms of movement system impairments, body tissues affected, and specific structures. Treatments include therapeutic (corrective) exercises, neuromuscular reeducation, gait training, functional training, and physical agents (ultrasound, electrical stimulation, and others). In management of chronic disease and persistent pain, clinicians need to add psychosocial expertise. This section discusses interprofessional pain clinics, PNE, specific screening tools, outcome measures, and other evidence-based topics.

Interdisciplinary/Multidisciplinary Pain Clinics

The interprofessional pain clinic has strong research support. One case study even goes back to the 1800s, describing Clara Schumann's chronic right upper extremity pain that interrupted her piano performances for over a year. Her interprofessional treatment included medication, physical therapy, activity modification, and psychotherapy, resulting in complete recovery from the overuse injury.[78] Generally, an interprofessional program includes "individual and group-based therapies such as physical and occupational therapy, pain psychology, relaxation therapy, counseling, vocational rehabilitation services, nursing education, and aerobic conditioning" in one facility.[79]

Multiple systematic reviews and meta-analyses describe the benefits of pain clinics:

- **Programs that include physical therapy, when not limited by managed-care policies, improve depressive symptoms, pain, physical and mental function, coping styles, and disability, while saving at least $1 billion over 19 years in the United States.**[80]
- In a Cochrane review, **interventions including "education, exercise, psychological therapies, occupational interventions, and review of pain medicines"** are slightly superior to physical therapy alone for short-term pain and intermediate-term disability levels, and **are equivalent in results to surgery for non-specific cLBP.**[81]
- Medicine is shifting toward a biopsychosocial perspective on pain. A review of several systematic reviews and meta-analyses shows that **multidisciplinary pain management programs have better results, and potentially lower costs, than traditional medical care.**[82]
- In management of medically complex patients, primary care providers usually place chronic pain control in the top 3 issues to address 77% of the time, otherwise referring to a specialist. They **benefit from training and access to multidisciplinary pain clinics.**[83]

Lower-level evidence also supports the widespread use of pain clinics:

- A month-long worker's compensation rehabilitation program, at 32 hours per week, focused on individual and group interventions, including "pain psychology, physical therapy, occupational therapy, relaxation training/biofeedback, aerobic conditioning, pool therapy, vocational counseling, patient education and medical management."[84] An impressive 91% of participants were released to return to work (with 80% allowed full-time work). Although only half of these actually returned to work, participants had significantly reduced depression, pain intensity, and catastrophizing.

- An integrated pain management program in a nursing home included staff education (regarding assessment, medication, and non-pharmacological strategies for pain control) and activities (including gardening and physical therapist-guided therapeutic exercise). It improved staff knowledge and attitudes as well as resident pain control and mood symptoms.[85]
- A 3-week interprofessional outpatient program included physical and occupational therapy, CBT, and medication management services. Interventions included moderate-intensity physical activity, time management, energy conservation, activity modification, weaning off opioids, and management of psychosocial symptoms. This program improved endurance (measured by 6-Minute Walk Test distance) and occupational performance.[86]
- In a hospital outpatient setting, nurses led a team offering physical therapy and CBT for an 8-week program that improved pain severity, pain interference, and health-related quality of life.[87]
- In Kosovo, a resource-poor country, 10 weekly sessions of CBT were combined with biofeedback and group physical therapy. Clients had undergone torture in a war. One-third of PTSD cases were resolved, and employment status and disability improved. The intervention, however, had inconsistent effects on mental health symptoms, anger, and hatred.[88]
- A program including physical and occupational therapy, education, and clinical psychology used goal attainment scaling to improve mobility, pain quality and intensity, disability, general health, and impairment in over three-quarters of patients, even at 6-month follow-up. Goal attainment scaling was defined as an individually-relevant and patient-directed process of defining goals for therapy in terms of true therapist-patient collaboration.[89]

IPE in the classroom and clinic can increase economic feasibility of interprofessional pain clinics. Ethical considerations include cost and coverage, the research support for condition-specific treatments, and variation of population and service characteristics.[90] A set of four 4-hour IPE sessions for health care providers (including physical therapists, anesthetists, nurses, and palliative care professionals) improved patients' pain levels in one pilot study from 2.9 to 2.0 on the 0 to 10 rating scale, but with less confidence on the clinician's part for persistent vs acute pain.[91] A caveat is that the minimal clinically important difference on the 0 to 10 rating scale is 2 points, less than the 0.9-point average decrease noted.

Other considerations for pain clinics include stakeholders' expectations, engagement of each patient's social support, and the patient's goals. Broad, holistic teams for services in "psychology, self-management, physiotherapy, peripheral nervous system stimulation, complementary therapies and comprehensive pain-management programmes [sic]" focus more on rehabilitation of function and quality of life than on a cure.[92] Social support is vital, especially in cases of pediatric chronic pain. Adherence to program components for parents and these children ranges from 46.7% to 100%, especially if the child was active before the onset of pain; the best adherence rates were found for physical therapy in one study.[93]

Finally, the provider must consider diversity of patient goals: return to professional life, a career in athletics, or a more comfortable position in a wheelchair. Frustrating, persistent pain complicates these goals. Pain's long-term effects on the brain, influenced by a number of unsuccessful coping strategies, cause major lifestyle changes, which can cause mental health issues, including depression and suicide attempts.[94]

While pain clinics may have inconsistent staffing and practice standards depending on the geographic area,[95] they are nevertheless one of the best tools in the physical therapist's set of strategies for persistent pain management. A guidance article on primary care models for osteoarthritis highlights a physical therapist's optimal position to provide evidence-based care. Such care includes weight management, aerobic exercise, strength training, electrical stimulation (transcutaneous electrical nerve stimulation [TENS]), joint braces, manual therapy, local thermotherapy, and assistive device prescription. As physical therapists already have such knowledge, their involvement may be more efficient than adding the same material to medical school curricula. All of these non-pharmacological treatments are first-line recommendations by the National Institutes of Health and Clinical Excellence guidelines.[96]

Pain Neuroscience Education

PNE is a relatively new approach to pain; it focuses on biological and psychological perspectives to explain pain. This helps many patients who have tried other approaches for their persistent pain, since pain changes their thought processes and is influenced by incomplete knowledge of how pain works. Physical therapists have traditionally been taught the gate control theory (ie, that non-noxious sensory stimuli can block the transmission of noxious stimuli to prevent pain) and, since the 1990s, the concept of the pain neuromatrix (ie, the neurological structures and pathways responsible for pain). However, their knowledge of PNE has thus far not consistently translated into better outcomes.[97] Research into the areas of "true behavior change, including health care utilization and cost, along with societal effects" for today's environment is in its infancy.

The book *Explain Pain* by Butler and Moseley is an excellent resource for patients and clinicians. Additionally, Lotze and Moseley provide basic concepts for persistent pain rehabilitation. Such rehabilitation involves "reconceptualizing the pain itself ... careful and intentional observation of the person in pain, and the strategic and constant communication of safety."[98] It contrasts with treatment (exercise to relieve pain) and management (therapy to maintain function, despite pain). The following is a list of **5 key points to remember**:

1. Pain is a stimulus to protect the body against real or perceived danger.
2. Neuroplasticity can go wrong with central sensitization, where the brain treats more and more areas as "injured" and needing the protection of a pain response and physical inactivity.
3. Graded motor imagery can retrain the brain for desensitization.
4. Since pain does not equal injury, rehabilitation does not need to avoid pain, given appropriate education.
5. Drive rehabilitation with the clinician-patient relationship.

Several studies showed positive effects of PNE on persistent pain. Given somewhat limited evidence on graded motor imagery and mirror therapy, either intervention might be better than standard physical therapy alone for persistent pain.[99] A case report, of a 31-year-old patient with brachioradialis myofascial pain syndrome, complicated by centrally generated pain due to self-diagnosis via the internet, found that 3 sessions of PNE followed by 3 more sessions of dry needling and therapeutic exercise reversed the syndrome.[100] Continued research and research translation are needed for susceptible populations, including older adults and young adults. While geriatric clients often state an intention to cope with long-lasting back pain, younger clients exhibit the maladaptive behavior of catastrophizing.[101] This is one facet addressed specifically by PNE, since catastrophic thought patterns change the brain's function.

Screening Tools and Outcome Measures

Besides common functional tests and patient self-report measures, this section examines other tools supported by research for assessing the movement system in people with chronic disease and persistent pain. For assessing pain intensity, the Numeric Pain Rating Scale is often complicated by medication seeking behaviors because patients report their pain as a constant 10/10 despite a lack of objective pain behaviors. One option is the Wong-Baker Faces scale, which is sensitive to change and also has good reliability and validity for measuring musculoskeletal pain intensity.[102] To discern chronic stress-related causes of pain and illness, the clinician can use the Social Readjustment Rating Scale,[34] available at www.acc.com/aboutacc/newsroom/pressreleases/upload/srrs.pdf.

Fear of pain and pain pressure sensitivity are 2 other aspects. The original Fear of Pain Questionnaire is appropriate for adults, with modified forms for children and adolescents or a parent proxy report. Fear is important to measure because it causes secondary impairments of "disuse, disability, and depression."[103] Pressure pain thresholds are a clinical measure of pain sensitization, one aspect of persistent pain in conditions such as knee osteoarthritis. Unfortunately, this method is currently unreliable due to high measurement error.[104]

Two valid measures relevant to persistent pain, as well as chronic disease and fatigue, are the Global Physiotherapy Examination (GPE-52) and the 26-item Activity Pacing Questionnaire. The GPE-52 examines posture, respiration, movement, muscle, and skin integrity. However, the GPE-52 may be better as a screen than as a measure of change over time because minimal clinically important differences exist only for the total score and movement and respiration subsections.[105] The 26-item Activity Pacing Questionnaire, a more valid and concise form than the original Activity Pacing Questionnaire, has good measurement properties for persons with persistent pain and fatigue. It clearly describes activity pacing, a recommended "coping strategy to manage long-term conditions."[106,107]

Physiological tests of muscle strength and exercise capacity are also appropriate, but must be used judiciously for valid results in persons with persistent pain. The single-limb stance test measures fall risk, but does not correlate with low back pain or that pain's associated weakness of the gluteus medius muscle.[108] For aerobic capacity, maximal (fatiguing) exercise tests can be used only if the patient is able to safely perform the test and give maximal effort. Due to fear of pain and other adverse effects, as well as low pain tolerance, many patients with persistent pain or chronic disease (especially persons over 65 years old) may limit effort due to fear of pain and other adverse effects.[109]

Other Opportunities for Physical Therapist Practice to Promote Health and Wellness

Many niches exist for physical therapists to fill, both in the United States and internationally, to promote health and wellness in their clients with persistent pain and illness. These include exercise adherence initiatives, judicious use of modalities, integration of CBT principles, and coordination with CAM methods. One study found that few pain-management programs for the geriatric population exist in Germany. Barriers to such programs include clients' fear of movement (kinesiophobia); polypharmacy, which complicates safe exercise prescription; and medical complexity of the clients. Resources for program development include group-based techniques for motivation and choosing activities relevant to the older client's interests and activities of daily living.[110]

Exercise Adherence

Regardless of the program, activity, modality, or other intervention, managing the patient's chronic condition requires adhering to interventions and recommendations, especially exercise during and after a physical therapy episode of care. A study of exercise maintenance in persons with rheumatoid arthritis found that self-efficacy, being able "to exercise in different settings," and developing an internal locus of control (where the person believes he or she can control outside events, rather than be controlled by them) helped patients adapt to barriers to good exercise habits.[111] Older women with osteoporosis saw physical activity as preserving their health. Patients may have more difficulty adhering if they have low levels of responsibility or challenging socioeconomic or cultural backgrounds.[112]

Another study found complex influences on a patient's exercise adherence[113]:

- When pain or disability appear, patients consider their illness-related beliefs, personal prognosis, exercise outcome expectations, and whether adherence will help them.
- When pain or disability decrease, patients weigh their perceived barriers (time, fatigue, memory, side effects, other medical conditions), social support (family and social interaction), physical environment (fun aspects of exercise), and self-efficacy.
- When pain or disability disappear for a while, patients consider their odds of relapse and what level of adherence will achieve a good cost-benefit ratio for them.

While a Cochrane review found that there are major knowledge gaps as to what fosters exercise adherence, each patient's preference for a given mode of exercise (eg, a gym membership vs a home resistance band program), along with therapist-provided options, may play a role. Safety comes first when choosing the mode of exercise. **Options to increase long-term adherence include activity logs, exercise contracts, referral to local group programs, and referral to chronic disease self-management programs.**[114]

Types of Activity

Aerobic exercise is well-supported by the literature for most, if not all, mental and physical chronic conditions, including pain. In an animal model of widespread hypersensitivity to pain, researchers found that as little as 3 weeks of moderate-intensity aerobic exercise improved sensitivity and promoted the production of a nerve growth factor in specific muscle types.[115] For persons with cLBP, a 12-week program of high-intensity aerobic exercise improved pain, disability, and psychological burden more than 12 weeks of pain modalities alone.[116]

Activity pacing, or energy conservation, is also important in chronic conditions, since these conditions and associated medications often cause fatigue. Physical therapists view activity pacing as a management tool and not a cure for the pain; they also combine activity pacing instruction with approaches including reflective listening.[117] In an underdiagnosed condition, such as chronic fatigue syndrome (or myalgic encephalomyelitis), aerobic and cognitive deficits respond to graded exercise (progressing from anaerobic to aerobic), instruction in pacing and self-management of physical activity, and use of the rating of perceived exertion scale (0 to 10, with 10 being the exertion following a person's hardest possible activity). Therapists can refer patients for diagnosis of potential chronic fatigue syndrome by noting the following[118]:

- Duration of symptoms of at least 6 months; postexertion fatigue lasts more than 24 hours
- Autonomic symptoms, including orthostatic hypotension, pallor, irritable bowels, and dyspnea on exertion
- Neuroendocrine symptoms, including inability to tolerate temperature extremes or stress flare-ups
- Immune symptoms, including new substance sensitivities and lymphadenopathy

Self-management of chronic disease incorporates activity pacing and other techniques. Richardson et al[119] developed START, the Self-Management and Task-Oriented Approach to Rehabilitation Training, for persons who have had a stroke but remain motivated and cognitively intact while receiving home physical therapy. This tool emphasizes functional training and early supported discharge to home for appropriate patients.[119] Bennell et al developed a pain coping skills training intervention for persons with knee osteoarthritis in Australia; the study protocol included education about the disease, progression of pain coping skills, and use of an activity log. The results of this study were not available at the time of this text's writing.[120]

Examining chronic disease and persistent pain self-management more broadly, Richardson et al[121] noted that many components of programs for osteoarthritis, chronic obstructive pulmonary disease, and chronic pain were based on social cognitive and self-efficacy theories. While physical therapists focused on "disease-specific education, fatigue, posture, and pain management," occupational therapists focused on "joint protection, fatigue, and stress management."[121] Cederbom et al[122] looked at cognitively intact, community-dwelling older women who had persistent pain but no immediate social support, thus increasing risk for physical dependence. In the feasibility study, adding a behavioral component to undefined "standard physical therapy" did not change outcomes.[122]

Modalities

While active interventions are a more natural choice from the physical therapist's perspective, modalities of electricity, heat, cold, and other substances or forces (eg, menthol gel on painful knees with osteoarthritis) can be adjuncts in the plan of care for a person with chronic illness, persistent pain, and associated movement dysfunctions.[123,124] This section covers evidence related to sensory discrimination and tactile acuity training, affective images, TENS, and noxipoint therapy.

Alone, sensory discrimination training has uncertain efficacy for reversing the sensory changes caused by cLBP. This technique focuses on "tactile discrimination and sensorimotor retraining [for] recognition of the location and the type of stimuli by the patient,"[125] since the brain's reorganization in persistent pain distorts how the person perceives normal sensation. Similarly, tactile acuity training is only as effective as a placebo for correcting inaccurate sensory representation of the person's body parts affected by pain; another person also needs to apply this training.[126]

In the geriatric population, patients often try to bear their pain without asking for pain medication. A pilot study about affective (emotionally-connected) images used 6 weeks of pictures eliciting certain emotions as an adjunct to physical therapy. This intervention took place in China, where Tse et al[127] selected culturally relevant images to promote reminiscence to the patient's childhood. Results indicated a positive effect on health-related quality of life and pain ratings.[127]

TENS is used by health care providers to relieve acute and persistent pain. It is generally effective and safe if precautions are followed, including avoiding use in persons with pacemakers, impaired sensation, markedly impaired cognition, and poor skin integrity. Fuentes et al[128] found that adding a strong therapeutic alliance increases the single-session effects of TENS; such an alliance includes the provider asking questions about the patient's lifestyle and symptoms, actively listening, using a collaborative vocal tone, and expressing empathy. In older clients, clinicians might consider starting with a conventional setting of TENS for comfort before trying another setting.[129]

A novel form of electrotherapy, called *noxipoint therapy*, incorporates brief immobilization of the body part with precise surface electrical stimulation to the point of soreness or dull pain. One study comparing noxipoint therapy to conventional TENS, with both groups also receiving standard physical therapy, found that the novel technique dramatically improved persistent pain. Additional benefits included joint flexibility and quality of life; however, little research exists examining this new technique.[130]

Cognitive Behavioral Therapy

CBT and its subtypes are discussed in Chapter 4. However, this section highlights studies on treatment of chronic conditions and persistent pain. Training home health physical therapists in CBT interventions resulted in good patient recall of the techniques taught.[131] These included "pain theory, goal setting, general relaxation, deep breathing, visual imagery, pleasant activity scheduling, activity pacing, progressive muscle relaxation, sleep tips, [and] dealing with pain flare-ups."[132]

In another study, adults who had had spinal laminectomy, who were first screened for kinesiophobia, were referred to a CBT-based intervention 6 weeks after surgery. The physical therapy significantly improved pain, disability, health, and physical performance at a 3-month follow-up.[133] According to a US-based survey, physical therapists have a large opportunity for learning CBT because the desire and need are present, but incorporation into clinical practice is currently limited.[134]

Other Psychosocial Considerations

Many populations in the United States do not know or follow best practices for management of their persistent pain; health care providers need to educate the public and promote universal access to safe exercise spaces. For example, a survey of Hispanic persons with persistent non-cancer pain living in southwestern states found that people with low income typically used prescription pain medication at 4 times the rate of using exercise.[135]

Regardless of treatment setting, mindful movement helps to better link the mind and body, which can attenuate chronic conditions. Norwegian psychomotor physical therapy is one such technique that "claims that posture, respiration, and muscle tension are closely related to emotional states."[136] This technique incorporates massage and corrective therapeutic exercises as well, after a comprehensive patient examination (see Chapters 5 through 7 for more information).

Spirituality and religious convictions are an important aspect of a person's makeup and personality. Although most physical therapists recognize the impact that a patient's belief system can have on chronic illness and pain coping, many hesitate to address faith issues due to insufficient time, training, and comfort. Therapist students, however, believed that faith could positively influence hope and coping skills according to one study.[137] Therapists enhanced rapport by knowing the patient's faith background and sharing their own; experience in faith-related discussions begot comfort in bringing up topics.

Physical therapists can also explore the mind-body connection by coordinating with activity therapists, whose scope includes dance, drama, games, and hobbies. For persistent, psychological-based pain in adolescents, parental buy-in to therapy may be difficult. One study of a multidisciplinary intervention found that "physiotherapy ... relaxation training, hypnotherapy, systemic and cognitive-behavioural approaches," added to drama and movement therapy, helped 2 teenage girls undergoing pain treatment.[138] Besides reducing pain, the treatment improved verbal expression, function, and emotional health. However, one caution is that pain relief may not necessarily improve mood symptoms, which may be challenging when working with the unpleasant patient![139]

Complementary and Alternative Medicine

Reimbursement is a constant concern in the clinician's mind. Certain treatments, whether considered traditional or alternative, need advocacy to gain appropriate payment. A survey of New York, New Jersey, and Connecticut in 2000 found that although most insurance systems paid for chiropractic services, less than one-half paid for acupuncture, and very few for isolated massage: "other CAM services receive negligible coverage."[140] Ongoing surveys and reform of health insurance systems are needed.

Ventegodt et al[141] found strong support for several classes of CAM treatments including chemicals, physical therapy (without joint manipulation), psychotherapy, spiritual therapy, mind-body medicine, holistic medicine, and shamanism with hallucinogenic drugs. Principles of CAM include salutogenesis (healing the whole person); similarity (trying to access the patient's subconscious for getting at the root of persistent symptoms); Hering's law of cure (following the opposite order for healing vs injury); resources (replenishing whatever resources were depleted); and the use of minimal force to avoid harming the patient.

Yoga and hypnotherapy are 2 CAM techniques gaining more literature support; their success may be affected by the patient's temperament. For example, the author's grandfather could not be hypnotized with repeated attempts, influenced by his mental strength and desire to remain in control of his mind. Sulenes et al[142] note that yoga is under-prescribed for patients with chronic illness, persistent pain, and mental health disorders, but that occupational therapists and physician's assistants are the professionals most likely to ask patients to try yoga. Hypnotherapy is also rarely used, but has promising results for persistent pain, with studies requiring larger sample sizes and long-term follow-up.[143,144]

Summary

Long-lasting mental and physical illness and pain affect many people, especially those seeking physical therapy for movement system limitations. While this chapter could not cover the entire breadth of resources, data, and opportunities available, it gives the reader a framework to explore areas of interest. Treatment options for the clinician span the psychosocial as well as the physical, with the bottom line being the importance of a listening ear. Not only can skilled physical therapy significantly impact patients' lives regarding pain and associated functional limitation, but it can achieve these results in a cost-effective way.

Key Points

- Have a repository of cost-effectiveness studies to show insurance representatives, as needed, to gain reimbursement for physical therapy.
- Prevention is primary (risk factor-targeted), secondary (disease prevention), or tertiary (secondary effect prevention). Physical inactivity is a prevalent risk factor for all lifestyle-related diseases.
- The American Geriatrics Society includes physical therapy among pharmacologic pain management recommendations for persons over age 65.
- Manage persistent pain with patient engagement, emphasis on function and mobility, weight management, substance use training, and careful medication prescription.
- Interdisciplinary pain clinics, including physical therapy, are shown to save money while improving outcomes on mental health symptoms, pain, coping, and disability, superior to surgical outcomes.
- PNE emphasizes pain's role as a protective stimulus, with potential for maladaptive neuroplasticity that responds to graded motor imagery and education.
- Exercise adherence options include activity logs, written contracts, referral to local group programs, and referral to chronic disease self-management programs.

Review Questions

- According to Hensley and Courtney,[23] what are 3 proposed mechanisms for how chronic (persistent) pain develops?
  - What are the risk factors associated with each?
  - How might your knowledge from this chapter influence how you would address your next patient who presents with persistent pain? If desired, discuss with classmates or colleagues.
- Describe several options you read about in this chapter for addressing chronic pain.
  - Which ones are you less familiar with?
  - How will you evaluate the emerging literature to determine whether you should try a given option for a patient with persistent pain?
  - In your own words, restate the key principles of PNE so that you can educate your patients who have persistent pain.
- What are some opportunities in your geographic area for health promotion and primary or secondary prevention? What are some factors (economic, demographic, etc) that influence how feasible these opportunities may be to implement?

- Recall a patient, real or hypothetical, with several comorbid chronic conditions.
  - What are your considerations for the patient interview and examination?
  - What are the effects of the patient's medication and substance use on the plan of care?
  - In what ways did the patient's comorbidities influence each other's courses?
  - How might you adapt your treatment approach if you saw this patient again?

Case Studies: First Impressions

As you review the following case studies, you may want to consider these questions for thought or discussion:

- What standardized tests and measures (including psychiatric, for example, a depression screen) would you select for this patient? Why?
- Based on available data, what short- and long-term goals would you write for your plan of care? Consider using the acronyms SMART (specific, measurable, attainable, realistic, and timely) or ABCDE (actor, behavior, conditions, degree, and expected time frame) to guide your goal writing.
- What elements (procedures, psychosocial aspects, communication aspects, etc) would you make sure to include or omit in your plan of care for this patient? Why?
- What are your anticipated needs, if any, for consultation and referral for this patient?
- How will you transition this patient toward lasting health behavior change following discharge (eg, recommending a YMCA membership trial)?

Case 1

A 43-year-old female was referred to outpatient physical therapy by the instructor of her group fitness class because of increased difficulty in completing stretching exercises. Her goal is to participate in classes as fully as possible while working as a home health aide.

- Social history: she lives in a single-story house with her husband while her child is attending college out of state. She is frequently called on to complete double shifts if another home health aide cancels; her clients' houses frequently have stairs to enter.
- Medical/psychiatric history: postpartum depression (18 years ago, after the birth of her only child), ankylosing spondylitis (diagnosed 10 years ago), overweight, and prehypertension
- Impairments, activity limitations, and participation restrictions found on initial interview and examination
  - Mild shortness of breath after walking 100 feet into the building from the parking lot
  - Reports increased stiffness in her low back, hips, and knees
  - Unable to get on and off the floor in fitness class without holding onto a chair
  - Standing tolerance limited to 15 minutes by pain and shortness of breath

Case 2

A 27-year-old female self-referred to outpatient physical therapy for an exacerbation of juvenile rheumatoid arthritis (diagnosed 10 years ago). Her goal is to reduce pain and inflammation with physical therapy and medication adjustment in order to return to playing recreational volleyball.

- Social history: she lives with her parents in a 2-story house; her parents both work full time on first shift. The patient works third shift as a cardiopulmonary intensive care unit nurse.
- Medical/psychiatric history: social anxiety disorder, asthma, and insomnia

- Impairments, activity limitations, and participation restrictions found on initial interview and examination
  - Pain in hands and knee joints rated 8/10, especially with weightbearing activity
  - Unable to lift backpack to shoulders immediately after exiting her car
  - Increased time required to ascend stairs to her bedroom, with shortness of breath noted
  - Impaired proprioception as determined by the "foam and dome" test, which examines visual and proprioceptive input into balance

Case 3

A 61-year-old male was hospitalized 2 days ago for exacerbation of congestive heart failure, but he is stable enough for you to evaluate him in the hospital today. His goals are to return home with his wife and take walks in their neighborhood.

- Social history: he lives with his wife in a 2-story house; his wife works part time as a church secretary and purchased an alert pendant for him when he was diagnosed with Alzheimer's disease.
- Medical/psychiatric history: hypertension, obesity, type 2 diabetes, lower extremity lymphedema, mid-stage Alzheimer's disease (diagnosed 6 months ago), and suspected mild depression (though he has so far refused a psychiatrist evaluation)
- Impairments, activity limitations, and participation restrictions found on initial interview and examination
  - Unable to name or state the use for any of his home medications
  - Requires 50% assistance to complete supine to sitting or sitting to standing with a 2-wheeled walker (previously he was ambulatory without a device, but required initiation cues for activities of daily living)
  - Disoriented to place and time
  - Repeatedly asks where his father is (deceased for 4 years)
  - Standing tolerance 15 seconds, limited by the patient impulsively sitting
  - Blood pressure rises from 132/86 supine to 158/92 standing

Case 4

An 80-year-old male was referred to home health physical therapy by his physician at the request of his daughter, who noticed increased losses of balance during her visit to his ALF 3 weeks prior. His goal is to walk more quickly around the facility to visit friends.

- Social history: he lives with his wife in an ALF that has inclined hallways between apartment clusters; his wife is independent from a motorized wheelchair level and is non-ambulatory. His daughter is unable to assist with home exercises due to rheumatoid arthritis and lack of readily available transportation.
- Medical/psychiatric history: Parkinson's disease (diagnosed 15 years ago), recurrent aspiration pneumonia, history of falls, medication-induced schizophrenia, cLBP, and orthostatic hypotension
- Impairments, activity limitations, and participation restrictions found on initial interview and examination
  - Requires multiple attempts and increased time to stand up from sitting in a standard (18 inches seat height) chair with armrests
  - Decreased ankle strategy noted with posterior sway in static standing
  - Forward functional reach 3 inches indicating a high fall risk

- Gait speed 0.2 m/second indicating physical dependence and a high fall risk (community gait speed norm is 1.0 m/second)
- Stooped posture with lack of lumbar lordosis
- Shuffling gait with a 4-wheeled walker
- Decreased carryover of safety precautions
- Unable to walk more than 50 feet due to light-headedness and low back pain

Case 5

A 93-year-old female was referred to physical therapy by the nurse practitioner in a skilled nursing facility due to a decline in ability to transfer and an increase in reports of persistent pain for the past month. Her goals are to perform transfers independently for toileting and participate in facility meals in the dining room.

- Social history: she has lived in the long-term care facility for 8 years. Her family members come to visit several times per week.
- Medical/psychiatric history: dementia with visual/tactile hallucinations (insects), obesity, abdominal surgery (30 years prior), stage 3 chronic kidney disease, congestive heart failure, multijoint osteoarthritis, bilateral knee replacements (20 years prior), major depressive disorder, and generalized anxiety disorder
- Impairments, activity limitations, and participation restrictions found on initial interview and examination
    - Abdominal pain rated 10/10 at evaluation, but requires cues to request pain medication
    - Sitting tolerance 5 minutes at edge of bed with upper extremity support
    - Shortness of breath in supine, mildly increased in sitting
    - Gross lower extremity muscle strength 3-/5 (moves full range against gravity but is unable to hold the test position for 5 seconds)
    - Gross upper extremity muscle strength 4-/5 (withstands light to moderate resistance)
    - Requires 90% assistance to stand from the bed using a 2-wheeled walker
    - Unable to pivot transfer at time of evaluation (previously able to transfer herself and walk short distances with the 2-wheeled walker and contact-guard assistance)

References

1. Fry S. Mind out. *The Old Friary: Stephen Fry.* http://www.stephenfry.com/2011/09/mind-out/. Published September 21, 2011. Accessed May 3, 2018.
2. Dean E, Greig A, Murphy S, et al. Raising the priority of lifestyle-related noncommunicable diseases in physical therapy curricula. *Phys Ther.* 2016;96(7):940-948.
3. Bürge E, Monnin D, Berchtold A, Allet L. Cost-effectiveness of physical therapy only and of physical therapy added to usual care for various health conditions: systematic review. *Phys Ther.* 2016;96(6):774-786.
4. Siemonsma PC, Stuive I, Roorda LD, et al. Cognitive treatment of illness perceptions in patients with chronic low back pain: A randomized controlled trial. *Phys Ther.* 2013;93(4):435-448.
5. Bertozzi L, Gardenghi I, Turoni F, et al. Effect of therapeutic exercise on pain and disability in the management of chronic nonspecific neck pain: systematic review and meta-analysis of randomized trials. *Phys Ther.* 2013;93(8):1026-1036.
6. Freburger JK, Carey TS, Holmes GM. Effectiveness of physical therapy for the management of chronic spine disorders: a propensity score approach. *Phys Ther.* 2006;86(3):381-394.
7. Cottrell E, Roddy E, Foster NE. The attitudes, beliefs and behaviours of GPs regarding exercise for chronic knee pain: a systematic review. *BMC Family Practice.* 2010;11:4.
8. Fouche C, Kenealy T, Mace J, Shaw J. Practitioner perspectives from seven health professional groups on core competencies in the context of chronic care. *J Interprof Care.* 2014;28(6):534-540.

9. Laliberté M, Feldman DE. Patient prioritization preferences among physiotherapy entry-level students: the importance of chronic pain. *Physiother Can.* 2013;65(4):353-357.
10. Ali N, Thomson D. A comparison of the knowledge of chronic pain and its management between final year physiotherapy and medical students. *Eur J Pain.* 2009;13(1):38-50.
11. Hirsh AT, Hollingshead NA, Bair MJ, Matthias MS, Kroenke K. Preferences, experience, and attitudes in the management of chronic pain and depression. *Clin J Pain.* 2014;30(9):766-774.
12. Adillón C, Lozano E, Salvat I. Comparison of pain neurophysiology knowledge among health sciences students: a cross-sectional study. *BMC Res Notes.* 2015;8:592.
13. Merikangas KR, Ames M, Cui L, et al. The impact of comorbidity of mental and physical conditions on role disability in the US adult household population. *Arch Gen Psychiatry.* 2007;64(10):1180-1188.
14. Scott-Dempster C, Toye F, Truman J, Barker K. Physiotherapists' experiences of activity pacing with people with chronic musculoskeletal pain: an interpretative phenomenological analysis. *Physiother Theory Pract.* 2014;30(5):319-328.
15. Miller EW, Ross K, Grant S, Musenbrock D. Geriatric referral patterns for physical therapy: a descriptive analysis. *J Geriatr Phys Ther.* 2005;28(1):20.
16. Campos AA, Amaria K, Campbell F, McGrath PA. Clinical impact and evidence base for physiotherapy in treating childhood chronic pain. *Physiother Can.* 2011;63(1):21-33.
17. Breivik H, Collett B, Ventafridda V, Cohen R, Gallacher D. Survey of chronic pain in Europe: prevalence, impact on daily life, and treatment. *Eur J Pain.* 2006;10(4):287-333.
18. Deyo RA, Dworkin SF, Amtmann D, et al. Report of the NIH Task Force on Research Standards for Chronic Low Back Pain. *Phys Ther.* 2015;95(2):e1-e18.
19. Lundy-Ekman L. *Neuroscience: Fundamentals for Rehabilitation.* 3rd ed. St. Louis, MO: Saunders; 2007.
20. Fowler EG, Kolobe THA, Damiano DL, et al; Section on Pediatrics Research Summit Participants; Section on Pediatrics Research Committee Task Force. Promotion of physical fitness and prevention of secondary conditions for children with cerebral palsy: Section on Pediatrics Research Summit Proceedings. *Phys Ther.* 2007;87(11):1495-1510.
21. Young G, Tachdjian R, Baumann K, Panopoulos G. Comprehensive management of chronic pain in haemophilia. *Haemophilia.* 2014;20(2):e113-e120.
22. Denlinger CS, Ligibel JA, Are M, et al.; National Comprehensive Cancer Network. Survivorship: pain version 1.2014: clinical practice guidelines in oncology. *J Natl Compr Canc Netw.* 2014;12(4):488-500.
23. Hensley CP, Courtney CA. Management of a patient with chronic low back pain and multiple conditions using a pain mechanisms-based classification approach. *J Orthop Sports Phys Ther.* 2014;44(6):403-414.
24. Dickson SK. Including parents in the treatment of pediatric complex regional pain syndrome. *Pediatr Nurs.* 2017;43(1):16-21.
25. Kvarén C, Johansson E. Pain experience and expectations of physiotherapy from a cultural perspective. *Adv Physiotherapy.* 2004;6(1):2-10.
26. Fishbain DA, Bruns D, Disorbio JM, Lewis JE, Gao J. Exploration of the illness uncertainty concept in acute and chronic pain patients vs community patients. *Pain Med.* 2010;11(5):658-669.
27. Pulles WLJA, Oosterman JM. The role of neuropsychological performance in the relationship between chronic pain and functional physical impairment. *Pain Med.* 2011;12(12):1769-1776.
28. Hankin HA, Spencer T, Kegerreis S, Worrell T, Rice JM. Analysis of pain behavior profiles and functional disability in outpatient physical therapy clinics. *J Orthop Sports Phys Ther.* 2001;31(2):90-95.
29. Haggman SP, Sharpe LA, Nicholas MK, Refshauge KM. Attentional biases toward sensory pain words in acute and chronic pain patients. *J Pain.* 2010;11(11):1136-1145.
30. Parra DC, Bradford ECH, Clark BR, Racette SB, Deusinger SS. Population and community-based promotion of physical activity: a priority for physical therapy. *Phys Ther.* 2017;97(2):159-160.
31. Hatch J, Lusardi MM. Impact of participation in a wellness program on functional status and falls among aging adults in an assisted living setting. *J Geriatr Phys Ther.* 2010;33(2):71-77.
32. Deshpande AD, Dodson EA, Gorman I, Brownson RC. Physical activity and diabetes: opportunities for prevention through policy. *Phys Ther.* 2008;88(11):1425-1435.
33. Benner JL, Hilberink SR, Veenis T, et al. Long-term deterioration of perceived health and functioning in adults with cerebral palsy. *Arch Phys Med Rehabil.* 2017;98(11):2196-2205.
34. Haber D. *Health Promotion and Aging: Practical Applications for Health Professionals.* 4th ed. New York, NY: Springer; 2007.
35. Lentz TA, Harman JS, Marlow NM, George SZ. Application of a Value Model for the Prevention and Management of Chronic Musculoskeletal Pain by physical therapists. *Phys Ther.* 2017;97(3):354-364.
36. Sullivan MJL, Adams H, Rhodenizer T, Stanish WD. A psychosocial risk factor-targeted intervention for the prevention of chronic pain and disability following whiplash injury. *Phys Ther.* 2006;86(1):8-18.
37. McCallum CA. Access to physical therapy services among medically underserved adults: a mixed-method study. *Phys Ther.* 2010;90(5):735-747.
38. Dossa A, Capitman JA. Implementation challenges and functional outcome predictors for elder community-based disability prevention programs. *J Geriatr Phys Ther.* 2012;35(4):191-199.

39. Cohn R. Economic realities associated with diabetes care: opportunities to expand delivery of physical therapist services to a vulnerable population. *Phys Ther.* 2008;88(11):1417-1424.
40. Hill ML, Craig KD. Detecting deception in facial expressions of pain: accuracy and training. *Clin J Pain.* 2004;20(6):415-422.
41. Pincus T, Anwar S, McCracken L, et al.; OBI Trial Management Team. Testing the credibility, feasibility and acceptability of an optimised behavioural intervention (OBI) for avoidant chronic low back pain patients: protocol for a randomised feasibility study. *Trials.* 2013;14:172.
42. Katz JD, Shah T. Persistent pain in the older adult: what should we do now in light of the 2009 American Geriatrics Society Clinical Practice Guideline? *Pol Arch Med Wewn.* 2009;119(12):795-800.
43. Angell M. The quality of mercy. *N Engl J Med.* 1982;306(2):98-99. DOI: 10.1056/NEJM198201143060210.
44. Hollingshead NA, Matthias MS, Bair MJ, Hirsh AT. Impact of race and sex on pain management by medical trainees: a mixed methods pilot study of decision making and awareness of influence. *Pain Med.* 2015;16(2):280-290.
45. Weimer MB, Macey TA, Nicolaidis C, et al. Sex differences in the medical care of VA patients with chronic noncancer pain. *Pain Med.* 2013;14(12):1839-1847.
46. Stålnacke BM, Haukenes I, Lehti A, et al. Is there a gender bias in recommendations for further rehabilitation in primary care of patients with chronic pain after an interprofessional pain team assessment? *J Rehabil Med.* 2015;47(4):365-371.
47. Joelsson M, Bernhardsson S, Larsson MEH. Patients with chronic pain may need extra support when prescribed physical activity in primary care: a qualitative study. *Scand J Prim Health Care.* 2017;35(1):64-74.
48. Liebschutz J, Beers D, Lange A. Managing chronic pain in patients with opioid dependence. *Curr Treat Options Psychiatry.* 2014;1(2):204-223.
49. Morasco BJ, Duckart JP, Dobscha SK. Adherence to clinical guidelines for opioid therapy for chronic pain in patients with substance use disorder. *J Gen Intern Med.* 2011;26(9):965-961.
50. Dorflinger L, Moore B, Goulet J, et al. A partnered approach to opioid management, guideline concordant care and the stepped care model of pain management. *J Gen Intern Med.* 2014;29(suppl 4):S870-S876.
51. Rosenberger PH, Kerns R. Implementation of the VA Stepped Care Model of Pain Management. *Ann Behav Med.* 2012;43(suppl 1):S265.
52. Baert V, Gorus E, Mets T, Bautmans I. Motivators and barriers for physical activity in older adults with osteoporosis. *J Geriatr Phys Ther.* 2015;38(3):105-114.
53. Workman EA, Hubbard JR, Felker BL. Comorbid psychiatric disorders and predictors of pain management program success in patients with chronic pain. *Prim Care Companion J Clin Psychiatry.* 2002;4(4):137-140.
54. George SZ, Coronado RA, Beneciuk JM, et al. Depressive symptoms, anatomical region, and clinical outcomes for patients seeking outpatient physical therapy for musculoskeletal pain. *Phys Ther.* 2011;91(3):358-372.
55. Avluk OC, Gurcay E, Gurcay AG, et al. Effects of chronic pain on function, depression, and sleep among patients with traumatic spinal cord injury. *Ann Saudi Med.* 2014;34(3):211-216.
56. Hadjistavropoulos HD, LaChapelle DL. Extent and nature of anxiety experienced during physical examination of chronic low back pain. *Behav Res Ther.* 2000;38(1):13-29.
57. Orr RM, Bennett N. Posttraumatic stress disorder management: a role for physiotherapists and physical training instructors. *J Mil Vet Health.* 2012;20(3):37-43.
58. Plagge JM, Lu MW, Lovejoy TI, Karl AI, Dobscha SK. Treatment of comorbid pain and PTSD in returning veterans: a collaborative approach utilizing behavioral activation. *Pain Med.* 2013;14(8):1164-1172.
59. Galantino MLA, Kietrys DM, Parrott JS, et al. Quality of life and self-reported lower extremity function in adults with HIV-related distal sensory polyneuropathy. *Phys Ther.* 2014;94(10):1455-1466.
60. Cade WT, Peralta I, Keyser RE. Aerobic exercise dysfunction in human immunodeficiency virus: a potential link to physical disability. *Phys Ther.* 2004;84(7):655-664.
61. Maharaj SS, Yakasi AM. Does a rehabilitation program of aerobic and progressive resisted exercises influence HIV-induced distal neuropathic pain? *Am J Phys Med Rehabil.* 2018;97(5):364-369. doi: 10.1097/PHM.0000000000000866.
62. Gomes-Neto M, Ogalha C, Andrade AM, Brites C. A systematic review of effects of concurrent strength and endurance training on the health-related quality of life and cardiopulmonary status in patients with HIV/AIDS. *BioMed Res Int.* 2013;ArticleID 319524. doi: 10.1155/2013/319524.
63. Cade WT, Reeds DN, Mondy KE, et al. Yoga lifestyle intervention reduces blood pressure in HIV-infected adults with cardiovascular disease risk factors. *HIV Med.* 2010;11(6):379-388.
64. Mgbemena O, Westfall AO, Ritchie CS, et al. Preliminary outcomes of a pilot physical therapy program for HIV-infected patients with chronic pain. *AIDS Care.* 2015;27(3):244-247.
65. Merlin JS. Chronic pain in patients with HIV infection: what clinicians need to know. *Top Antivir Med.* 2015;23(3):120-124.
66. Segatto AFM, Junior IFF, dos Santos VR, et al. Lipodystrophy in HIV/AIDS patients with different levels of physical activity while on antiretroviral therapy. *Revista da Sociedade Brasil de Med Trop.* 2011;44(4):420-424.
67. Bauer LO, Wu Z, Wolfson LI. An obese body mass increases the adverse effects of HIV/AIDS on balance and gait. *Phys Ther.* 2011;91(7):1063-1071.

68. Lima ALLM, Zumiotti AV, Camanho GL, et al. Osteoarticular complications related to HIV infection and highly active antiretroviral therapy. *Br J Infect Dis.* 2007;11(4):426-429.
69. O'Brien KK, Bayoumi AM, Strike C, Young NL, Davis AM. Exploring disability from the perspective of adults living with HIV/AIDS: development of a conceptual framework. *Health Qual Life Outcomes.* 2008;6:76.
70. Dean E, Al-Obaidi S, De Andrade AD, et al. The first Physical Therapy Summit on Global Health: implications and recommendations for the 21st century. *Physiother Theor Pract.* 2011;27(8):531-547.
71. Mills EJ, Bärnighausen T, Negin J. HIV and aging—preparing for the challenges ahead. *N Engl J Med.* 2012;366(14):1270-1273.
72. Baillieu N, Potterton J. The extent of delay of language, motor, and cognitive development in HIV-positive infants. *J Neurol Phys Ther.* 2008;32(3):118-121.
73. Sankar A, Nevedal A, Neufeld S, Berry R, Luborsky M. What do we know about older adults and HIV? A review of social and behavioral literature. *AIDS Care.* 2011;23(10):1187-1207.
74. DiazGranados CA, Saavedra-Trujillo CH, Mantilla M, et al. Chagasic encephalitis in HIV patients: common presentation of an evolving epidemiological and clinical association. *Lancet Infect Dis.* 2009;9(5):324-330.
75. O'Brien K, Wilkins A, Zack E, Soloman P. Scoping the field: identifying key research priorities in HIV and rehabilitation. *AIDS Behav.* 2010;14(2):448-458.
76. Myezwa H, Stewart A, Solomon P, Becker P. Topics on HIV/AIDS for inclusion in a physical therapy curriculum: consensus through a modified Delphi technique. *J Phys Ther Educ.* 2012;26(2):50-62.
77. Van Derbur M. *Miss America by Day: Lessons Learned From Ultimate Betrayals and Unconditional Love.* Denver, CO: Oak Hill Ridge Press; 2003.
78. Altenmüller E, Kopiez R. Suffering for her art: the chronic pain syndrome of pianist Clara Wieck-Schumann. *Front Neurol Neurosci.* 2010;27:101-118.
79. Stanos S. Focused review of interprofessional pain rehabilitation programs for chronic pain management. *Curr Pain Headache Rep.* 2012;16(2):147-152.
80. Robbins H, Gatchel RJ, Noe C, et al. A prospective one-year outcome study of interdisciplinary chronic pain management: compromising its efficacy by managed care policies. *Anesth Analg.* 2003;97(1):156-162.
81. Saragiotto BT, de Almeida MO, Yamato TP, Maher CG. Multidisciplinary biopsychosocial rehabilitation for nonspecific chronic low back pain. *Phys Ther.* 2016;96(6):759-763.
82. Noe C, Williams CF. The benefits of interdisciplinary pain management: studies show equal or better clinical outcomes compared with standard treatments, low risk, and reduced costs of care. *J Fam Pract.* 2012;61(suppl 4):S5-S16.
83. Mitchinson AR, Kerr EA, Krein SL. Management of chronic noncancer pain by VA primary care providers: when is pain control a priority? *Am J Manag Care.* 2008;14(2):77-84.
84. Gagnon CM, Stanos SP, van der Ende G, Rader LR, Harden N. Treatment outcomes for workers compensation patients in a US-based interprofessional pain management program. *Pain Pract.* 2013;13(4):282-288.
85. Tse MMY, Ho SSK. Pain management for older persons living in nursing homes: a pilot study. *Pain Manag Nurs.* 2013:14(2):e10-e21.
86. Kurklinsky S, Perez RB, Lacayo ER, Sletten CD. The efficacy of interprofessional rehabilitation for improving function in people with chronic pain. *Pain Res Treat.* 2016. doi: 10.1155/2016/7217684.
87. Dysvik E, Kvaløy JT, Furnes B. Evaluating physical functioning as part of a Cognitive Behavioural Therapy approach in treatment of people suffering from chronic pain. *J Clin Nurs.* 2013;22(5-6):806-816.
88. Wang SJ, Bytyçi A, Izeti S, et al. A novel bio-psycho-social approach for rehabilitation of traumatized victims of torture and war in the post-conflict context: a pilot randomized controlled trial in Kosovo. *Confl Health.* 2017;10:34.
89. Fisher K, Hardie RJ. Goal attainment scaling in evaluating a multidisciplinary pain management programme. *Clin Rehabil.* 2002;16(8):871-877.
90. Gilligan CJ, Borsook D. The promise of effective pain treatment outcomes: rallying academic centers to lead the charge. *Pain Med.* 2015;16(8):1457-1466.
91. Carr ECJ, Brockbank K, Barrett RF. Improving pain management through interprofessional education: evaluation of a pilot project. *Learning in Health and Social Care.* 2003;2(1):6-17.
92. Mills S, Torrance N, Smith BH. Identification and management of chronic pain in primary care: a review. *Curr Psychiatry Rep.* 2015;18(2):22.
93. Simons LE, Logan DE, Chastain L, Cerullo M. Engagement in multidisciplinary interventions for pediatric chronic pain: parental expectations, barriers, and child outcomes. *Clin J Pain.* 2010;26(4):291-299.
94. Parhar HS. A hospital-based multidisciplinary approach to chronic pain management. *University of British Columbia Medical Journal.* 2013;5(1):30-32.
95. Peng P, Stinson JN, Choiniere M, et al. Role of health care professionals in multidisciplinary pain treatment facilities in Canada. *Pain Res Manag.* 2008;13(6):484-488.
96. Dziedzic KS, Hill JC, Porcheret M, Croft PR. New models for primary care are needed for osteoarthritis. *Phys Ther.* 2009;89(12):1371-1378.
97. Louw A, Puentedura EJ, Zimney K, Schmidt S. Know pain, know gain? A perspective on pain neuroscience education in physical therapy. *J Orthop Sports Phys Ther.* 2016;46(3):131-134.

98. Lotze M, Moseley GL. Theoretical considerations for chronic pain rehabilitation. *Phys Ther.* 2015;95(9):1316-1320.
99. Bowering KJ, O'Connell NE, Tabor A, et al. The effects of graded motor imagery and its components on chronic pain: a systematic review and meta-analysis. *J Pain.* 2013;14(1):3-13.
100. Anandkumar S. Effect of pain neuroscience education and dry needling on chronic elbow pain as a result of cyberchondria: a case report. *Physiother Theory Pract.* 2015;31(3):207-213.
101. Cabak A, Dąbrowska-Zimakowska A, Truszczyńska A, et al. Strategies for coping with chronic lower back pain in patients with long physiotherapy wait time. *Med Sci Monit.* 2015;21:3913-3920.
102. Dogan SK, Ay S, Evcik D, Kurtais Y, Öztuna DG. The utility of faces pain scale in a chronic musculoskeletal pain model. *Pain Med.* 2012;13(1):125-130.
103. Simons LE, Sieberg CB, Carpino E, Logan D, Berde C. The fear of pain questionnaire (FOPQ): assessment of pain-related fear among children and adolescents with chronic pain. *J Pain.* 2011;12(6):677-686.
104. Skou ST, Simonsen O, Rasmussen S. Examination of muscle strength and pressure pain thresholds in knee osteoarthritis: test-retest reliability and agreement. *J Geriatr Phys Ther.* 2015;38(3):141-147.
105. Kvåle A, Skouen JS, Ljunggren AE. Sensitivity to change and responsiveness of the Global Physiotherapy Examination (GPE-52) in patients with long-lasting musculoskeletal pain. *Phys Ther.* 2005;85(8):712-726.
106. Antcliff D, Campbell M, Woby S, Keeley P. Assessing the psychometric properties of an activity pacing questionnaire for chronic pain and fatigue. *Phys Ther.* 2015;95(9):1274-1286.
107. Antcliff D, Keeley P, Campbell M, Oldham J, Woby S. The development of an activity pacing questionnaire for chronic pain and/or fatigue: a Delphi technique. *Physiotherapy.* 2013;99(3):241-246.
108. Penney T, Ploughman M, Austin MW, Behm DG, Byrne JM. Determining the activation of gluteus medius and the validity of the single leg stance test in chronic, nonspecific low back pain. *Arch Phys Med Rehabil.* 2014;95(10):1969-1976.
109. Snell CR, Stevens SR, Davenport TE, Van Ness JM. Discriminative validity of metabolic and workload measurements for identifying people with chronic fatigue syndrome. *Phys Ther.* 2013;93(11):1484-1492.
110. Kuss K, Laekeman M. Aktivierende Physiotherapie bei chronischen Schmerzen älterer Patienten [in German]. *Schmerz.* 2015;29(4):402-410.
111. Swärdh E, Biguet G, Opava CH. Views on exercise maintenance: variations among patients with rheumatoid arthritis. *Phys Ther.* 2008;88(9):1049-1060.
112. Dohm IM, Ståhle A, Roaldsen KS. "You have to keep moving, be active": perceptions and experiences of habitual physical activity in older women with osteoporosis. *Phys Ther.* 2016;96(3):361-370.
113. Medina-Mirapeix F, Escolar-Reina P, Gascón-Cánovas JJ, Montilla-Herrador J, Collins SM. Personal characteristics influencing patients' adherence to home exercise during chronic pain: a qualitative study. *J Rehabil Med.* 2009;41(5):347-352.
114. Crandall S, Howlett S, Keysor JJ. Exercise adherence interventions for adults with chronic musculoskeletal pain. *Phys Ther.* 2013;93(1):17-21.
115. Sharma NK, Ryals JM, Gajewski BJ, Wright DE. Aerobic exercise alters analgesia and neurotrophin-3 synthesis in an animal model of chronic widespread pain. *Phys Ther.* 2010;90(5):714-725.
116. Chatzitheodorou D, Kabitsis C, Malliou P, Mougios V. A pilot study of the effects of high-intensity aerobic exercise versus passive interventions on pain, disability, psychological strain, and serum cortisol concentrations in people with chronic low back pain. *Phys Ther.* 2007;87(3):304-312.
117. Scott KM, Von Korff M, Alonso J, et al. Mental-physical co-morbidity and its relationship with disability: results from the World Mental Health Surveys. *Psychol Med.* 2009;39(1):33-43.
118. Davenport TE, Stevens SR, VanNess MJ, et al. Conceptual model for physical therapist management of chronic fatigue syndrome/myalgic encephalomyelitis. *Phys Ther.* 2010;90(4):602-614.
119. Richardson J, DePaul V, Officer A, et al. Development and evaluation of Self-Management and Task-Oriented Approach to Rehabilitation Training (START) in the home: case report. *Phys Ther.* 2015;95(6):934-943.
120. Bennell KL, Ahamed Y, Bryant C, et al. A physiotherapist-delivered integrated exercise and pain coping skills training intervention for individuals with knee osteoarthritis: a randomised controlled trial protocol. *BMC Musculoskelet Disord.* 2012;13:129.
121. Richardson J, Loyola-Sanchez A, Sinclair S, et al. Self-management interventions for chronic disease: a systematic scoping review. *Clin Rehabil.* 2014;28(11):1067-1077.
122. Cederbom S, Rydwik E, Söderlund A, et al. A behavioral medicine intervention for older women living alone with chronic pain--a feasibility study. *Clin Interv Aging.* 2014;9:1383-1397.
123. Topp R, Brosky JA, Pieschel D. The effect of either topical menthol or a placebo on functioning and knee pain among patients with knee OA. *J Geriatr Phys Ther.* 2013;36(2):92-99.
124. Wu PI, Meleger A, Witkower A, Mondale T, Borg-Stein J. Nonpharmacologic options for treating acute and chronic pain. *PM R.* 2015;7(suppl 11):S278-S294.
125. Kälin S, Rausch-Osthoff AK, Bauer CM. What is the effect of sensory discrimination training on chronic low back pain? A systematic review. *BMC Musculoskel Disord.* 2016;11:143.
126. Ryan C, Harland N, Drew BT, Martin D. Tactile acuity training for patients with chronic low back pain: a pilot randomised controlled trial. *BMC Musculoskel Disord.* 2014;15:59.

127. Tse MMY, Pun SPY, Benzie IFF. Affective images: relieving chronic pain and enhancing quality of life for older persons. *CyberPsychol Behav.* 2005;8(6):571-580.
128. Fuentes J, Armijo-Olivo S, Funabashi M, et al. Enhanced therapeutic alliance modulates pain intensity and muscle pain sensitivity in patients with chronic low back pain: an experimental controlled study. *Phys Ther.* 2014;94(4):477-489.
129. Barr JO, Weissenbuehler SA, Cleary CK. Effectiveness and comfort of transcutaneous electrical nerve stimulation for older persons with chronic pain. *J Geriatr Phys Ther.* 2004;27(3):93.
130. Koo CC, Lin RS, Wang TG, et al. Novel noxipoint therapy versus conventional physical therapy for chronic neck and shoulder pain: multicentre randomised controlled trials. *Sci Rep.* 2015;5:16342.
131. Beissner K, Bach E, Murtaugh C, et al. Implementing a cognitive-behavioral pain self-management program in home health care, part 1: program adaptation. *J Geriatr Phys Ther.* 2013;36(3):123-129.
132. Bach E, Beissner K, Murtaugh C, Trachtenberg M, Reid MC. Implementing a cognitive-behavioral pain self-management program in home health care, part 2: feasibility and acceptability cohort study. *J Geriatr Phys Ther.* 2013;36(3):130-137.
133. Archer KR, Devin CJ, Vanston SW, et al. Cognitive-behavioral based physical therapy for patients with chronic pain undergoing lumbar spine surgery: a randomized controlled trial. *J Pain.* 2016;17(1):76-89.
134. Beissner K, Henderson CR Jr, Papaleontiou M, et al. Physical therapists' use of cognitive-behavioral therapy for older adults with chronic pain: a nationwide survey. *Phys Ther.* 2009;89:456-469.
135. Turner BJ, Rodriguez N, Valerio MA, et al. Less exercise and more drugs: how a low income population manages chronic pain. *Arch Phys Med Rehabil.* 2017;98(11):2111-2117.
136. Dragesund T, Råheim M. Norwegian psychomotor physiotherapy and patients with chronic pain: patients' perspective on body awareness. *Physiother Theory Pract.* 2008;24(4):243-254.
137. Sargeant DM, Newsham KR. Physical therapist students' perceptions of spirituality and religion in patient care. *J Phys Ther Educ.* 2012;26(2):63-72.
138. Christie D, Hood D, Griffin A. Thinking, feeling, and moving: drama and movement therapy as an adjunct to a multidisciplinary rehabilitation approach for chronic pain in two adolescent girls. *Clin Child Psychol Psychiatry.* 2006;11(4):569-577.
139. Sator-Katzenschlager SM, Schiesser AW, Kozek-Langenecker SA, et al. Does pain relief improve pain behavior and mood in chronic pain patients? *Anesth Analg.* 2003;97(3):791-797.
140. Cleary-Guida MB, Okvat HA, Oz MC, Ting W. A regional survey of health insurance coverage for complementary and alternative medicine: current status and future ramifications. *J Altern Complement Med.* 2001;7(3):269-273.
141. Ventegodt S, Andersen NJ, Kandel I, Merrick J. Effect, side effects and adverse effects of non-pharmaceutical medicine. A review. *Int J Disabil Hum Dev.* 2009;8(3):227-235.
142. Sulenes K, Freitas J, Justice L, et al. Underuse of yoga as a referral resource by health professions students. *J Altern Complement Med.* 2015;21(1):53-59.
143. Jensen M, Patterson DR. Hypnotic treatment of chronic pain. *J Behav Med.* 2006;29(1):95-125.
144. Elkins G, Jensen MP, Patterson DR. Hypnotherapy for the management of chronic pain. *Int J Clin Exp Hypn.* 2007;55(3):275-287.

Caregiving, Domestic Violence, Abuse, and Neglect

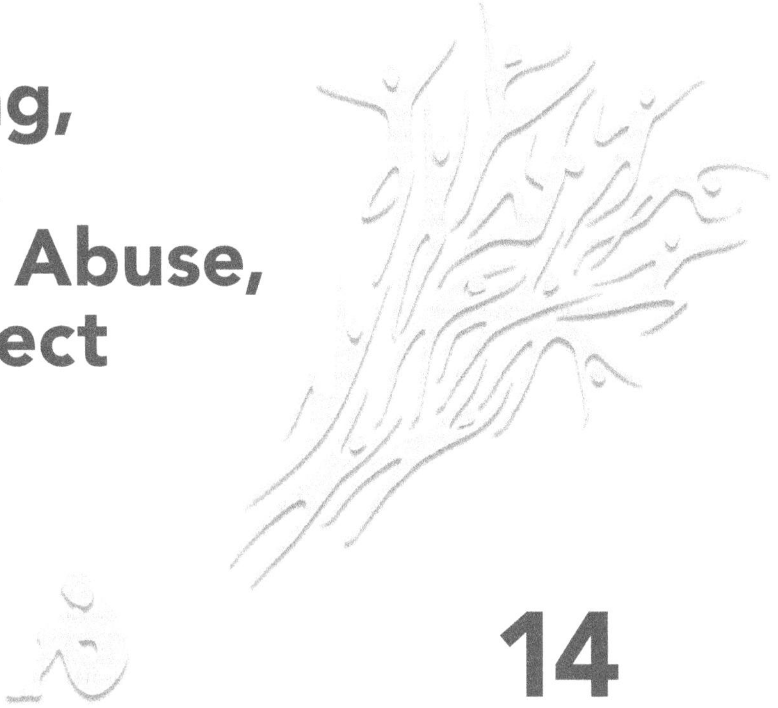

14

Outline

- Family Caregiving for Persons With Disabilities
- Family Systems
- Scope and Classification of Domestic Violence
- Risk Factors
- Secondary Medical and Psychosocial Issues
- Specific Clinical Approaches to Improve Physical Therapy Outcomes
  - Direct Approaches by the Clinician
  - Indirect Approaches: Referral by the Clinician for Counseling
- Summary
- Key Points
- Review Questions
- Case Studies: First Impressions

Learning Objectives

- Differentiate between types and manifestations of domestic violence based on patient characteristics in the clinical setting
- Craft patient interview questions that sensitively determine whether someone may be undergoing domestic violence or abuse, and know where to refer for help
- Articulate adaptations to interventions to address comorbidities and functional limitations/participation restrictions related to domestic violence

Johnson H.
Psychosocial Elements of Physical Therapy: The Connection of Body to Mind (pp 237-249).

If we are to fight discrimination and injustice against women we must start from the home, for if a woman cannot be safe in her own house, then she cannot be expected to feel safe anywhere.

—Aysha Taryam[1]

Domestic violence, also called *domestic abuse* or *intimate partner violence* (IPV), is a widespread worldwide problem. Its direct and indirect consequences on the victim are widespread, and it is likely clinicians will encounter many patients with a history of IPV. This chapter seeks to improve background knowledge, awareness, attitudes,[2] intervention, and readiness for referral of providers encountering persons who have been abused in any way, including neglect and exploitation (both prevalent in the aging population). As with many psychosocial issues, the key is to be a sensitive, compassionate, and active listener.

Family Caregiving for Persons With Disabilities

When patients are discharged home from an acute or subacute rehabilitation setting, they may need part- or full-time help due to physical or cognitive deficits. Additionally, many persons with preexisting conditions, such as intellectual or developmental disability (IDD) or acquired disability, require caregivers for safety. Family members fill many of these roles, and it is critical to involve them in a patient's rehabilitation for carryover, as well as acknowledge their presence as "an emerging public health issue involving complex and fluctuating roles" across the lifespan.[3] An online fact sheet describes characteristics of family caregivers in the United States.[4] Because of chronic and acute stress associated with caregiving, family caregivers can benefit from community resources for care coordination and mental health, with research beginning to develop frameworks to better target the areas of greatest need.[5-7]

In families with children with congenital or acquired disability, caregiving can be physically and emotionally demanding. One study compared a hospital-based exercise program to a community-based one to evaluate family cohesiveness and the quality of life of children with burns who required day hospitalization. The community-based program had better results; it is important to give parents enough information to help them make an informed choice about what is best for them and their children.[8] Also, health care providers should avoid unwarranted assumptions about resilience in family caregivers; surveys of parents and caregivers of children with autism reveal higher levels of resilience than might be expected.[9]

As persons with IDD age into adulthood, they still require caregivers, often siblings or mothers. Mediating factors for becoming such a caregiver include female gender, close relationship, geographic proximity, and having no other siblings without disabilities.[10] As families of adults with IDD adapt to their needs, worse outcomes tend to occur in cultural minorities or families of persons with behavioral disturbances.[11] To relieve stress and decrease the risk of adverse health outcomes, including hypertension, obesity, and arthritis,[12] families of persons with IDD seek respite by vacations, where basic needs can be met and good health can be appreciated; sometimes the person with IDD is placed in a skilled nursing facility (SNF) during this time.[13]

A final common scenario for family caregiving is for persons with mental illness. Over the last several decades, deinstitutionalization of persons with conditions such as schizophrenia has increased the burden of care on families and society because such persons are hospitalized frequently and lose productivity over a lifetime.[14] The concept of *burden of care* can include stigma by friends and coworkers, depression, and anxiety.[15,16] Recommended interventions include access to quality treatment options, advocacy, preventive services, and multicomponent treatments; in addition to decreasing the burden of care, such treatments can also delay SNF placement.[17]

Family Systems

Especially within the last several generations, the nuclear family system of parents and biological or adopted children has become less the norm and more of one system among many possible types of families; also, family systems research increasingly considers economic and political effects on family units.[18] While the moral and ethical debate around this cultural shift is far beyond the scope of this text, readers should have a basic awareness of family systems, which is applicable to all populations seen by physical therapists. Family psychologists, like physical therapists, use biopsychosocial theory in combination with family systems theory to improve patient-family relationships and health. Two overarching goals in family psychology are (1) patient empowerment to make good choices in response to illness, including domestic violence and mental illness; and (2) relationship strengthening to combat deterioration due to disability.[19] Part of psychology and other counseling includes attention to how closed or open the communication boundaries are between various family members; generally, more open boundaries prove more advantageous.[20]

As life expectancy increases and the average age of persons in the United States approaches the *silver tsunami* of 65 years old and beyond, older family members are involved in many ways. The "sandwich generation" consists of adults who care for both aging parents and younger children. Overall, members of different generations have long-term relationships with each other; grandparents can sometimes help their children and grandchildren socially, if not physically and cognitively.[21] However, if grandparents require help themselves or are more physically and socially isolated from their adult children, they are at a higher risk for depression.[22]

Another increasingly common phenomenon, due to demographic shifts, is the use of children, especially older girls, as "language brokers" for their immigrant parents. In this capacity, they are often called upon to translate oral and written language too complex for their cognitive and linguistic developmental level. If the children thus learn more about the new culture and language subtleties, they gain power over their parents, causing disequilibrium in the family system.[23] In a sample of undocumented immigrants from Mexico, Bacallao and Smokowski[24] found that other family system changes after immigration included decreased family time, increased child loneliness and risk-taking, and a more authoritarian style of parenting. Coping strategies included a continued focus on family and cultural heritage.[24]

Another challenge that the physical therapist should be aware of is the effects of divorce. In the United States, 50% of first marriages end in divorce, with remarriage frequent within 5 years. Communication boundaries in such blended families can range from closed to open, with individualized rules for interaction between selected family members. Cooperation between new spouses is essential to avoid conflicting loyalties and the false expectation that the new spouse will replace the old one.[25] One study found long-term effects of divorce on children at a 20-year follow-up. Depending on the emotional climate of the divorce and whether parents remarried, children indicated that a remarriage of either parent was highly stressful. "No single factor contributed more to children's self-reports of well-being after divorce than the continuing relationship with their parents."[26]

Finally, major acute or long-term trauma, including homelessness, can challenge family system integrity. About one-third of homeless individuals in the United States are family members. Because homelessness is a barrier to mental health care, a common cycle includes "poverty, mental illness, trauma, and substance abuse," which can disrupt families by children being placed in foster care while the recovering parent seeks residential treatment.[27] Variations of families in homeless populations include single or distant parents, different rates of employment and shelter placement, exposure of children to illness and violence, and the need for external resources to manage subsequent behavioral challenges. Trauma, however, can be turned to growth by a shift in focus to the family's strengths. In applying the posttraumatic growth model, individuals and families avoid posttraumatic stress disorder (PTSD) by viewing the trauma as an opportunity for positive transformation.[28,29]

Scope and Classification of Domestic Violence

Domestic violence spans all ages and clinical settings. Little is documented on it in rehabilitation literature, hence the need to draw from resources outside the profession for related knowledge and skills. Though most physical therapists can easily identify or suspect battering (ie, IPV), very few habitually ask their patients about being physically abused. Therapists need to know, for example, "that battering injuries are more likely to occur in a central pattern (head, neck, chest, abdomen)."[30] Statistics show that up to one-third of separated and divorced women, and up to one-half of all women, have experienced IPV. Additionally, over 90% of victims are women hurt by men, one-quarter of women in the emergency room have experienced domestic violence, 17% of pregnant women are abused, and one-quarter of women in primary care (where the physical therapist is the first health care professional the patient sees) have been abused.[31]

Not only women, but other vulnerable groups, experience abuse. The geriatric population is at risk due to higher proportion of physical dependence on others, cognitive factors more prevalent with age, and other attributes. DeFrancesco[32] describes the case of a physical therapist working in a wellness setting with a gentleman with an inability to walk, hemiparesis, and decreased verbal communication skills due to a prior stroke. The therapist followed up with the local Elder Abuse Hotline and Adult Protective Services about a cluster of signs, including decreased motivation and participation in the wellness program, client reports of his home health aide being on vacation, observed verbal aggressiveness in his wife, and reports by others that the wife was neglecting him. The reporting resulted in an abuse investigation and ongoing monitoring of the man's situation.[32]

Ample statistics and analysis exist regarding the stereotypical depiction of domestic violence: a man harming a woman. Shorey et al[33] investigated the prevalence of psychological conditions in men arrested for domestic violence, and found that common coexisting mental health problems in these men included PTSD, depression, generalized anxiety disorder, social phobia, panic disorder, and substance use disorders (SUDs). Each of these problems could predispose the aggressor to more aggression.[33]

Rees et al[34] looked at another side: how women who experienced violence because they were women were affected mentally and psychosocially. The Australian-based article's definition of such gender-based violence also included stalking along with direct physical harm to the woman. Findings indicated that, in the one-quarter of women reporting gender-based violence, many also had a mood disorder, SUDs (see Chapter 12), PTSD (see Chapter 6), and suicide attempts (see Chapter 7). These women also had higher physical and mental disability, poorer quality of life, and the likelihood of having at least 3 lifetime disorders.[34]

Risk Factors

Abuse is an anger problem on the part of the abuser.[35] Risk for abuse increases when a potential abuser is present, and if the potential abused person is vulnerable to the abuse. Tina Zahn[35] profiles a typical abuser: angry, emotionally labile, manipulative in personality, unable to respect interpersonal boundaries, possessive, hardworking, and seeking to be in a position of authority. The victim often has a previous trusting relationship with the abuser and may not know that abuse is happening until it is too late (eg, a person with dementia may not realize that his or her child is financially exploiting him or her). Or, if the person knows that abuse is happening, he or she may not be in a position to escape it.

Specific risk factors for child abuse noted in the literature include parental hostility, financial problems, and antisocial personality. These were noted for family systems with adopted toddlers.[36] Both child and elder abuse have estimated 3% to 4% prevalence in the United States. Research has found specific factors influencing elder abuse and neglect as well. In the community, persons with cognitive, physical, and psychiatric impairment, as well as low income and a history of trauma, are at higher risk.[37] In SNF residents, risk factors include institution understaffing, lack of appropriate supervision, care staff with burnout, paternalistic attitude, a history of SUDs or psychological issues, and a history of being abused themselves.[38,39] About one-quarter of all at-risk older adults will experience physical or psychological abuse, without adequate detection or psychometrically sound measurement tools for abuse.[40]

Home health care agencies and other entities require annual training in recognizing and reporting abuse, including the Elder Justice Act. One study found that the vast majority of experienced physical therapists and physical therapist assistants were familiar with identification and reporting requirements, but they identified many barriers to reporting:

> [F]ear of retaliation, lack of confidence in the system, uncertainty of suspicions, potential for escalation of abuse, patient fear of going to live in a nursing home, and concern that patient or family would avoid seeking future medical care.[41]

One case study illustrates the complexities of the clinical reasoning skills needed to identify abuse or recognize that abuse may not be the cause of the problems. Miller and Mangione[42] describe a 93-year-old female who had fallen, been hospitalized, and had multiple medical conditions. Receiving home health therapy, she was progressing well until a 2-week break in home care services. After this break, she showed an abrupt decline in condition, including pallor, urinary incontinence, confusion, fatigue, and declines in cognition, function, and balance. The treating therapist reviewed body systems to correctly identify this as caused by delirium and not by abuse, and referred the patient to the primary care provider and family members for treatment.[42]

Secondary Medical and Psychosocial Issues

In situations of captivity the perpetrator becomes the most powerful person in the life of the victim, and the psychology of the victim is shaped by the actions and beliefs of the perpetrator.

—Judith Lewis Herman[43]

Many psychological and secondarily medical conditions can arise from domestic abuse. In the United States, the likelihood of a physical therapist encountering a person in the clinical setting who has undergone abuse is high. Such abuse involves repeated trust and boundary violations, causing a perceived loss of control, potential for dissociative disorder as a coping strategy (see Chapter 10), and an impaired mind-body relationship.[44]

Other long-term sequelae of abuse include:

> [H]ypervigilance ... objectification ... difficulty with trust ... conditioning to be passive ... experience of body pain related to abuse ... difficulty with unfamiliar physical environment, with privacy issues, disrobing, touch, certain body positions, particular exercises ... dissociative reactions to stressful situations.[44]

All of these can detract from the patient's success in physical therapy, barring sensitive clinical approaches.

Medical issues due to abuse include direct physical harm (bruising, broken bones), suicide attempts, depressive symptoms, and secondary effects.[45] Due to high stress levels, the victim can develop metabolic syndrome, irritable bowel syndrome, chronic pain, and other diseases related to sustained high levels of the stress hormone cortisol and associated inflammation. Treating the sources of stress is essential and needs interdisciplinary team/interprofessional team intervention due to the interwoven mental health and safety concerns, especially if the person is still in an abusive relationship.

Literature specifically notes secondary effects of physical and sexual abuse on children and on older adults. In children, the following can occur:

- Fractures that cannot be otherwise accounted for[46]
- Disorders in sexual, behavioral, medical, and psychological domains[47]
- SUDs, suicide, and behavior resulting in sexually transmitted infections[48]
- Lifetime diagnosis of PTSD, anxiety, depression, and eating or sleep disorders[49]

In older adults, documented secondary effects were as follows:

- Malnutrition, pressure injuries, dehydration, and death, especially in SNFs[38]
- Mood disorders and PTSD, especially with premorbid mood symptoms[50,51]

As a case example, Zahn[35] is a person who underwent years of abuse by her stepfather. Her complex medical and psychiatric history stemming from that includes years of sexual abuse, subsequent chronic and incapacitating back and shoulder pain (managed with physical therapy and a home transcutaneous electrical nerve stimulation unit), anxiety, 2 abortions (followed by years of hiding that fact from her family), postpartum depression, severe medication-induced fatigue, lack of healthy boundaries with important people in her life, being a people pleaser, denial, and repressed anger. Her autobiography describes the **effects of sexual abuse on children**, so that providers can be aware for screening and referral as needed[35]:

- Clinical signs: pain and redness in the genital area, dysuria, and constipation
- Behavioral signs: suicide gestures, phobias, aggression, PTSD, depression, anxiety, pyromania, dissociation, multiple personalities, and SUDs
- Emotional signs: fear, anger, isolation, sadness, guilt, shame, and confusion

Specific Clinical Approaches to Improve Physical Therapy Outcomes

Direct Approaches by the Clinician

At minimum, students and clinicians should screen for, identify, and properly report suspected cases of abuse. Concrete suggestions for such screening include:

- Ask the patient "Do you ever feel unsafe at home?" and "Has anyone at home hit you or tried to injure you in some way?"[31]
- Note the presence of cuts and bruises "on the head, face, and neck" or forearms. These can be due to physical abuse and defensive injuries, respectively.[31]

The Elder Justice Act is one example of legislation in which therapists working with geriatric clients are regularly trained.[41] This law limits time frames between the reasonable suspicion of abuse formed by the observer and the required reporting of that suspicion. One study of physical therapists in Michigan found that facility-based training strongly influenced therapists' action on suspected elder abuse. About a quarter of therapists thought that one or more of their older clients was being abused (financially, physically, or emotionally), but fewer than half of those reported the suspicion. Nationally, about one-fifth of suspected elder abuse cases are reported, primarily in persons with disabilities that make them dependent in mobility or activities of daily living.[52]

Especially before graduation, education and a supportive environment can help students to identify and report potential abuse. MacDonnell et al[53] asked students from medical, pharmacy, physical therapy, social work, and nursing programs to collaborate in using a standardized interview of a patient presenting with "a cut on the hand" that was actually related to domestic violence. Many students did not use team members as resources to give insight into the issue of IPV, but all students knew their own roles and responsibilities on the team. Debriefing during interprofessional education (IPE), following sessions such as this one, can introduce students to ways of increasing their ability to recognize and report abuse.

One way to assist doctor of physical therapy students, and potentially novice clinicians with mentors, is the ECHOWS tool. **This rubric for patient interviews includes the following areas** for the interviewer[54]:

- E: establishing rapport with the patient
- C: determining the chief complaint (why the patient is coming to physical therapy)
- H: obtaining health history, which includes licit substance use and any abuse history
- O: obtaining the patient's psychosocial perspective of the health issue(s)
- W: wrapping up with pointers to the direction of the episode of care
- S: summary of performance, which includes non-verbal behaviors and attentive listening

After the interview, recorded with the patient's permission, the mentor can review with the interviewer to make sure all components were addressed and give constructive feedback.

Behavioral anti-abuse interventions for clinical, support, and community staff are diverse. Many societal institutions, including churches, can partner with abuse prevention organizations to improve the systematic training of staff in how to deal with domestic abuse. "Abuse is an anger problem, not a marriage counseling problem. Most pastors are trained to work toward reconciliation and don't always think about the safety of the wife and children."[35]

In a therapy clinic, clinicians and staff should[44]:

- Establish an atmosphere of safety
- Maintain therapeutic rapport with patients
- Share control with patients, always leaving the option for the patient to say "no"
- Share information regularly, within the boundaries of Health Insurance Portability and Accountability Act
- Ask if the patient wants to be seen by a therapist of a particular sex
- Educate the patient, verbally and by modeling, about self-care and knowledge of the body
- Treat the whole person

Treating the whole person should involve a team because professionals can then pool their knowledge and resources for addressing the patient's problems. Treatment options include medications (for mood and behavioral symptoms), electroconvulsive therapy for appropriate patients, strong social support, music, and faith. In Zahn's[35] case, 9 women from her church prayed for her throughout her recovery after her attempted suicide, which was the culmination of her history of abuse and subsequent mental health issues. Psychiatric medications should be used only with caution, with every team member responsible for monitoring for side effects and medication interactions.

Indirect Approaches: Referral by the Clinician for Counseling

Although the scope of physical therapy practice encompasses the entire human movement system (parts of all body systems that contribute to or are influenced by physical movement), it is dynamic and influenced by many outside factors. These include practice specialty (eg, orthopedics or geriatrics), local environment and access to other health care providers, and legislation. For example, the Wisconsin legislature recently passed a law allowing qualified therapists to order x-rays for patients vs requiring referral to a physician for the imaging order.[55] Thus, a service that physical therapists previously were required to ask another professional to address, may become part of the therapist's expected skill set.

Routinely, the clinician needs to determine whether a patient's needs require another medical or other professional. Especially in a psychosocially complex situation, the clinician should be ready to refer a patient to a psychiatrist, psychologist, social worker, or community resource for counseling for mental health needs outside of the therapist's education, training, experience, and job description. This is a particular need in cases of known or suspected domestic abuse. Useful texts for helping the therapist make this distinction include Boissonnault's[31] *Primary Care for the Physical Therapist* and Goodman and Snyder's[56] *Differential Diagnosis for Physical Therapists*. Counseling and other psychosocial interventions for persons with comorbid severe mental illness and SUD are supported by a systematic review.[57]

When considering a course of action that may include referral, therapists should have a basic background knowledge of literature regarding effective interventions for child and elder abuse. Specifically for child abuse:

- Checklists applied in emergency departments can improve detection rates.[58]
- In high-income countries especially, risk and incidence can be reduced by home visits, prevention of abusive head trauma, and education of parents.[59]

Specifically for elder abuse, however:

- A review of over 20 programs to educate health professionals on abuse indicated a lack of outcome measures for program effectiveness.[60]
- Another review found poor methodological quality of intervention studies, with major outcomes of possibly higher recurrence rates of abuse, and relocation rates that can sacrifice autonomy and friendship for safety.[61]

While physical therapists can and should participate in health promotion for patients and members of the community, this may require in-team referral to other professionals. In a study of Chicago-area physical therapists serving geriatric clients in inpatient, outpatient, or home health settings, therapists indicated that their one-on-one time with patients significantly helped them consistently promote health. Areas included chronic disease management, smoking cessation, and alcohol and drug use. Facilitators for health promotion included therapists' experience and knowledge of community-based resources, professional organization resources, and the individual clinic's or facility's resources (eg, an academic hospital would have trained mental health counselors). Barriers included time constraints, lack of reimbursement for health promotion activities, and lack of ownership by the patient and family. These may influence the therapist's decision to refer or educate.[62]

A final influence in a physical therapist's decision to refer a patient for counseling may be the attitudes of local health care professionals toward interprofessional work. Although the health care landscape is moving toward a team-based norm, many professionals may still practice in silos, depending on prior education and work experience. Curricula and professional organizations' educational offerings can help to address potential deficits in students' and clinicians' attitudes toward IPE and interprofessional practice. One such profession is that of the physician assistant. A recent study of physician assistant students used the Readiness for Interprofessional Learning Scale to find out that these students do not display as strong a preference toward IPE and interprofessional practice as do other professional students who have had experience in health care via being or knowing a patient.[63]

Summary

Abuse, whether physical, emotional, sexual, or financial, is a common worldwide problem. After examining related aspects such as caregiving for persons with disabilities and family systems, this chapter focused on physical abuse in a domestic context, as an example of what to look for and what questions to ask if the physical therapist suspects a patient may be abused. Poor mental health is a large component of abuse and neglect, for both abusers and victims. It is a clinician's social responsibility to protect patients' health; this chapter offers some tools for that process. In any situation, the therapist should strive to embody the profession's core values of compassion and respect for the individual patient's dignity.

Key Points

- Children undergoing sexual abuse display clinical, behavioral, and emotional signs, including dysuria, constipation, aggression, depression, sadness, and confusion.
- Use the ECHOWS rubric to guide patient interviewing: establishing rapport, determining the chief complaint, obtaining health history, obtaining the patient's psychosocial perspective, wrapping up, and summary of performance.

Review Questions

- Recall a patient case, if applicable, where you or a classmate/colleague encountered a patient who displayed signs and symptoms consistent with domestic violence, abuse, or neglect.
  - What was the treatment setting?
  - What signs and symptoms led to your suspicion of domestic violence, abuse, or neglect?
  - What was the course of action you or your classmate/colleague took? What was the outcome?
  - What was the clinical reasoning process behind that course of action?
- Craft several patient interview questions that sensitively determine whether someone is likely undergoing domestic violence or abuse.
- Given the patient case you described in the first question, what specific changes to the physical therapy plan of care and treatment approach would you make if you encountered this patient a second time?
- Brainstorm, with classmates or colleagues if desired, strategies to reduce the fear that commonly prevents laypersons or health professionals from promptly reporting suspected domestic violence.
- Research to develop a list of resources in your community to which you can refer patients who are current or former victims of domestic violence.

Case Studies: First Impressions

As you review the following case studies, you may want to consider these questions for thought or discussion:

- What standardized tests and measures (including psychiatric, for example, a depression screen) would you select for this patient? Why?
- Based on available data, what short- and long-term goals would you write for your plan of care? Consider using the acronyms SMART (specific, measurable, attainable, realistic, and timely) or ABCDE (actor, behavior, conditions, degree, and expected time frame) to guide your goal writing.
- What elements (procedures, psychosocial aspects, communication aspects, etc) would you make sure to include or omit in your plan of care for this patient? Why?
- What are your anticipated needs, if any, for consultation and referral for this patient?
- How will you transition this patient toward lasting health behavior change following discharge (eg, recommending a YMCA membership trial)?

Case 1

A 26-year-old female was referred to outpatient physical therapy 1 week after a left ankle sprain. Her goal is to return to recreational sports, especially soccer, in her neighborhood association.

- Social history: she lives alone in a second-floor apartment but mentions having a significant other. She works in a restaurant kitchen full time, which involves standing and walking frequently.
- Medical/psychiatric history: asthma, recurrent bilateral ankle sprains, and generalized anxiety disorder
- Impairments, activity limitations, and participation restrictions found on initial interview and examination
  - Left lower extremity weightbearing-as-tolerated order from the referring physician
  - Noted quiet demeanor and apparent discomfort in speaking with male staff
  - Bruising visible on bilateral forearms
  - Pain in lateral left ankle rated 7/10
  - Impaired single-leg standing balance bilaterally
  - Increased postural sway with eyes closed on both firm and foam surfaces
  - Increased respiratory rate and report of anxiety during supine lower extremity strength and range-of-motion testing (mild weakness in hip extensors/abductors and moderate weakness noted in all left ankle musculature)
  - Reports difficulty concentrating on therapist directions and statements
  - Asymmetric gait with a single crutch to offload the affected ankle
  - Unable to manage the flight of stairs to reach her apartment

Case 2

A 41-year-old female was admitted to subacute rehabilitation following a 4-day hospitalization for an exacerbation of multiple sclerosis, complicated by stage 3 sacral pressure injury (tendon/muscle visible). Her goal is to return home as soon as possible to pursue part-time work.

- Social history: she lives with her husband and 2 children in a lower duplex. Her husband works full time commuting to a major city, and her children help with outdoor chores after school.
- Medical/psychiatric history: schizoaffective disorder, history of pressure injuries, history of falls, bilateral drop-foot, osteopenia, and frequent upper respiratory infections
- Impairments, activity limitations, and participation restrictions found on initial interview and examination
  - Mild cognitive deficits in memory and problem solving
  - Standing tolerance 2 minutes unsupported, with increased postural sway in any test position (Romberg, sharpened Romberg, eyes open or closed)
  - Shortness of breath with short-distance ambulation, requiring 25% assistance for safety
  - Stated "I have a sore on my bottom right now because they just let me sit at home"
  - Primary mode of locomotion is with a single-point cane and bilateral ankle-foot orthoses, using a lightweight wheelchair for community distances

Case 3

A 68-year-old male was seen in acute care immediately following hospitalization for aspiration pneumonia. His goal is to become independent in transfers and wheelchair mobility for return home.

- Social history: he is widowed (1 year) and lives in a ranch house with a ramp to enter. His daughter-in-law is his paid caregiver. His son has financial power of attorney, while his younger brother has health care power of attorney. The hospital social worker indicates that there is an open elder abuse situation regarding the patient and his primary caregiver (daughter-in-law).
- Medical/psychiatric history: right (dominant side) hemiparesis and cognitive/visual deficits following 2 strokes that happened 2 years previously, type 2 diabetes, hypertension, recurrent lower and upper extremity cellulitis, bipolar II disorder (diagnosed 40 years ago), and urinary incontinence
- Impairments, activity limitations, and participation restrictions found on initial interview and examination
  - Limited ability to provide his own social and medical history
  - Pain behavior noted with passive or active motion of right upper and lower extremity
  - Currently requires 75% assistance for all functional mobility tasks (was previously independent in pivot transfers and wheelchair propulsion)
  - Requires 50% assistance for maintaining sitting balance due to posterior lean and increased extensor tone, with possible poor safety awareness (previously required cues and 25% assistance for all activities of daily living)

References

1. Taryam A. *The Opposite of Indifference: A Collection of Commentaries.* Sharjah, United Arab Emirates: Dar Al Khaleej Printing & Publishing; 2011.
2. Aktaş D. Attitudes of university students towards domestic violence against women. *Clin Invest Med.* 2016;39(6):S173-S178.
3. Talley RC, Crews JE. Framing the public health of caregiving. *Am J Public Health.* 2007;97(2):224-228.
4. Family Caregiver Alliance. Fact sheet: selected caregiver statistics. *Family Caregiver Alliance: National Center on Caregiving.* https://circlecenterads.info/documents/FCAPrint_SelectedCaregiv...pdf. Published September 21, 2010. Accessed February 28, 2018.
5. Schulz R, Sherwood PR. Physical and mental health effects of family caregiving. *Am J Nurs.* 2008;108(suppl 9):23-27.
6. Chang HY, Chiou CJ, Chen NS. Impact of mental health and caregiver burden on family caregivers' physical health. *Arch Gerontol Geriatr.* 2010;50(3):267-271.
7. Cameron JI, Gignac MA. "Timing it right": a conceptual framework for addressing the support needs of family caregivers to stroke survivors from the hospital to the home. *Patient Educ Couns.* 2008;70(3):305-314.
8. Peña R, Suman OE, Rosenberg M, et al. A 1 year comparison of a community based exercise program versus a day-hospital based exercise program on quality of life and mental health in severely burned children. *Arch Phys Med Rehabil.* 2017;pii: S0003-9993(17):31384-31389. DOI: 10.1016/j.apmr.2017.10.023.
9. Bayat M. Evidence of resilience in families of children with autism. *J Intellect Disabil Res.* 2007;51(9):702-714.
10. Burke MM, Taylor JL, Urbano R, Hodapp RM. Predictors of future caregiving by adult siblings of individuals with intellectual and developmental disabilities. *Am J Intellect Devel Disabil.* 2012;117(1):33-47.
11. Heller T, Caldwell J, Factor A. Aging family caregivers: policies and practices. *Ment Retard Dev Disabil Res Rev.* 2007;13(2):136-142.
12. Yamaki K, Hsieh K, Heller T. Health profile of aging family caregivers supporting adults with intellectual and developmental disabilities at home. *Intellect Devel Disabil.* 2009;47(6):425-435.
13. Mactavish JB, MacKay KJ, Iwasaki Y, Betteridge D. Family caregivers of individuals with intellectual disability: perspectives on life quality and the role of vacations. *J Leisure Res.* 2007;39(1):127-155.
14. Awad AG, Voruganti LNP. The burden of schizophrenia on caregivers: a review. *Pharmacoeconomics.* 2008;26(2):149-162.

15. Mak WWS, Cheung RYM. Affiliate stigma among caregivers of people with intellectual disability or mental illness. *J Appl Res Intellect Disabil.* 2008;21(6):532-545.
16. Cooper C, Balamurali TBS, Livingston G. A systematic review of the prevalence and covariates of anxiety in caregivers of people with dementia. *Int Psychogeriatr.* 2008;19(2):175-195.
17. Etters L, Goodall D, Harrison BE. Caregiver burden among dementia patient caregivers: a review of the literature. *J Am Acad Nurs Pract.* 2008;20(8):423-428.
18. Menaghan EG. Review of: Family Systems and Life-Span Development. (Kreppner K, Lerner RM, eds.). *J Marriage Fam.* 1992;54(1):243-244.
19. McDaniel SH, LeRoux P. An overview of primary care family psychology. *J Clin Psychol Med Settings.* 2007;14(1):23-32.
20. Distelberg BJ, Blow A. Variations in family system boundaries. *Family Business Review.* 2011;24(1):28-46.
21. Becker OA, Steinbach A. Relations between grandparents and grandchildren in the context of the family system. *Comparative Population Studies.* 2012;37(3-4):543-566.
22. Taqui AM, Itrat A, Qidwai W, Qadri Z. Depression in the elderly: does family system play a role? A cross-sectional study. *BMC Psychiatry.* 2007;7:57.
23. Weisskirch RS. Child language brokers in immigrant families: an overview of family dynamics. *MediAzioni.* 2010;10.
24. Bacallao ML, Smokowski PR. The costs of getting ahead: Mexican family system changes after immigration. *Family Relations.* 2007;56(1):52-66.
25. Dupuis S. Examining the blended family: the application of systems theory toward an understanding of the blended family system. *J Couple Relatsh Ther.* 2010;9(3):239-251.
26. Ahrons CR. Family ties after divorce: long-term implications for children. *Fam Process.* 2007;46(1):53-65.
27. Paquette K, Bassuk EL. Parenting and homelessness: overview and introduction to the special section. *Am J Orthopsychiatry.* 2009;79(3):292-298.
28. Berger R, Weiss T. The posttraumatic growth model: an expansion to the family system. *Traumatology.* 2009;15(1):63-74.
29. Calhoun LG, Tedeschi RG. (Eds.) *Handbook of Posttraumatic Growth.* Mahway, NJ: Lawrence Erlbaum; 2006.
30. Clark TJ, Smith McKenna L, Jewell MJ. Physical therapists' recognition of battered women in clinical settings. *Phys Ther.* 1996;76(1):12-18.
31. Boissonnault WG. *Primary Care for the Physical Therapist: Examination and Triage.* 2nd ed. St. Louis, MO: Saunders Elsevier; 2011.
32. DeFrancesco A. Recognizing the signs and symptoms of elder abuse in a wellness setting. *J Geriatr Phys Ther.* 2001;24(1):20.
33. Shorey RC, Febres J, Brasfield H, Stuart GL. The prevalence of mental health problems in men arrested for domestic violence. *J Fam Violence.* 2012;27(8)741-748.
34. Rees S, Silove D, Chey T. Lifetime prevalence of gender-based violence in women and the relationship with mental disorders and psychosocial function. *JAMA.* 2011;306(5):513-521.
35. Zahn T, Dyson W. *Why I Jumped: A Dramatic Story of Finding Hope Beyond Depression.* Grand Rapids, MI: Pilgrim Feet; 2006.
36. Stover CS, Connell C, Leve LD, et al. Fathering and mothering in the family system: linking marital hostility and aggression in adopted toddlers. *J Child Psychol Psychiatry.* 2012;53(4):401-409.
37. Johannesen M, LoGiudice D. Elder abuse: a systematic review of risk factors in community-dwelling elders. *Age Ageing.* 2013;42(3):292-298.
38. Lindbloom EJ, Brandt J, Hough LD, Meadows SE. Elder mistreatment in the nursing home: a systematic review. *J Am Med Dir Assoc.* 2007;8(9):610-616.
39. Thornberry TP, Knight KE, Lovegrove PJ. Does maltreatment beget maltreatment? A systematic review of intergenerational literature. *Trauma Violence Abuse.* 2012;13(3):135-152.
40. Cooper C, Selwood A, Livingston G. The prevalence of elder abuse and neglect: a systematic review. *Age Ageing* 2008;37(2):151-160.
41. Wooton CR, Williams NQ, Harrison AL, Teaster PB. An examination of the knowledge base of home health professionals regarding elder mistreatment. *J Geriatr Phys Ther.* 2006;29(3):127-128.
42. Miller AH, Mangione KK. Does delirium need immediate medical referral in a frail, homebound elder? *J Geriatr Phys Ther.* 2006;29(2):57.
43. Herman JL. *Trauma and Recovery: the Aftermath of Violence—From Domestic Abuse to Political Terror.* New York, NY: BasicBooks; 1992.
44. Schachter CL, Stalker CA, Teram E. Toward sensitive practice: issues for physical therapists working with survivors of childhood sexual abuse. *Phys Ther.* 1999;79(3):248-261.
45. Devries KM, Mak JY, Bacchus LJ, et al. Intimate partner violence and incident depressive symptoms and suicide attempts: a systematic review of longitudinal studies. *PLoS Med.* 2013;10(5):e1001439.
46. Kemp AM, Dunstan F, Harrison S, et al. Patterns of skeletal fractures in child abuse: systematic review. *BMJ.* 2008;337:a1518.

47. Maniglio R. The impact of child sexual abuse on health: a systematic review of reviews. *Clin Psychol Rev.* 2009;29(7):647-657.
48. Norman RE, Byambaa M, De R, Butchart A, Scott J, Vos T. The long-term health consequences of child physical abuse, emotional abuse, and neglect: a systematic review and meta-analysis. *PLoS Med.* 2012;9(11):e1001349.
49. Chen LP, Murad MH, Paras ML, et al. Sexual abuse and lifetime diagnosis of psychiatric disorders: systematic review and meta-analysis. *Mayo Clin Proc.* 2010;85(7):618-629.
50. Cook JM, Dinnen S, O'Donnell C. Older women survivors of physical and sexual violence: a systematic review of the quantitative literature. *J Women Health.* 2011;20(7):1075-1081.
51. Dong X, Chen R, Chang ES, Simon M. Elder abuse and psychological well-being: a systematic review and implications for research and policy - a mini review. *Gerontology.* 2013;59(2):132-142.
52. Saliga S, Adamowicz C, Logue A, Smith K. Physical therapists' knowledge of physical elder abuse—signs, symptoms, laws, and facility protocols. *J Geriatr Phys Ther.* 2004;27(1):5.
53. MacDonnell C, George P, Nimmagadda J, Brown S, Gremel K. A team-based practicum bringing together students across educational institutions and health professions. *Am J Pharmaceut Educ.* 2016;80(3):49.
54. Boissonnault JS, Evans K, Tuttle N, et al. Reliability of the ECHOWS tool for assessment of patient interviewing skills. *Phys Ther.* 2016;96(4):443-455.
55. PT In Motion. New Wisconsin law allows PTs to order X-rays. *PT In Motion.* http://www.apta.org/PTinMotion/News/2016/4/25/WisconsinXRays/. Published April 25, 2016. Accessed February 28, 2018.
56. Goodman CC, Snyder TEK. *Differential Diagnosis for Physical Therapists: Screening for Referral.* 5th ed. St. Louis, MO: Saunders Elsevier; 2013.
57. Drake RE, O'Neal EL, Wallach MA. A systematic review of psychosocial research on psychosocial interventions for people with co-occurring severe mental and substance use disorder. *J Subst Abuse Treat.* 2008;34(1):123-138.
58. Louwers ECFM, Affourtit MJ, Moll HA, de Koning HJ, Korfage IJ. Screening for child abuse at emergency departments: a systematic review. *Arch Dis Child.* 2010;95(3):214-218. DOI: 10.1136/adc.2008.151654.
59. Mikton C, Butchart A. Child maltreatment prevention: a systematic review of reviews. *Bull World Health Organ.* 2009;87(5):353-361.
60. Alt KL, Nguyen AL, Meurer LN. The effectiveness of educational programs to improve recognition and reporting of elder abuse and neglect: a systematic review of the literature. *J Elder Abuse Negl.* 2011;23(3):213-233.
61. Ploeg J, Fear J, Hutchison B, MacMillan H, Bolan G. A systematic review of interventions for elder abuse. *J Elder Abuse Neglect.* 2009;21(3):187-210.
62. Healey WE, Broers KB, Nelson J, Huber G. Physical therapists' health promotion activities for older adults. *J Geriatr Phys Ther.* 2012;35(1):35-48.
63. Hertweck ML, Hawkins SR, Bednarek ML, et al. Attitudes toward interprofessional education: comparing physician assistant and other health care professions students. *J Physician Assist Educ.* 2012;23(2):8-15.

Acronyms

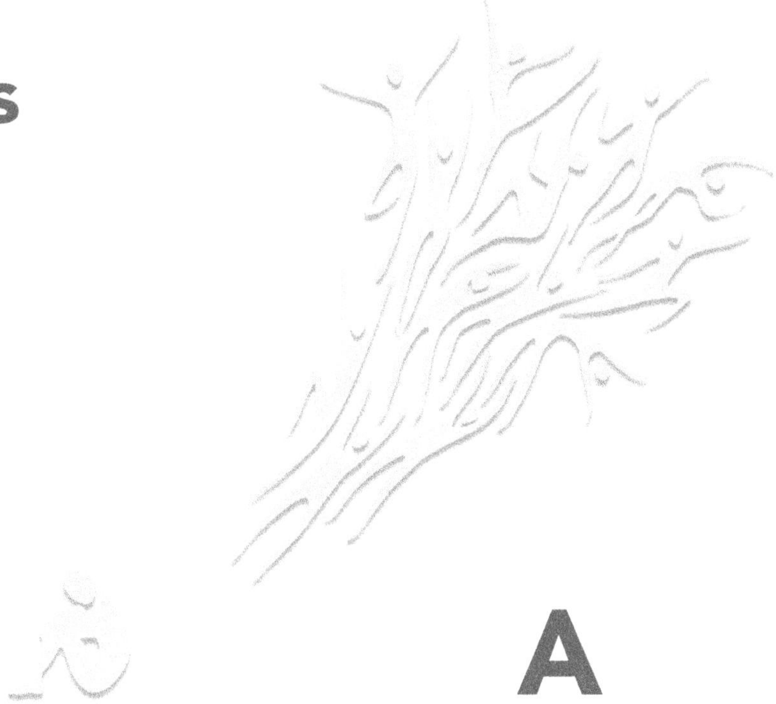

A

AAA	Area Agency on Aging
ABCDE	actor, behavior, conditions, degree, and expected time frame
ABN	advanced beneficiary notice
ABPTS	American Board of Physical Therapy Specialties
ACA	Affordable Care Act
ACE	angiotensin-converting enzyme
ACh	acetylcholine
ACSM	American College of Sports Medicine
AD	Alzheimer's disease
ADHD	attention-deficit hyperactivity disorder
ADL	activity of daily living
ADRC	Aging and Disability Resource Center
AGPT	Academy of Geriatric Physical Therapy
AIDES	acknowledge and affirm the person you are meeting, introduce yourself, define the duration of the session, explain the flow of and expectations for the session, and set the tone with a stated intention to collaborate
AMA	against medical advice
ANS	autonomic nervous system
APTA	American Physical Therapy Association
ARB	angiotensin receptor blocker

Johnson H.
Psychosocial Elements of Physical Therapy: The Connection of Body to Mind (pp 251-256).

B

BBAT	basic body awareness therapy
BBS	Berg Balance Scale
BD	bipolar disorder
BDI	Beck Depression Inventory
BDNF	brain-derived neurotrophic factor
BESTest	Balance Evaluation Systems Test
BMI	body mass index
BPD	borderline personality disorder
BPH	benign prostatic hypertrophy
BPSD	behavioral and psychological symptoms of dementia

C

CAD	coronary artery disease
CAM	complementary and alternative medicine/Confusion Assessment Method
CBT	cognitive behavioral therapy
CCB	calcium channel blocker
CEEAA	Certified Exercise Expert for the Aging Adult
CESDS	Center for Epidemiologic Studies Depression Scale
CHD	coronary heart disease
CHF	congestive/chronic heart failure
CI	clinical instructor
CKD	chronic kidney disease
CNS	central nervous system
COPD	chronic obstructive pulmonary disease
COX	cyclooxygenase enzyme
CPG	clinical practice guideline
CSDD	Cornell Scale for Depression in Dementia
CSF	cerebrospinal fluid
CT	cognitive therapy
CVA	cerebrovascular accident

D

DBT	dialectical behavior therapy
DEARS	develop discrepancy, express empathy, avoid argumentation, roll with resistance, and support self-efficacy
DLB	dementia with Lewy bodies/Lewy body dementia
DRS	Delirium Rating Scale
DSM-5	*Diagnostic and Statistical Manual of Mental Disorders, 5th edition*

E

ECHOWS	establishing rapport with the patient, determining the chief complaint, obtaining health history, obtaining the patient's psychosocial perspective of the health issue(s), wrapping up with pointers to the direction of the episode of care, summary of performance
ECM	extracellular matrix
ECT	electroconvulsive therapy
ER	emergency room

F

FAST	Functional Assessment Staging Tool
FES	functional electrical stimulation
5TSTS	5 Times Sit to Stand
FTD	frontotemporal dementia

G

GAD	generalized anxiety disorder
GCS	Geriatric Clinical Specialist
GDS	Geriatric Depression Scale/Global Deterioration Scale
GERD	gastroesophageal reflux disease
GMWT	Groningen Meander Walking Test

H

HbA1c	hemoglobin A1c type, indicating control of blood glucose levels over several months
HD	Huntington's disease
HDL	high-density lipoprotein
HEP	home exercise program
HIPAA	Health Insurance Portability and Accountability Act
HRR	heart rate reserve
HTN	hypertension
HVLA	high-velocity, low-amplitude (joint manipulation)

I

ICF	*International Classification of Functioning, Disability and Health*
ICU	intensive care unit
IDT/IPT	interdisciplinary team/interprofessional team
IOPTMH	International Organization of Physical Therapists in Mental Health
IPE	interprofessional education
IPTOP	International Association of Physical Therapists working with Older People

J

JAMCO	judgment, affect, memory, cognition, and orientation

L

LDL	low-density lipoprotein

M

MAOI	monoamine oxidase inhibitor
MBSR	mindfulness-based stress reduction
MBTI	Myers-Briggs Type Indicator
MCID	minimal clinically important difference
MDC	minimal detectable change
MDD	major depressive disorder
MDS	minimum data set
MI	motivational interviewing
MMSE	Mini-Mental State Exam
MoCA	Montreal Cognitive Assessment
MRI	magnetic resonance imaging

N

N4A	National Association of Area Agencies on Aging
NAMI	National Alliance on Mental Illness
NDT	neurodevelopmental treatment
NLP	neurolinguistic psychology
NPH	normal pressure hydrocephalus
NPRS	Numeric Pain Rating Scale
NSAID	non-steroidal anti-inflammatory drug
NWB	non-weightbearing

O

OCD	obsessive-compulsive disorder
ODD	oppositional defiant disorder

P

P&P	policies and procedures
PACE	Program of All-Inclusive Care for the Elderly
PAINAD	Pain Assessment in Advanced Dementia

PD	Parkinson's disease
PHI	patient health information
PHQ-2	Patient Health Questionnaire, 2-question version
PHQ-9	Patient Health Questionnaire, 9-question version
PMDD	premenstrual dysphoric disorder
PPT	Physical Performance Test
PRE	progressive resistance exercise
PRIME-MD	Primary Care Evaluation of Mental Disorders Procedure
PST	problem-solving therapy
PT-CRT	Physical Therapy Clinical Reasoning and Reflection Tool
PTSD	posttraumatic stress disorder

R

RCT	randomized controlled trial
REBT	rational emotive behavior therapy
RUG	resource utilization group

S

SBAR	situation, background, assessment, recommendations
SF-36	Short Form, 36-question version
SIADH	syndrome of inappropriate antidiuretic hormone
SIG	special interest group
6MWT	6-Minute Walk Test
SMART	specific, measurable, attainable, realistic, and timely
SMI	severe mental illness
SNF	skilled nursing facility
SNRI	serotonin/norepinephrine reuptake inhibitor
SNS	sympathetic nervous system
SSRI	selective serotonin reuptake inhibitor
ST	schema therapy

T

TBI	traumatic brain injury
TCA	tricyclic antidepressant
TUG	Timed Up and Go

U

UTI	urinary tract infection

V

VAD	vascular-associated dementia
VAS	visual analogue scale
VO_2max	maximal voluntary oxygen consumption

W

WCPT	World Confederation of Physical Therapy
WKS	Wernicke-Korsakoff syndrome

Glossary

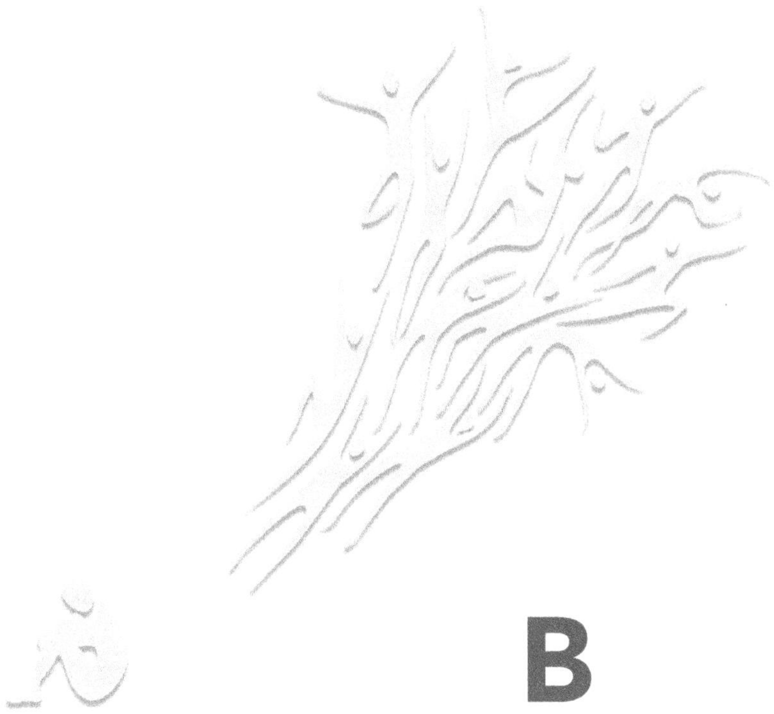

B

A

Action: the fourth stage of behavior change; a sustained demonstration of change by the patient, usually over 3 to 6 months.

Addictive behavior: involving "the pursuit of short-term gratification at the expense of long-term harm."[1]

Affect: "the patient's prevailing emotional tone as observed by the [clinician] during the interview."[2]

Agoraphobia: the fear of being in public or open places, especially with risk of embarrassment.

Agreeableness: a Big-5 model personality trait that allows the person to be cooperative, trusting, and potentially perceived as submissive. Its opposite is competitiveness.

Alexithymia: "difficulty naming and describing emotions"[2]; a negative symptom of schizophrenia

Alogia: lack of normal flow and quantity of speech during conversation; a negative symptom of schizophrenia and other disorders.

Alzheimer's disease: a type of dementia that progresses slowly to impair memory, thinking, behavior, word-finding, environmental navigation, and motor control.

Anhedonia: is the "inability or decreased ability to experience pleasure, joy, intimacy, and closeness"[2]; it is a negative symptom of schizophrenia and depression.

Antisocial personality disorder: marked by "disregard for social obligations … a low tolerance to frustration and a low threshold for discharge of aggression, including violence [and] a tendency to blame others."[3]

Anxiety: "a diffuse, vague apprehension associated with feelings of uncertainty and helplessness. This emotion has no specific object."[2]

Anxiety disorder: one of several conditions with an excessive duration or intensity of fear or anxiety.

Johnson H.
Psychosocial Elements of Physical Therapy: The Connection of Body to Mind (pp 257-264).

Apathy: "lack of feelings, emotions, interest, or concern"[2]; it is a negative symptom of schizophrenia and other disorders.

Avoidant personality disorder: marked by "tension and apprehension, insecurity, and inferiority ... [and] a hypersensitivity to rejection and criticism."[3]

Avolition: lack of motivation, initiative, interest, and engagement in goal-oriented behavior; it is a negative symptom of schizophrenia and other disorders.

Axis I: clinical disorders, or the primary diagnosis related to mental health (eg flare-up of panic disorder).

Axis II: personality disorders and developmental disorders, including borderline personality disorder.

Axis III: general medical conditions (ie, the person's potentially relevant medical comorbidities).

Axis IV: psychosocial and environmental problems (ie, stressors the person has recently encountered).

Axis V: global assessment and functioning, rated on a 0 to 100 scale, with higher scores indicating better function psychosocially.

B

Behavioral activation: "increased activity, aggression, sleep disturbance, disinhibition, and subjective feelings of increased energy" related to antidepressant medication treatment.[4]

Behavioral and psychological symptoms of dementia: non-cognitive manifestations that include aggression, agitation, combativeness, and resistance to care.

Bipolar disorder: mood disorder with alternating episodes of mania and depression.

Bipolar I disorder: depression with at least one manic episode.

Bipolar II disorder: depression with at least one hypomanic episode.

Body dysmorphic disorder: "a person with a normal appearance is concerned about having a physical defect."[2]

Borderline personality disorder: marked by impulsive actions, as well as "disturbances in self-image, aims, and internal preferences, by intense and unstable interpersonal relationships, and by a tendency to self-destructive behavior."[3]

Bradykinesia: a movement symptom of Parkinson's disease that involves slow, fatiguing movement.

Burnout: "to fail, wear out, or become exhausted by making excessive demands on energy, strength, or resources."[5]

C

Catatonia: a range of abnormal movement patterns including stereotypic movements, echopraxia, and impulsive movements. Movement may be increased (hyperkinesia), decreased (hypokinesia), or absent altogether (akinesia).[3]

Circumstantial: thought process with "excessive and unnecessary detail that is usually relevant to a question."[2]

Cognitive behavioral therapy: a set of psychotherapeutic techniques and principles that address a patient's erroneous patterns of thought, which in turn influence habits.

Complementary and alternative medicine: non-pharmacological interventions, which are typically based in ancient theories and practices, that seek to heal the whole person naturally.

Conscientiousness: a Big-5 model personality trait that allows the person to be organized, planned, and goal-oriented. Its opposite is spontaneous and seen as sloppy.

Contemplation: the second stage of behavior change; ambivalence toward behavior change due to analyzing risks and rewards.

Conversion disorder: a disorder "in which a loss or alteration of physical functioning occurs."[2]

Critical illness: one or more medical conditions requiring a stay in the intensive care unit.

Cyclothymic disorder: alternating hypomanic and hypodepressive episodes.

D

Delirium: a "nonspecific cerebral organic syndrome" including simultaneous impairments in "consciousness and attention, perception, thinking, memory, psychomotor behaviour [sic], emotion, and the sleep-wake schedule" that fluctuate over hours to days.[3]

Delusion: a "false belief that is firmly maintained even though it is not shared by others and is contradicted by social reality".[2] Delusions are categorized as grandiose, paranoid, thought broadcasting, and thought insertion or withdrawal.

Dementia (neurocognitive disorder): a typically chronic, slowly progressive collection of symptoms demonstrating impaired "memory, thinking, orientation, comprehension, calculation, learning capacity, language, and judgment" with frequent "deterioration in emotional control, social behaviour [sic], or motivation."[3]

Dependent personality disorder: marked by "pervasive passive reliance on other people to make major and minor life decisions, great fear of abandonment, feelings of helplessness … [and] passive compliance with the wishes of elders and others."[3]

Depersonalization: a "feeling of having lost self-identity."[2]

Depression: "an abnormal extension or overelaboration of sadness and grief."[2]

Depressive disorder: "the presence of sad, empty, or irritable mood, accompanied by somatic and cognitive changes that significantly affect the individual's capacity to function."[6]

Determination: the third stage of behavior change; commitment to change regardless of how adamant the patient is externally.

Disruptive mood dysregulation disorder: a persistent angry or irritable mood beyond what parents or teachers see as typical child moodiness.

Dysthymia: a chronic depressed mood over several years, which is not severe enough to be classified as major depression.

E

Echopraxia: a "pathologic imitation of the movements or gestures of another, usually semi-automatic in nature"[3]; a movement symptom of schizophrenia.

Evidence-based practice: "the conscientious, explicit, and judicious use of the best evidence from systematic research to make decisions about the care of individual patients."[2]

Executive function: a set of organizational and regulatory cognitive functions that allow goal-directed behavior. These include attention, abstract thinking, self-control, and stimulus monitoring.[7]

Extraversion: a Big-5 model personality trait that allows the person to be outgoing, sociable, and talkative. Its opposite is a reserved quality.

F

Flight of ideas: a thought process that includes "rapid shifting from one topic to another and fragmented ideas."[2]

Frontotemporal dementia: an early-onset dementia that impairs safety regarding food and causes increased continuous walking until late in the disease.

G

Generalized anxiety disorder: excessive, ongoing, uncontrollable worry about day-to-day matters. These patients may have insomnia, headaches, irritability, and fatigue.

Grandiose delusion: with "exaggerated notions of capacities, possessions, and esteem which in delusional form are associated with mania, schizophrenia, and cerebral organic psychoses."[3]

H

Hallucination: "false sensory impressions or experiences."[2]

Histrionic personality disorder: marked by "self-dramatization, theatricality, exaggerated expression of emotions, suggestibility, egocentricity, self-indulgence, [and] lack of consideration for others."[3] The person will also crave "appreciation, excitement, and attention."[3]

Human movement system: "the anatomic structures and physiologic functions that interact to move the body or its component parts."[8]

Hypochondriasis: "somatic over-concern with ... details of body functioning."[2]

I

Ideas of reference: "incorrect interpretation of casual incidents ... as having direct personal references."[2]

Illusions: "false perceptions or false responses to a sensory stimulus."[2]

Insight: "patient's understanding of the nature of the illness."[2]

Interdisciplinary team/interprofessional team: the collaboration of at least 2 health care providers to improve individualized care for a patient or group of patients.

J

Judgment: "making decisions that are constructive and adaptive."[2]

L

Dementia with Lewy bodies/Lewy body dementia: a type of dementia caused by abnormal accumulations of proteins within the brain's substantia nigra and associated with variable cognition and alertness, fainting, falls, and Parkinsonian signs that worsen if anti-Parkinson's disease medications are administered.

Locus ceruleus: a brainstem region involved in production of norepinephrine and contributory to physiological symptoms of stress and panic.

Loose associations: thought process with a "lack of a logical relationship between thoughts and ideas."[2]

M

Magical thinking: the "belief that thinking equates with doing."[2]

Maintenance: the fifth stage of behavior change; the preservation of a new habit past 6 months.

Major depressive disorder: intense and prolonged depressive symptoms without a manic phase.

Mania: "characterized by an elevated, expansive, or irritable mood."[2]

Medical complexity: having a greater number of chronic diseases, personal and psychosocial factors, and mental illnesses that require expert care coordination by the health care provider.

Mood: "the patient's self-report of the prevailing emotional state and reflects the patient's life situation."[2]

Mood disorder: "a mood disturbance such as severe depression or depression alternating with mania."[6]

Motivational interviewing: a communication technique developed to advance patients through the stages of behavior change to form new and better habits.

N

Narcissistic personality disorder: marked by "an exaggerated sense of self-importance, an exhibitionistic need for attention and admiration, feelings of entitlement [and] envy, lack of empathy, and exploitation of others while disregarding their rights and feelings."[3]

Neologisms: thought process with "new word or words created by [the] patient, often a blend of other words."[2]

Neurolinguistic psychology: a framework for improving communication based on responses; this incorporates matching, pacing, and leading in interpersonal interactions.

Neuroticism: a Big-5 model personality trait that allows the person to be emotionally unstable and experience negative emotions more easily. Its opposite is emotional stability.

Nihilistic ideas: "thoughts of nonexistence and hopelessness."[2]

Normal pressure hydrocephalus: a type of dementia caused by ventricular impingement on key areas of the cerebral cortex, causing urinary incontinence, behavioral changes, and unsteady wide-based gait.

Norwegian psychomotor physical therapy: a treatment approach incorporating specific movement-training exercises, massage, and validation of a patient's subjective experiences of mood disorders.

O

Obsession: especially present in anxiety disorders, obsession is an "idea, emotion, or impulse that repetitively and insistently forces itself into consciousness, although it is unwelcome."[2]

Obsessive-compulsive disorder: uncontrollable thoughts causing repetitive actions (eg, hoarding, hand-washing, or arranging objects) that attempt to decrease the thought-induced anxiety. Patients usually recognize the irrationality of their obsessions, but this may make them feel more helpless.

Obsessive-compulsive personality disorder: marked by "personal insecurity and doubt leading to excessive conscientiousness, stubbornness, caution, and rigidity," but not severe enough to be diagnosed as obsessive-compulsive disorder.[3]

Openness to experience: a Big-5 model personality trait that allows the person to be creative, curious, and prefer variety. Its opposite is pragmatic and seen as dogmatic.

P

Pain disorder: where "psychological factors play an important role in the onset, severity, or maintenance of the pain."[2]

Panic attack: "a discrete period of intense fear or discomfort in which at least four of the following symptoms develop abruptly and reach a peak within 10 minutes": tachycardia, sweating, trembling, shortness of breath, choking, angina, nausea, light-headedness, feelings of unreality or detachment from self, fear of losing control or going crazy, fear of dying, paresthesias, chills or hot flashes.[2]

Panic disorder: typically occurring with agoraphobia (fear of open or public spaces), this includes 5 to 10 minute panic attacks involving intense fear and sympathetic nervous system arousal. Patients may have fear of panic attacks themselves, elevated heart rate, dizziness, and shortness of breath.

Paranoid delusion: where the patient is consumed by themes including "persecution, love, hate, envy, jealousy, honour [sic], litigation, grandeur, and the supernatural."[3]

Paranoid personality disorder: marked by "excessive sensitivity to setbacks, unforgiveness of insults, suspiciousness, a tendency to distort experience ... and a combative and tenacious sense of personal rights."[3]

Perseveration: "involuntary, excessive continuation or repetition of a single response, idea, or activity."[2]

Personality disorder: "enduring, inflexible, and maladaptive patterns of behavior that are severe enough to cause either dysfunctional behavior or profound distress."[2]

Phobia: "a persistent and irrational fear of a specific object, activity, or situation that is excessive and unreasonable, given the reality of the threat."[6] In anxiety disorders, it is "a morbid fear associated with extreme anxiety."[2]

Polypharmacy: when an individual has over 4 medications prescribed and taken regularly.

Posttraumatic stress disorder: hypervigilance, nightmares, and unwanted flashbacks following an extremely traumatic event.

Precontemplation: the first stage of behavior change; "reluctance, rebellion, resignation, and rationalization" toward changing an undesirable or addictive behavior.[1]

Premenstrual dysphoric disorder: extreme mood shifts including depressive moods for several days prior to each menstrual period.

Psychoneuroimmunology: "a field that explores the interactions among the central nervous system, the endocrine system, and the immune system; the impact of behavior or stress on these interactions; and how psychological and pharmacological interventions may modulate these interactions."[2]

S

Schizoaffective disorder: including "both affective and schizophrenic symptoms" such that the condition qualifies as neither schizophrenia, nor depression, nor mania.[3]

Schizoid personality disorder: marked by "withdrawal from affectional, social, and other contacts, with preference for fantasy, solitary activities, and [introspection]."[3] The person is unable to express feelings (alexithymia) or experience joy (anhedonia).

Schizophrenia: "a serious, persistent brain disease that results in psychotic behaviors, concrete thinking, and difficulties in information processing, interpersonal relationships, and problem solving."[2]

Schizotypal personality disorder: marked by lack of schizophrenic disturbances, but with "eccentric behaviour [sic] and anomalies of thinking and affect which resemble those seen in schizophrenia."[3]

Selective mutism: an anxiety disorder involving the person choosing not speak to or around certain people.

Severe mental illness: defined legally, and in several articles throughout the text, as including schizophrenia, paranoia, bipolar spectrum disorders, and major depressive disorders.

Social cognition or intelligence: "a theory of personality that refers to the expertise people bring to their experience of life tasks."[6]

Social phobia: a specific phobia related to situations requiring social interaction.

Somatization disorder: wherein "the person has many physical complaints."[2]

Somatoform disorder: a group of symptoms without any somatic impairment.[2] This group includes somatization disorders, conversion disorders, hypochondriasis, body dysmorphic disorders, and pain disorders.

Spaced retrieval: a therapeutic memory technique that incorporates consistent verbal prompts that elicit a specific motor action, with the goal of increasing time between successful prompt-action trials to enhance long-term memory.

Stereotypic movement disorder: marked by "voluntary, repetitive, stereotyped, non-functional (and often rhythmic) movements that do not form part of any recognized psychiatric or neurologic condition [including] body-rocking, head-rocking, hair-plucking ... and hand-flapping [if non-self-injurious] and head-banging, face-slapping, [or] eye-poking" if self-injurious.[3]

T

Tangential: a thought process "similar to circumstantial, but [the] patient never returns to [the] central point and never answers [the] original question."[2]

Tardive dyskinesia: a side effect of many antipsychotic drugs after prolonged use, marked by "abnormal, involuntary, slow, irregular movements of the tongue, lips, mouth, and trunk, and by choreoathetoid movements of the extremities.[3] Remission ranges from 5% to 90% depending on severity of the initial dyskinesia.

Therapeutic nihilism: a lack of belief in the efficacy of therapy (medical, rehabilitation, or other) for a condition such as dementia.

Thought blocking: a "sudden stopping in the train of thought or in the midst of a sentence."[2]

Thought broadcasting delusion: "the experience that one's thoughts are somehow immediately shared with other people or otherwise made public knowledge."[3]

Thought content: "the specific meaning expressed in the patient's communication,"[2] including delusions.

Thought insertion or withdrawal: a paranoid delusion involving "the individual's experience of (1) thoughts recognized as alien intruding into his or her mental processes; (2) his or her own thoughts being taken away or otherwise appropriated by an external agency."[3]

Thought process: "the 'how' of the patient's self-expression ... observed through speech."[2]

V

Vascular dementia: a late effect of stroke that involves stepwise cognitive deterioration, early gait abnormalities, urinary incontinence, and personality changes.

W

Waxy flexibility: present in schizophrenia with catatonia. This is the tendency of a person to stay in the posture placed by another, without initiating movement him- or herself.

Wernicke-Korsakoff syndrome: a type of dementia caused by vitamin B deficiency, with symptoms including confabulation, a manipulative personality, ataxic slow gait, and severely impaired memory.

Word salad: a "series of words that seem completely unrelated."[2]

References

1. Miller WR, Rollnick S. *Motivational Interviewing: Preparing People to Change Addictive Behavior.* New York, NY: Guilford;1991.
2. Stuart GW. *Handbook of Psychiatric Nursing.* 6th ed. St. Louis, MO: Elsevier Mosby; 2005.
3. World Health Organization. *Lexicon of psychiatric and mental health terms.* 2nd ed. World Health Organization. http://apps.who.int/iris/bitstream/10665/39342/1/924154466X.pdf. 1994. Accessed February 19, 2018.
4. Bradshaw DM, Young-Walker L. An 11-year-old girl with suicidal thoughts, hallucinations. *Psych Annals.* 2011;41(8), 386-389. DOI: 10.3928/00485713-20110727-03.
5. Davis CB. *Clinical geriatric neurology.* [Course notes.] Great Seminars & Books;2014.
6. American Psychiatric Association. *Diagnostic and Statistical Manual of Mental Disorders.* 5th ed. Washington, DC: American Psychiatric Association; 2013.
7. Regents of UCSF. Executive functions. *UCSF Memory and Aging Center.* http://memory.ucsf.edu/ftd/overview/biology/executive/single. Updated 2018. Accessed February 19, 2018.
8. American Physical Therapy Association. 'Movement system' is our professional identity. *APTA.* http://www.apta.org/NEXT/News/2015/6/6/MovementSystem/. Published June 8, 2015. Accessed May 3, 2018.

Tests and Measures

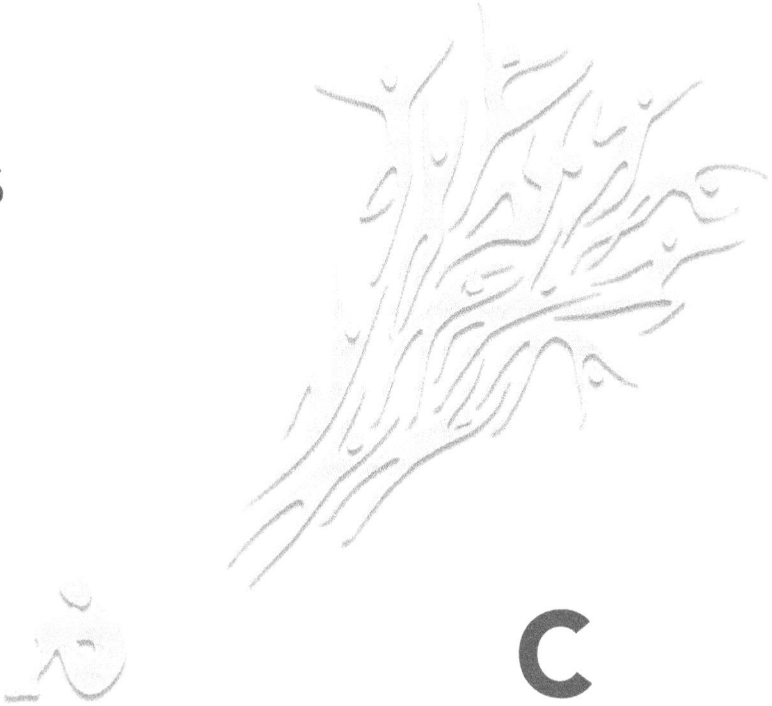

C

A

- Activity Pacing Questionnaire
    - Abstract available at www.ingentaconnect.com/content/wk/cjpn/2017/00000033/00000003/art00003?crawler=true&mimetype=application/pdf
- Allen Cognitive Level Test
    - Information and purchase at https://allencognitive.com
- Apparent Emotions Rating
    - Purchase article at www.tandfonline.com/doi/abs/10.1300/J018v18n04_03?journalCode=wcli20

B

- Balance Evaluation Systems Test
    - Found at www.sralab.org/rehabilitation-measures/balance-evaluation-systems-test
- Barthel Index
    - Found at www.sralab.org/rehabilitation-measures/barthel-index
- Beck Depression Inventory
    - Found at www.sralab.org/rehabilitation-measures/beck-depression-inventory
- Beers criteria
    - Found at www.dcri.org/beers-criteria-medication-list
- Berg Balance Scale
    - Found at www.sralab.org/rehabilitation-measures/berg-balance-scale

Johnson H.
Psychosocial Elements of Physical Therapy: The Connection of Body to Mind (pp 265-268).

C

- Center for Epidemiologic Studies Depression Scale
  - Found at www.sralab.org/rehabilitation-measures/center-epidemiological-studies-depression-scale-ces-d
- Chair Rise Test (30-Second Sit to Stand)
  - Found at www.sralab.org/rehabilitation-measures/30-second-sit-stand-test
- Confusion Assessment Method
  - Found at www.icudelirium.org/delirium/monitoring.html
- Cornell Scale for Depression in Dementia
  - Found at http://geropsychiatriceducation.vch.ca/docs/edu-downloads/depression/cornell_scale_depression.pdf

D

- Delirium Rating Scale
  - Email for permission at https://www.americandeliriumsociety.org/resources/tools
- Doloplus-2
  - Found at http://prc.coh.org/PainNOA/Doloplus%202_Tool.pdf

F

- Fear of Pain Questionnaire (child and adult proxy versions)
  - Short form available at https://www.researchgate.net/publication/6349751_The_Fear_of_Pain_Questionnaire_-_Short_Form_FPQ-SF_Factorial_validity_and_psychometric_properties
- 5 Times Sit to Stand
  - Found at www.sralab.org/rehabilitation-measures/five-times-sit-stand-test
- Functional Assessment Staging Tool
  - Found at http://geriatrics.uthscsa.edu/tools/FAST.pdf

G

- Gait speed
  - Found at www.cgakit.com/fr-1-gait-speed-test
- Geriatric Depression Scale (15 and 30)
  - Multiple versions at http://web.stanford.edu/~yesavage/GDS.html
- Global Deterioration Scale
  - Found at https://www.fhca.org/members/qi/clinadmin/global.pdf
- Global Physiotherapy Examination
  - Article found at https://www.researchgate.net/publication/7698161_Sensitivity_to_Change_and_Responsiveness_of_the_Global_Physiotherapy_Examination_GPE-52_in_Patients_With_Long-Lasting_Musculoskeletal_Pain
- Groningen Meander Walking Test
  - Article found at https://academic.oup.com/ptj/article/94/2/262/2735458

H

- Hamilton Anxiety Rating Scale
  - Found at https://dcf.psychiatry.ufl.edu/files/2011/05/HAMILTON-ANXIETY.pdf
- Hamilton Depression Rating Scale
  - Found at www.assessmentpsychology.com/HAM-D.pdf

M

- Mini-BESTest
  - Found at www.sralab.org/rehabilitation-measures/mini-balance-evaluation-systems-test
- Mini-Cog
  - Found at http://www.alz.org/documents_custom/minicog.pdf
- Mini-Mental State Exam
  - Found at www.uml.edu/docs/Mini%20Mental%20State%20Exam_tcm18-169319.pdf
- Montreal Cognitive Assessment
  - Available by subscription at http://www.mocatest.org

N

- Numeric Pain Rating Scale
  - Found at www.sralab.org/rehabilitation-measures/numeric-pain-rating-scale

O

- 1-Minute Verbal Fluency for Animals
  - Found at www.ncbi.nlm.nih.gov/pmc/articles/PMC3711831

P

- Pain Assessment in Advanced Dementia
  - Found at http://dementiapathways.ie/_filecache/04a/ddd/98-painad.pdf
- Patient Health Questionnaire-9
  - Found at www.sralab.org/rehabilitation-measures/patient-health-questionnaire-phq-9
- Physical Performance Test
  - Found at http://www.brightonrehab.com/wp-content/uploads/2012/02/Physical-Performance-Test-PPT.pdf
- Primary Care Evaluation of Mental Disorders
  - Found at https://instruct.uwo.ca/kinesiology/9641/Assessments/Social/PRIME-MD.html

S

- Sharpened Romberg
  - Found at www.sralab.org/rehabilitation-measures/sharpened-romberg
- Short Form, 36 question version
  - Found at www.sralab.org/rehabilitation-measures/medical-outcomes-study-short-form-36
- 6-Minute Walk Test
  - Found at www.sralab.org/rehabilitation-measures/6-minute-walk-test

T

- 10-Meter Walk Test
  - Found at www.sralab.org/rehabilitation-measures/10-meter-walk-test
- Timed Up and Go Test
  - Found with norms at http://www.unmc.edu/media/intmed/geriatrics/nebgec/pdf/frail-elderlyjuly09/toolkits/timedupandgo_w_norms.pdf

V

- Visual Analogue Scale for pain
  - Found at www.blackwellpublishing.com/specialarticles/jcn_10_706.pdf and www.physiotherapyalberta.ca/files/pain_scale_visual_and_numerical.pdf

W

- Wong-Baker FACES Scale
  - Information at http://wongbakerfaces.org

Z

- Zung Self-Rating Depression Scale
  - Found at www.specialtybehavioralhealth.com/wp-content/Zung%20Self-Rating%20Depression%20Scale.pdf

Index

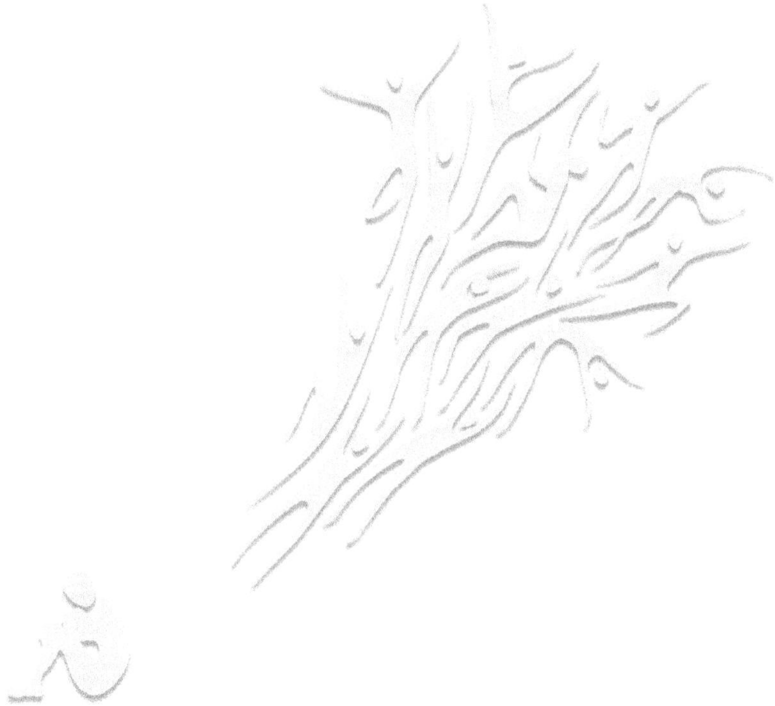

Printed in the USA
CPSIA information can be obtained
at www.ICGtesting.com
LVHW060547170924
791293LV00006B/629

9 781630 915537